What Experts Are Saying About This Book

"The sex education myths of the past may have brainwashed a generation, but now the truth is out! Josh McDowell has composed a masterpiece that can benefit school children for generations to come."

Coleen Kelly Mast
Author, *Sex Respect*

"Josh McDowell has pulled together research that exposes the agenda of special interest groups targeting our schools. It must be read by all who implement education programs for adolescents. Teachers, nurses, counselors, administrators, school board members and legislators should read THE MYTHS OF SEX EDUCATION."

Dinah Richard, Ph.D.
Author, *Has Sex Education Failed Our Teenagers? A Research Report*

"We are profoundly grateful for this extensive analysis of THE MYTHS OF SEX EDUCATION. It provides the greatest compilation available of documentation and evidence to refute the widespread, mistaken claims made about school-based sex ed. It is our earnest plea that this book awaken caring parents nationwide to the **counterproductive** effects of 'comprehensive' birth control/sex education programs in the schools—and avoid a repeat of the Virginia debacle."

Anne Marie Morgan
Legislative and Political Reporter
Capital Radio News

"This is the time to rally for our children who are being taught sex education without morals. THE MYTHS OF SEX EDUCATION will be of great importance to the children in our schools."

Beverly LaHaye, President
Concerned Women for America

More research for parents and teachers from JOSH McDOWELL

"The Myths of Sex Education"
(LifeSounds Audio Album)

"Why Wait?" What You Need to Know About the Teen Sexuality Crisis

The Dad Difference

Teens Speak Out: "What I Wish My Parents Knew About My Sexuality"

And Josh's newest bestseller: *A READY DEFENSE*
(available in both book and LifeSounds Audio Album)

JOSH McDOWELL

THE MYTHS OF SEX EDUCATION

Josh McDowell's Open Letter to His School Board

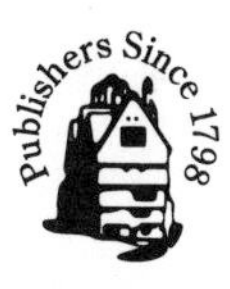

THOMAS NELSON PUBLISHERS
Nashville

Acknowledgments

Like my other books, *The Myths of Sex Education* is the result of combined efforts of a great many people. To Bill Wilson, Anne Schaefer and Marcus Maranto for extensive research; to Terri Childs and Debi Suchecki for putting much of the manuscript into the computer; to Duane Zook for his tireless and extensive efforts in coordinating all the computer work; to Harry Yates for extensive library work on the documentation; to Ed Stewart for honing volumes of rough writings into a presentable manuscript; to Jean Bryant of Here's Life Publishers for massive final editing and interior design, making it ready to print; and to all those – too numerous to list – who critiqued the content . . .

My heartiest thanks, every one of you!
Josh

First Printing, September 1990
Second Printing, January 1991

Published by
HERE'S LIFE PUBLISHERS, INC.
P. O. Box 1576
San Bernardino, CA 92402

Printed by Dickinson Press, Inc., Grand Rapids, Michigan
Cover design by Cornerstone Graphics

Library of Congress Cataloging-in-Publication Data
McDowell, Josh.

The myths of sex education : startling research that deserves a close look from parents and teachers / Josh McDowell.
p. cm.
ISBN 0-89840-287-5

1. Sex instruction – United States. 2. Teenagers – United States – Sexual behavior. I. Title.
HQ57.5.A3M35 1990
306.7'0835 – dc20 90-37834
CIP

For More Information, Write:

Josh McDowell Ministries – P.O. Box 1000, Dallas, TX 75221
L.I.F.E. – P.O. Box A399, Sydney South 2000, Australia
Campus Crusade for Christ of Canada – Box 300, Vancouver, B.C., V6C 2X3, Canada
Campus Crusade for Christ – Pearl Assurance House, 4 Temple Row, Birmingham, B2 5HG, England
Lay Institute for Evangelism – P.O. Box 8786, Auckland 3, New Zealand
Campus Crusade for Christ – P.O. Box 240, Raffles City Post Office, Singapore 9117
Great Commission Movement of Nigeria – P.O. Box 500, Jos, Plateau State Nigeria, West Africa
Campus Crusade for Christ International – Arrowhead Springs, San Bernardino, CA 92414, U.S.A.

Contents

➧ Indicates **key sections** for busy parents.

PART THREE
Seven Strategies for Resolving the Teenage Sexuality Crisis

CHAPTER

PART FOUR
Resources for Evaluating Abstinence Education

CHAPTER

FOOTNOTES: The footnote references are at the end of each documented quote (e.g., 56/82). The number on the left of the diagonal (56) is the reference number of the source in the Documentations list, beginning on page 285. The number on the right (82) is the page of the source where the quote or information is found.

BOLDFACE: The boldface is to highlight the content of the quotation and does not indicate boldface type in the original source.

ABBREVIATIONS:

JAMA	Journal of the American Medical Association
CDC	Centers for Disease Control in Atlanta, GA (Notice the "Centers" is plural).
STD(s)	Sexually Transmitted Disease(s)
PPFA	Planned Parenthood Federation of America
SBHC	School-Based Health Clinic
CSE	Comprehensive Sex Education (For a thorough **definition** of *comprehensive sex education*, see page 80.)

The Letter Begins . . .

Dear Julian School Board Member:

You are important! As an elected board member, you have been given a tremendous responsibility for the education of the children in our community, including my children. You sought your position on the Julian School Board because you care about kids. (You definitely aren't doing it for the money!) Your commitment of time and effort has not gone unnoticed. Dottie and I, and the other parents in Julian, deeply appreciate your involvement in our community.

We enjoy living in Julian very much, and we count it a great privilege to be a part of this community. A portion of our joy comes from our interaction with those who teach and administrate the schools our four children attend. The education staff in our school district has done a wonderful job helping us with our children's education. I'm sure they receive criticism, but Dottie and I are thankful for the teachers, principals, superintendents and staff our children have had over the years. Everyone in the district has welcomed our involvement and has always encouraged us as the primary educators of our children. We really feel that the education community in Julian is here to help us. That's a great feeling!

I'm not writing only to express my appreciation to you and the Julian district. I also want to express my concern for the kids here in Julian and across this great nation. My concern springs from being the father of four children and from being involved with literally hundreds of thousands of teenagers for more than 25 years in the U.S. and abroad. At the heart of my concern is a crisis which seriously threatens the mental, emotional, spiritual and physical well-being of our teenagers, not just in the burgeoning population centers of Philadelphia, Chicago, Dallas, Los Angeles and New York, but also right here in Julian, California. I recently addressed a conference of educators in Seattle, Washington, about this crisis. I want to share with you some of what they said as they introduced me at the convention so you can understand my background and my concern for kids, which prompted me to write this letter:

> Josh McDowell is one of the most popular speakers on the world scene today. In the last twenty-three years he has given more than 18,000 talks to more than eight million students and faculty at a thousand universities and high schools in seventy-two countries. Josh is the author of thirty-two best-selling books

and has been featured in twenty-seven films and videos and two TV specials.

Josh graduated cum laude from Kellogg College and Wheaton College in economics and business. He finished graduate school magna cum laude with degrees in languages and theology. He is a member of two national honor societies and was selected by the Jaycees in 1976 as one of the "Outstanding Young Men in America." He holds three honorary doctorate degrees—in law, theology and literature.

Teens in Crisis

We face a teenage sexuality crisis. Many have cited the alarming statistics about teenage pregnancy—children having children. In 1976, Planned Parenthood Federation of America (PPFA) published an article titled, "11 Million Teenagers: What Can Be Done About the Epidemic of Adolescent Pregnancy in the United States?" The thrust of the article was that one million teens aged 15-19 would become pregnant that year. Things have only gotten worse since then.

More recently, many others have sounded the alarm. The *New York Times* reported: "Some studies indicate three-fourths of all girls have had sex during their teenage years and 15 percent have had four or more partners." 332 The *Washington Post* published this appalling news: "Half of U.S. girls have now had intercourse by the age of 15."

The *American Journal of Diseases of Children* reports on research by Indiana University and the Marion County Health Department. Dr. Donald P. Orr states that of the "677 seventh, eighth and ninth graders in a mostly white, lower-middle-class junior high in Indianapolis,

55% have had sex
18% have had one sexual experience
30% have had more than one experience
7% have had multiple partners
50+% of boys have had intercourse by the age of 13
50+% of girls have had intercourse by the age of 15." 333

The 1986 Lou Harris poll, commissioned by PPFA, showed:

28% aged 12-17 had sexual intercourse
4% of 12-year-olds
10% of 13-year-olds
46% of 16-year-olds
57% of 17-year-olds
50+% had sexual intercourse by the age of 17. 27/13

A 1987 study by the National Academy of Science discovered: "The attitude shift has been best documented among girls. From 1971 to

1982, the proportion of unmarried girls aged 15 to 19 who had had sexual intercourse at least once increased from 28 percent to 44 percent." 334/2 A Mark Clements Research study of 11 million teenage boys indicated:

> 66% had sex
> 15 years old, age of first sex
> 18 years old, on the average boys had sex with five girls. 335/16

The New York polling firm Audits and Surveys posed 41 questions to 1,300 students in 16 high schools around the U.S., 1,600 students in 10 colleges, and 500 parents of teens in 12 cities. They did not poll the impoverished inner-city or rural areas. They wanted to get a reading of the "mainstream" adolescent. They discovered:

> 57% lost virginity in high school
> 79% lost virginity by end of college
> 16.9 average age for sex
> 33% of high school students had sex once a month to once a week
> 52% of college students had sex once a month to once a week. 336

A December 1988 nationwide study in Canada reported:

> 31% of ninth-grade boys had sex
> 21% of ninth-grade girls had sex
> 49% of eleventh-grade boys had sex
> 46% of eleventh-grade girls had sex. 337/C1

The state of California, being quite perplexed about the teenage sexuality crisis, passed Senate Bill 2394 which cites the awesome reality of teen promiscuity in California:

a. Sixty-four percent of male teens and 44 percent of female teens have had sexual intercourse by the age of 18.

b. Each year, one in seven teens contracts a sexually transmitted disease.

c. The teen pregnancy rate for California's 15- to 19-year-olds—the sums of births, abortions and miscarriages—has increased by 32.9 percent in California from 1970 to 1985.

d. The abortion rate for teens 15 to 19 years of age has more than tripled from 1970 to 1985 and now exceeds the rate of births among California women under 20 by 38 percent.

e. California's abortion rate for 15- to 19-year-olds is 64 percent, 8 percent higher than the national average. 228

A federal survey by the National Center for Health Statistics indicates that America's teenage girls seem to be having sex sooner:

Women 15-19 having had sex:
1982 – 47% 1988 – 54% 338/E3

Speaking to the National School Board Association, former Secretary of Education William J. Bennett stated, "The statistics by which we measure how our children – how our boys and girls – are treating one another sexually are little short of staggering." 339/3 Then he reported some of the heartbreaking statistics:

- More than one million teenage girls in the United States become pregnant each year. Of those who give birth, nearly half are not yet 18.
- Teen pregnancy rates are at or near an all-time high. A 25-percent decline in birth rates between 1970 and 1984 is due to a *doubling* of the abortion rate during that period. More than 400,000 teenage girls now have abortions each year [emphasis mine].
- Unwed teenage births rose 200 percent between 1960 and 1980.
- Forty percent of today's 14-year-old girls will become pregnant by the time they are 19. 339/3

"These numbers," confessed Bennett, "are an irrefutable indictment of sex education's effectiveness in reducing teenage sexual activity and pregnancies." 339/3

Getting Worse Instead of Better

As Secretary Bennett's testimony suggests, attempts to resolve the teenage sexuality crisis through comprehensive sex education programs and school-based health clinics has only exacerbated the problem. Planned Parenthood and other so-called family planning groups have insisted for more than ten years that the crisis of teen pregnancies, abortions and sexually transmitted diseases (STDs) would be eased if we teach young people about sex, equip them with contraceptive methods and devices and encourage them to develop moral values and sexual practices which are "right for me." But it isn't working. Instead, the crisis has only escalated – more pregnancies, more abortions and a staggering epidemic of STDs.

Why has comprehensive sex education in our schools and communities failed so miserably to deliver on its promise to solve the crisis? I see at least two major reasons: **(1)** The sex educators and family planning groups do not understand the problem; consequently **(2)** they are foisting on us a faulty solution.

First, Planned Parenthood and other proponents of comprehensive sex education can't resolve the crisis because they don't correctly perceive the problem. They are operating under a number of false assumptions about teenage sexuality. In Part One of the pages ahead I want to share with you six false assumptions about teenage sexuality and explain how parents and educators who buy into these fantasies tend to make things worse for our kids instead of better.

Second, sex educators and family planning groups like Planned Parenthood can't resolve the crisis because they don't have the right solution. Their assumptions are flawed, so the solutions based on those assumptions are flawed and ineffective. They are operating under a number of myths about the effectiveness of sex education to reduce teen pregnancies, abortions and STDs. In Part Two I want to share with you six prevalent myths about comprehensive sex education and show you how these attempts are counterproductive in reducing the teen sexuality crisis.

A Hope-Filled Solution

If what you've read so far seems like only so much "gloom and doom," rest assured: I'm not writing to you just to rehash the problem and express my concern over the crisis. I'm also bringing some proposed solutions. In Part Three I want to share with you seven proven strategies for resolving the teen sexuality crisis in Julian and around the country. In Part Four I have included some additional resources to help you evaluate the core tenet of these strategies. That core tenet is: **abstinence-based sex education**.

These solutions aren't mine alone. The strategies presented here have been developed by concerned educators and parents across our country who have refused to yield to the persuasive argument that comprehensive sex education (see page 80, at the beginning of Part Two, for a full definition of this term) is the answer to our kids' problems. Programs implementing these strategies are presently in place and operating in numbers of school districts in America. And while the rates for teen pregnancies, abortions and STDs continue to climb in districts promoting comprehensive sex education, districts applying the strategies from Part Three are seeing a remarkable reduction in all three crisis areas.

I realize I may be at a disadvantage as I review for you the urgency of the problem and communicate to you solutions for our kids' sexuality crisis. I am an evangelical Christian. I know my Christian stance immediately clashes with biases and prejudices many people hold concerning evangelicals. I trust that won't be a problem for you.

I am also a conservative. Again, in many educational circles such an admission raises all kinds of red flags—some justifiable, but most not. Perhaps we all can benefit from the observations Senator David Carlin, Jr., made in his article, "Liberals, Conservatives and Sex Education," published in *America*. A self-proclaimed liberal, he writes:

My suggestion is that we liberals, instead of confining ourselves, as we do now, to ridicule and denunciation, ought to adopt a studious and respectful attitude toward the conservative prejudices inhabiting the souls of a great many of our fellow citizens. Behind the inadequate and often exasperating formulas popular conservatism uses when it tries to express itself, there usually exists a genuine insight—an insight it would profit liberalism to disengage, to appreciate and to incorporate within its own world view. . . .

[Usually] liberals favor sex education, holding that it will cut the alarming pregnancy rate among unmarried girls, that it will reduce venereal disease, and that schools have to take up the slack caused by the reluctance or inability of parents to educate their children in this area. Conservatives, by contrast, generally oppose it, contending that schools have no right to teach sexual views parents might disapprove of (an objection we liberals have a certain grudging sympathy for) and that sex education leads to an increase in premarital sex, hence an increase in venereal disease and teenage pregnancy. I do not say . . . the liberal camp should tolerate a taboo-based sexual morality or that we should abandon efforts to ground sexual rules on a rational foundation. But we should recognize that conservatives are not talking simple nonsense when they say sex education can lead to increases in premarital sex, along with its frequently unpleasant side effects. We ought to admit that there is a price the world has to pay—at times a very high price—for attempts to give sexual conduct a rational, moral basis. And though it is a price we liberals may be willing to see paid, we must not think too badly of our conservative friends when we find they think the price too high. . . .

Personally, I think the experiment of creating a rational sex ethic worthwhile; but it might be carried on more intelligently if we paused from time to time to consider the reservations, objections and criticisms of conservatives." 340/396-98

Conservatives are sometimes resistant to change when change is needed. Conservatives also are often guilty of holding to tradition for tradition's sake. Yet, in this case, virtually everyone is in agreement: There is a problem and something urgent must be done. Unfortunately, there is also broad disagreement among conservatives, liberals, evangelicals and non-evangelicals on the cause of the crisis and the nature of the solution. As you read these pages, I ask you not to judge the contents based on your biases for or against evangelicals or conservatives. Rather, please evaluate my comments and observations on their intrinsic merit.

My goal in sharing these thoughts with you is to make your job easier. My hope is that you, as a concerned school board member, will better understand the teenage sexuality crisis and the resources at our disposal to resolve it. I trust you will have the wisdom to make the right decisions about sex education in our schools. Remember: Our greatest resources as a nation are our children and families.

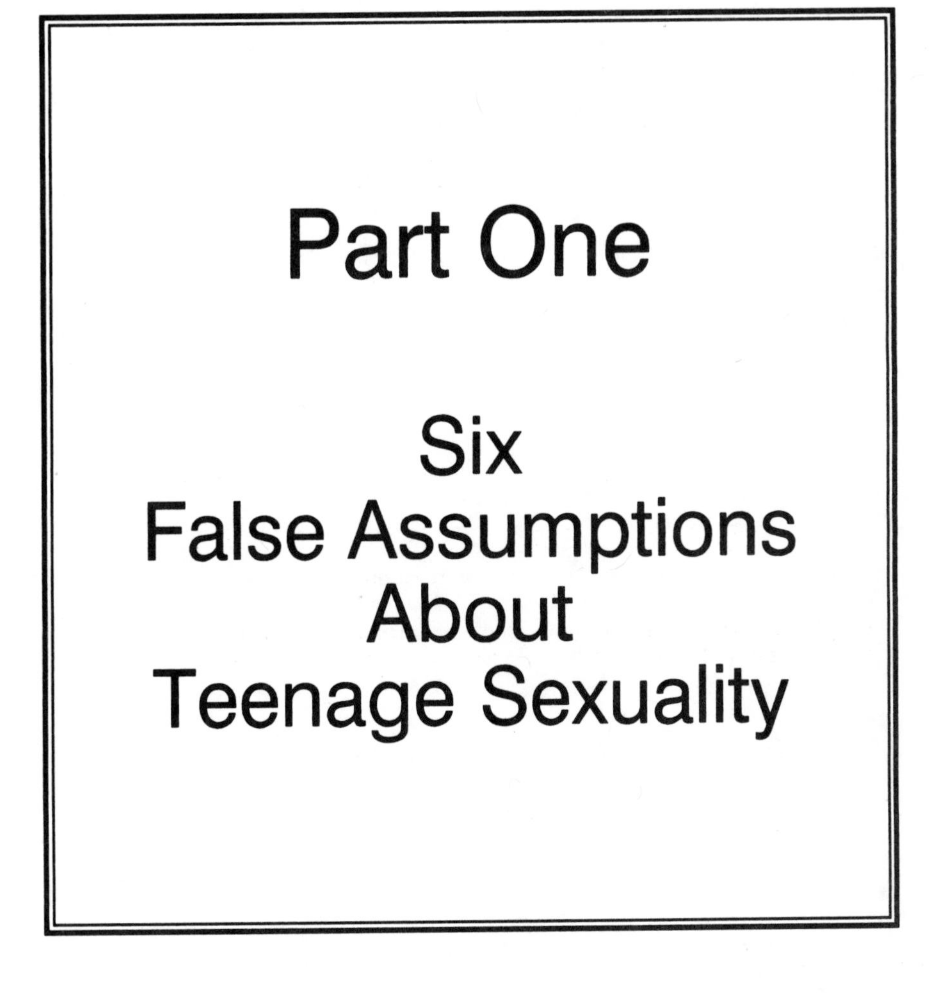

Part One

Six False Assumptions About Teenage Sexuality

CHAPTER 1

♦ A **key section** for busy parents.

False Assumption 1

"Teens Want Sex More Than They Want Love"

A staggering number of teenagers are sexually active today—there's no doubt about it—but we have been duped by the statistics into believing that sexual involvement is what they want most. That's not true. When you dig a little deeper, you discover that kids don't want to be sexually involved as much as they want to be loved. They want someone who really cares for them. A 16-year-old girl wrote to me after my last tour of England:

> *Josh, I want someone to love me (not physically). I want someone who cares. I want to love and be loved, and I don't know how to do either.*

We aren't experiencing a sexual revolution among our teenagers; we're experiencing a revolution in the search for intimacy. In a study conducted in the junior high schools of a major U.S. city, **67 percent of the kids said their greatest need in sex education was learning how to say no to sexual pressure.** 74 Young people today want close, caring relationships and mistakenly think that saying yes to sex means saying yes to intimacy.

♦ Two Deep Fears

Some college students are not noted for benevolence toward visiting speakers, especially speakers with conservative and/or Christian views. As I waited my turn to speak at the outdoor free speech platform at a secular university, I had butterflies in my stomach. I realized that what I said had better be right on or the crowd would shove it right back down my throat.

As I stepped up to speak, the crowd was noisy and not particularly hospitable. There was no public address system so I had to rely on old-fashioned lung power to be heard. I had only a few seconds to get their attention, so I called out to them, "Almost every one of you has two fears. First, you're afraid you'll never be loved. Second, you're afraid you'll never be able to love."

Suddenly everyone became very quiet. I wasn't surprised; it happens every time I make those statements. Our young people know that one of their deepest needs is for real love and intimacy.

Psychologists believe this "love famine" among kids is one reason many young girls become pregnant. Lisa, who is 16 and pregnant, would agree: "My mother kept asking, 'Why? Why?' I said, 'Because I wanted to be loved, that's why.' Is that so terrible? I just wanted someone to tell me that I'm pretty, and that he cared about me." The kind of love kids like Lisa want is not sex. They crave real love – love that expresses caring, transparency, vulnerability and intimacy.

♦ Love Is Learned

We don't grow up, or reach puberty, automatically knowing how to love. Love is not primarily a feeling; it's an action. Since it is first and foremost an action, it must be learned. Saying "I love you" has no meaning if it is not supported by loving action. We can't learn how to love in a classroom. We learn to give and receive love by experiencing it, by seeing it modeled and by responding to its expression.

God intends for us to learn love in the home by seeing our parents love each other and by experiencing their love for us. When the home breaks down and parental models cease to function, children grow up not knowing how to give or receive love. This is the story of our generation. One out of every two marriages ends in divorce, and many of the couples who remain married model hatred, distrust or apathy instead of love. No wonder so many kids today are unable to develop close, intimate relationships.

♦ Hungry for Love

Many young people are uncertain of their parents' love. Several thousand high school students were asked, "What one question would you like your parents to answer truthfully?" Fifty percent of them responded with the question, "Do you really love me?" 70/43 I personally know many parents who sincerely love their children, but whose actions don't always show it. One teenage girl wrote:

> *When I was eight years old, I first had sex with a boy of 15. I did it because I lacked love and attention from my parents. I need love, and my parents never show me any. Nothing really changed at home, and at 15 I became pregnant. My boyfriend blamed me and left. I had nowhere to turn; I was trapped, so I had an abortion. Now I'm afraid to date anyone, and I cry myself to sleep every night.* 71/5

The only foolproof solution to teenage pregnancy is prevention of sexual activity. This involves the relational aspect of a teenager's life, and that begins with parents spending time with their children long before hormones, peers and the media begin pressuring them about sex. Our children, whatever their age, are hungry for our love and attention. We need to give it to them by spending time with them and loving them with words and actions.

Fathers are often worse offenders than mothers in failing to communicate love. One reason is that some men have real problems showing their emotions. Many fathers hide their tender feelings by pretending to be cynical about love. They are uncomfortable discussing love seriously, and those who can't talk about love usually have difficulty expressing it. I truly believe that lots of hugs between fathers and their teen daughters would do more to stop the teen pregnancy epidemic than any other single factor.

♦ Lasting Relationships

One thing I've learned about teenagers is that they **would rather stay in love forty years than fall in love forty times.** They desperately want a relationship that will last. They are crying out for role models of married couples who have it together—in love, marriage, sex and family. They are looking for relationships that work. Sadly, young people today are seldom exposed to role models for loving, lasting relationships, so they don't know how to develop a loving relationship of their own. Instead they are reproducing in their relationships the heartache they have observed in the marriages of their parents and other negative adult role models.

Entertainer Olivia Newton-John was once asked why she hadn't married sooner than she did. She answered that she had been devastated by the divorce of her parents when she was 10 years old. Then she said something which is echoed in the lives of countless numbers of our young people today: "If you've never seen a relationship that lasts forever, you tend not to believe it's possible." 72/113

A child's greatest sense of security comes from knowing his or her parents love each other. One of the best gifts a father and mother can give their children is to love each other and let their children know it.

♦ A Happy Home Life

Do you know what today's young teens (13-15 years) really want? Success in college? Success in business or career? Not primarily. Studies show their number one desire is for a happy home life. Interestingly, teenage boys today want this even more than girls do. 73 More emphasis on closer family ties is desired by 86 percent of teens, with only slightly greater emphasis on this value noted among young women (90 percent) than among young men (82 percent).

A research institute study showed that out of a list of 24 values, the two most important to young adolescents in grades five through nine are to have a happy family life and to get a good job as an adult.

♦ The Devastation of Divorce

Is it any wonder that 75 percent of the teens surveyed about values felt it is too easy to get a divorce in this country? Of teens from divorced homes, 74 percent said that their parents didn't try hard enough to stay together. A survey conducted by *Children and Teens Today* asked readers, "What do you see as the major stresses/problems facing today's teenagers?" Nearly 75 percent responded: "Problems arising from parental divorce/remarriage." 75/1-2

One of the great fears of many young children and teenagers is the loss of a parent through divorce–with good reason, since 50 percent of all marriages end in divorce. When divorcing parents ask their children, "Do you want us to continue our painful relationship for your sake?" the answer is almost universally, "Yes, we do!" Young people today want to be part of a loving, lasting family relationship.

A few years ago when our son Sean was only six years old, he came home from school one day acting a little down. "What's wrong, Sean?" I asked.

"Aw, nothing, Dad."

Sean and I communicate pretty well, so I said, "Come on, Son. Share with me what you're feeling."

Sean hesitated, then asked, "Daddy, are you going to leave Mommy?" He explained that three of his friends' dads had just walked out on their wives and children. He was afraid I might do the same.

I had known Sean's question would come up someday. So I sat down with him, looked him straight in the eye and said, "I want you to know that I love your mother very much. I am committed to her, and I'll never leave her—period."

Our little six-year-old breathed a sigh of relief, smiled at me and said, "Thanks, Dad." At that point he didn't need reinforcement of my love for him; he needed the security that comes from knowing that his mother and I love each other and are committed to a permanent relationship. All young people need the security of knowing their parents have a lasting relationship.

♦ Dysfunctional Families

The emotional and social consequences of divorce on young people are negative and far-reaching. One counseling magazine lists these 21 reactions of teenagers to the divorce of their parents: discipline problems, dependence on boyfriend or girlfriend, rebellion, depression, grief, loss of self-confidence, guilt, resentment, insecure feelings, inability to concentrate, self-image problems, loneliness, anger, fear, emotional detachment, anxiety, inability to trust anyone, cynical attitude, close attachment to friends, shame, and embarrassment.

Children also experience negative consequences when they observe adultery in their parents' relationship. Dr. Frank Pittman discovered that "the impact of adulterous affairs on the children of the adulterers is profound. Children react negatively to reduced attentiveness by their parents and to furtive discussions behind closed doors. Small children show anxiety when they perceive that the family is somehow disintegrating." The above findings are published in Dr. Pittman's book, *Private Lies.* 370

The fact that male leadership is absent from the home because of divorce, separation or abandonment usually translates into bad news in the lives of the children. Dr. Rhoda L. Lorand reports on the clinical observations of 303 white teenage girls who attended an informative session on contraception. Almost all the girls had already had sexual intercourse. It was found that "a significantly larger portion of teenagers from households headed by females than from those headed by males had had their first experience of sexual intercourse at the age of 15 or younger (67 percent compared to 47 percent)." 57/4 Lorand continues: "The proportion who had had only one sexual partner was greater in male-headed households (22 percent versus 7 percent)." 57/4

In homes where both parents are present, but where caring and structure is lacking, children are also negatively affected. Dr. Lorand observed:

Adolescents who hang around with nothing to do, whose homes lack warmth and protectiveness, whose lives are empty of accomplishments which would promote self-esteem and self-confidence, who lack rewarding contact with adults, and who witness adult coitus, are vulnerable to environmental pressures to engage in sex. . . . A sociological study of 600 boys and girls with venereal disease, conducted by Celia Deschin, asked the question, "What do you do in your spare time?" The majority replied: "Nothing." These youngsters need programs of structured activities which will enable them to acquire knowledge and develop skills, hobbies, interests and competence in a wide variety of fields. While there is, to be sure, an overlapping of needs, boys especially require channels of sublimation for sexual energies and girls especially need to feel that someone cares about them. 57/7

♦ Starving for Affection

It is the great void of love and affection in our homes that prompts our kids into sexual activity. It's not so much that they want sex, but that they want the affection, acceptance and friendship they think sex will bring. Kim Cox, a health educator at Balboa High School in San Francisco, says kids are "moved to sex, many of them, not by compassion or love or any of the other urges that make sense to adults, but by a need for intimacy that has gone unfulfilled by their families. . . . Sex is an easy way to get it."

According to a *Seventeen* magazine survey, most girls opt for affection over sex. "Nearly two-thirds feel strongly that affection is much more important than sex in a relationship and another 29 percent agree somewhat. In fact only 1.1 percent assert that sex is more important." 17/107

One teenager confesses: "We are all running around needing to get hugged. . . . The dilemma for some . . . is that 'if I want to be touched, if I want to be held, I have to have sex.' " Robert Olson, health educator with the Department of Public Health, has said that "many pregnant teens say wanting 'a man to hold me' was their motivation rather than having sexual relations with someone." 78/1-2

♦ The Search for Intimacy

"Mr. McDowell, in the last five nights I've gone to bed with five different men." The young university woman was speaking to me over the phone from several hundred miles away. "Tonight," she said, "I got out of bed and asked myself, 'Is this all there is?' " Then she began crying. When she regained her composure enough to speak, she said, "Please tell me there's something more."

"There certainly is," I said. "It's called intimacy."

What is intimacy? A 15-year-old girl once described intimacy as "a place where it's safe to be real." A recent survey of 300 women aged 18 to 60 found that women of all ages want men with whom they can be close. "They want intimacy, which is more than just love and sex," according to psychologist Lois Leiderman Davidz of Columbia University. 80/D1

Shere Hite, internationally recognized cultural historian and researcher, discovered that "most women interviewed enjoyed hugging, kissing, cuddling, closeness and conversation as much as intercourse. Overall, intimacy was more important than orgasm." 36/30-31

Our main problem today is not sexual, it's relational. We have embarked on a fruitless quest for intimacy without understanding what real intimacy is. We have allowed our culture to convince us that the only way to find intimacy is through physical involvement. I am personally convinced that most young people use sex as a means of achieving intimacy. They don't want sex as much as they want closeness with another human being. The tragedy is that people, including our kids, are jumping from one bed to another in search of intimacy. At best all they find is a sense of caring which only lasts for the short duration of lovemaking and orgasm. When it's over they feel more lonely than before. "Another letdown," they sigh, "so I'll just have to try again."

Today we see people getting involved in sexual activity—often promiscuous sexual activity—for the simple reason that they don't understand what true intimacy is. Sexual experience becomes a substitute for intimacy. We use phrases like "making love" and "being intimate" in talking about sexual intercourse. Yet most sexual involvements outside the loving commitment of marriage express very little genuine love or closeness.

♦ Afraid of Intimacy

Not only do many people misunderstand real intimacy, but they also are afraid of it. Existential psychologist Rollo May said:

> There is so much use of the body as a substitute for psychological intimacy. It's much easier to jump into bed with somebody than it is to share your fears, your anxieties, your hopes . . . all that goes on in your psychological life. Because the body is used as kind of a buffer, the intimacy gets short-circuited and never becomes real intimacy. 81/56

Why do people fear intimacy? Because intimacy inevitably brings vulnerability. Emotional sharing requires self-disclosure, and for many of us, opening our innermost selves to another person is a scary prospect.

♦ A Father's Love

Often the media asks me to give one reason kids become sexually involved. Many pressures affect teenage sexuality, but if I had to give one reason, I would say **kids get sexually involved in search of a father's love.**

Recently I was in Phoenix speaking in high school assemblies. In four days we had nine assemblies with fantastic responses from the kids and teachers. During one outdoor noon assembly with more than 900 in attendance, six tough-looking punk rockers with wild hairdos, and wearing chains, stood near the boulder I was using as a platform. I kept thinking, *What are these guys up to?* They stared at me as if to say, "I dare you to try to influence me." It was obvious they didn't fit in with the rest of the students, but I was glad to have them there because they attracted a greater crowd.

As soon as I finished speaking and stepped down off the boulder, the leader of the punk rockers charged right up to me. The crowd of 900 gasped in anticipation of what might happen. He came within six inches of my nose, and I could see tears streaming down his cheeks. He said, "Mr. McDowell, would you give me a hug?" I said yes, but before I could get my arms up he threw his arms around me. He stood there in front of his peers for over a minute just holding me and weeping. When he finished, he stepped back and tearfully said, **"Mr. McDowell, my father has never told me 'I love you' or hugged me."**

We don't have a teenage sexual crisis–we have a teenage/parental relationship crisis. Teens are looking for intimacy from those who love them, particularly their fathers. And when they don't find it there, they turn to sexual activity to get it.

A letter I received from a 27-year-old single woman named Dottie sums it up best. She gave me permission to print it:

Dear Josh,

When I was only 14, I dated an 18-year-old boy. After a month or so of dating, he told me he loved me and had to have me. He said if I loved him, I would have sex with him, and if I wouldn't, he couldn't control his desire for me and would have to break up with me. I knew that sex before marriage was wrong, and I didn't want to lose my virginity. Yet I so desired to have a man love me.

I was insecure in my father's love because I always felt that I had to earn it. The better I was at home and at school, the more my father loved me. Now here was the boy I thought I loved telling me sex was the way to earn his love. I didn't want to lose his love so I finally gave in.

I felt so guilty afterwards. I can remember sobbing in my bed at night after having been with him. I wanted so much to have my virginity back, but it was gone forever. After two years I broke up with my boyfriend, but soon had another and then another. I was a puppet in the hands of any man who said, "I love you," for I desperately wanted someone to love me unconditionally.

One night a few months ago I wrote these lines in my diary summarizing my search for love:

> *"I felt lonely tonight, and I thought about the many times in my life I have felt this intense loneliness. I realized that I was lonely for a daddy, to be able to call him up when I hurt, have him listen to me and hear him say he understands. But I never had that special relationship with my dad as I grew up. So I'm lonely, without a link to my past. Then I thought about the young girl who will lose her virginity tonight because she is searching for love, her daddy's love. And I wanted to be able to stop her somehow and tell her that she'll never find it in another man. How my heart hurts when I think of this girl, and of myself, so many years ago. My life has been one big search for my daddy's love." (August 11, 1985)*

Dottie

♦ Please Love Me

Our kids don't want sex as much as they want to be loved. It's as true for sons as it is for daughters, girls like Dottie. They want someone who cares, who will listen and who will talk to them, and they want it to start with their fathers. This is the heartache of the broken home, whether through a legal divorce, an "emotional divorce" between parents and children or simply a lack of love and communication. Kids who are not loved at home will look for love in all the wrong places.

The following paragraphs, written by teens, further illustrate how they feel about their parents' love or lack of love:

Dad, I've always wanted to do things with you, but you never want to do anything. I know you're busy and you have a hard time keeping your head above water. But, if we both sacrifice a little, maybe things will get better between us. I love you very much and I hope we can do things together before it's too late.

* * *

Thank you for loving me and spending time with me as I was growing up. You gave me everything I ever wanted: your love and your time.

* * *

I think it started when I was very small. I grew up with a father who never spent time with me. For so long I didn't understand what was missing or why I was so insecure and afraid of people, especially men and authority figures. I don't know how to love anyone because no one ever showed me. I wish I had a father like you. I wish someone loved me like you love your family. If someone would just hold me for a minute–no strings, no games.

* * *

We went to church every time the doors were open and sometimes when they weren't. I had (and still have) good, godly parents, and they expected me to be the same way. I think it really hit home when I was about six. I had done something wrong, so I told my mother about it. After I poured out my soul to her, she just sat there and looked at me like she was really hurt. "Honey, we expect better than this from you. Mommy and Daddy want their little girl to be good. We're so disappointed in you!" I can still feel those words ringing in my ears. I decided right then that if I ever had a problem or did something wrong, I would **not** *tell my parents. I couldn't risk their being disappointed in me.*

♦ Deal With Problems Instead of Symptoms

Sexual promiscuity, pregnancy and abortion among teens are only symptoms, not the real problem. **Kids get involved sexually because they are hurting relationally.** The problem stems from the three sources of influence for sexual activity in kids' lives: their peers, their hormones and their parents.

The **first** influence is *pressure from boyfriends or girlfriends* whose love is available and who say sex is okay. When teens feel rejected at home and believe their folks don't care, the words "I love you" have a powerful impact when expressed by one of their friends. Kids may be confused about whether or not to have sex, but the power of feeling loved is often stronger than any conviction to wait until marriage.

The **second** influence is the blossoming *adolescent sex drive* which craves fulfillment. Teens develop faster today. *Newsweek* reports:

> Among teenage girls, part of the explanation for the trend is biological. In the past century, the age of menarche, or first menstruation, has dropped from about 17 years to 12.5. (For boys, puberty usually begins at 13.) Young people's sexual awareness thus runs breathlessly ahead of their emotional development–particularly now that the period of adolescent dependency has grown longer. 82/51

Kids can say no to their peers and control their hormones, though, if the **third** influence, their *relationship with their parents,* is positive.

Kids who find genuine self-worth in a loving, caring relationship with mom and dad are less likely to unleash their drives and give in to their peers in search of intimacy. When the home is devoid of this parental love, acceptance and intimacy, all three influences are against them. Without a solid love base at home, kids will believe anything and fall for anyone who promises them the love and acceptance they need.

The root of this desire to love and be loved is the need for self-acceptance which comes from feeling secure. **Only when kids have a healthy sense of self-worth can they freely give and receive love.** Otherwise they take rather than give. If their self-worth is not reinforced in the home, and if their need for love is not met there, they will seek security and affirmation elsewhere.

If security at home can only be achieved through performance—good grades, clean room, obedience, etc.—a teen's sense of self-worth will be minimal at best because he can't always perform well. Furthermore, the security-through-performance syndrome at home often finds its way into a teen's relationships as well. The girl hears, "If you love me you'll go to bed with me," and gives in because her self-worth is centered on her need for her boyfriend's acceptance. The boy, also needing love, hopes sex will provide the answer to his own need for self-esteem and value. Sadly, both will probably go away unfulfilled.

♦ Help Kids by Helping Parents

We will never solve the problems of teenage sexual involvement until we begin to meet the emotional, relational and spiritual needs of the teens through parental love and intimacy. Yet the preponderance of comprehensive sex education today, intended to help teens toward emotional stability and mental and physical health, deals only with the physical aspect of teenage promiscuity, pregnancy and abortion. If we really want to help kids, we must help their parents. If we don't, we will continue to send our teenagers down the road to self-destruction by advocating a solution that is based on a false premise (e.g., teen pregnancies will be reduced through more education about sex and greater access to contraceptives).

My father used to hammer home to me, "Son, a problem well defined is a problem half solved." **We aren't seeing solutions to our kids' sexual problems because we have failed to correctly define those problems.** So much of sex education today is based on wrong assumptions about young people. If we don't learn from the mistakes and devastating results of the last twenty years of sex education, may God have mercy on us as a culture and a nation, especially on our young people.

CHAPTER 2

False Assumption 2

"It's Unrealistic to Expect Teens to Wait"

The proponents of this assumption contend that no matter what we do, say or teach to the contrary, kids are going to be sexually involved. Organizations such as Planned Parenthood advise us to give our teenagers contraceptives, and instructions on how to use them, because it is unrealistic to expect the teenagers to wait until marriage to have sex.

One leading spokesperson for this position is Dr. Ruth Westheimer, the popular sex therapist. During a recent tour, I spoke to the student body at the University of Cincinnati two weeks after Dr. Ruth had addressed the same crowd. A Cincinnati television station videotaped interviews with Dr. Ruth when she was in town, and then with me two weeks later. They edited the two tapes into a debate format and broadcast the program as if Dr. Ruth and I were talking to each other—not a very intimate debate, but certainly interesting!

Dr. Ruth's message to the students in Cincinnati, and on other campuses across the country, about postponing sexual gratification until marriage is this: "Young people, it's unrealistic to expect you to wait. Your libido [i.e., your sex drive] is too strong." You might as well give in to your instincts because they are in control anyway.

♦ Instincts Versus Self-Control

If we are really the helpless victims of our libido and are bound to give in to our sexual instincts and urges as Dr. Ruth contends, why do we punish rapists? If a person commits rape and is caught, and then claims that he couldn't help himself, shouldn't we set him free? Of course not! Rape is immoral and illegal, and rapists must be punished. If we didn't believe it was possible to control sexual instincts, we would have to wipe all the laws against rape and other sex crimes off the books.

And if we are really the helpless victims of our sexual urges, why do we censure people like former presidential candidate Gary Hart for infidelity? After all, his libido was too strong. How can we blame him for giving in to something he couldn't control? The argument is nonsense, of course—but if we expect public figures to control their urges and remain faithful in marriage, is it unrealistic to expect kids to control their urges and remain chaste before marriage?

Nationally syndicated columnist William Raspberry published this statement in his column, purposely leaving "it" undefined: "Young people are going to do it anyway, so rather than waste time shouting a futile 'Don't,' maybe we ought to just teach them to do it responsibly: supply them with the information, the resources and the devices to eliminate the worst of the consequences of their doing it." 231

Raspberry then pointed out that many people would reluctantly agree with his statement if the "it" were teenage sex. But they would react with shock and indignation if the "it" were teen drug use. He concluded: "We remain . . . absolute when it comes to illicit drugs, while in matters of sex, we are rapidly adopting . . . a tendency to set rules, not on what we think is proper behavior, but on what people actually do." 231

Reflecting on Raspberry's observation, a report by the staff of the Department of Education to the President of the United States says:

> Regarding drugs, we are now sending an absolute message of "no" to our children. On sex, we're still stuck in the '60s, trying to make the best of unacceptable conduct. But if these two patterns of behavior are intimately related, if indeed they are two parallel expressions of the same eth-ical vacuum among many teens, we cannot address them in conflicting ways. We cannot hope to fill half a vacuum. Either we give young people a coherent, integrated approach to the temptations of modern life; or else they will apply the least common ethical denominator to all the moral questions that confront them." 277/26 and 225

If it's possible to say no to drugs, it's also possible to say no to sex.

♦ Human Versus Animal

Educator Coleen Mast asks a pertinent question on the subject of instincts versus self-control: "If our culture encourages self-control in so many other health-related areas—diet, exercise, stress management, alcohol, tobacco, drugs—why shouldn't it encourage self-control in sexual matters as well?" She emphasizes that those who insist our kids are the victims of their sexual instincts "reinforce the mentality that our young people are nothing more than animals, enslaved by the need to mate whenever they feel the urge." 202/547

Mast explains that, "unlike animals, humans are able to use their minds to control the urge for sexual intercourse–they can reason about the appropriateness, the consequences, and the meaning of their sexual behavior. A biological basis for this distinction between man and animal can be found in the physiology of the brain." 202/545

Mast learned in her graduate studies in health education:

> The human brain is composed of the hypothalamus (the "old brain" or "animal brain"), which is concerned primarily with the sensations of pain and pleasure, and the cerebral cortex, the center of reasoning. While the hypothalamus prompts the individual to seek immediate gratification, the cerebral cortex enables the individual to think about consequences and ramifications, to make choices based on self-sacrifice, commitment, delayed gratification, and love. Understanding sex as a controllable drive rather than an irresistible need undermines the pleasure ethic so prevalent in "value-free" sex education. Recreational sex (hedonism), by assuming that adolescents are interested in sex merely as an act, treats them as less than human. We need to teach our youth that because they are human, they can choose to respect their sexuality, using it to meet their true need of finding mutual fulfillment in love. 202/545

One of the most basic and crucial differences between the views of those people advocating the comprehensive sex education model and those advocating the abstinence model concerns the human versus animal contrast.

The *comprehensive sex education* model promotes the "philosophical view of man as just a higher animal (B. F. Skinner . . . Pavlov, etc.)." He "can't stop biological urges. . . . All one can hope for is to provide training (contraceptives) and a way out for mistakes (abortion)."

The *abstinence model* sees man as having a mind, intellect and spirit and as a rational being who can exercise self-discipline, think abstractly and make decisions based on future expectations. People have the capacity to dream, to choose and to love.

I wish Dr. Ruth, Planned Parenthood and others like them would get one thing straight: We're not talking about animal sexuality; we're talking about human sexuality. We're talking about young people created in the image of God with personal dignity, respect for themselves and others, and the capacity to say no and abide by it. We're talking about teenagers who, given the opportunity and encouragement, can make right moral choices and carry them out. The moment we surrender this truth about our kids, we put them in the same category as dogs in heat. It *is* realistic to expect our kids to wait. Our kids are not animals! They *can* control their hormones and desires.

♦ Say No to Sex

I received the following letter from a college junior who wants to be treated as a human instead of an animal:

Dear Josh,

I know you're really busy, but I thought I'd write this to tell you how one of your talks changed my life.

I was involved in a sexual relationship with a guy. I didn't want to be, but I just didn't think I had the right to tell him no. I came to your conference two years ago and heard you speak about . . . love and forgiveness, and my life changed. **Please don't stop telling people that they can say no** [emphasis added].

Lori

A rather obvious conclusion about helping kids avoid premarital sex is that "rather than presuming the teenagers are going to have sex anyway, our collective strategy for combatting teen pregnancy should be similar to the approach we have taken on curbing adolescent drug addiction, alcohol abuse, and smoking—we should encourage teens to say no." **6/7**

Will they listen? Some of them will. I cannot accept the idea that all young people are going to become sexually involved no matter what we do. Statistics bear out my conviction: "A recent national study found that even today nearly half of all 19-year-old females have never had premarital intercourse. The issue is whether current pregnancy rates can be reduced by discouraging unmarried teenagers from engaging in sexual activity." **6/4-6**

A survey of the top 5 percent of high school juniors and seniors (6.5 million in 1979-80) clearly shows that **many outstanding young people have not chosen to succumb. More than 75 percent of these leaders have not had sexual intercourse.** **7/9**

On January 23, 1984, the Associated Press carried the following news item: "A survey of 1,200 young people in Grady's Teen Services Program found 80 percent said they wanted to know more about how to say no. And testing of the program in Atlanta and Cleveland found numbers of young people who were 'tremendously relieved' to hear a supportive message telling them that it's okay to slow down while growing up." **8**

Eunice Kennedy Shriver, after visiting a center for teenage girls, reported that **when students were asked what they most wanted**

to discuss, they chose "how to say no to your boyfriend." They showed no interest in human biology or family planning." 232/11-12; 233/4

♦ Not Everyone Is Doing It

Not too long ago NBC broadcast a week of *Today* shows live from China. On Friday's show a woman reporter interviewed a group of Communist Chinese high school and college students on the topic of sex. Did she get frustrated! She didn't get the kind of answers she wanted to send back to the U.S.

The first question she asked was, "Do you believe that premarital sex is wrong?"

The entire group immediately responded, "Yes."

When the reporter asked why, the students replied, "It's immoral." They went on to explain that sex is to be saved for a husband and wife in marriage.

Perplexed, the reporter exclaimed, "Are you trying to tell me that all of you are going to wait until marriage to have sex?"

The students looked at each other and then answered in the affirmative with expressions which conveyed, "What a dumb question!"

The reporter came unglued as the ramifications of their responses began to dawn on her. She said, "Are you telling me that all of you are virgins?" They answered yes.

If you take seriously what Planned Parenthood, Dr. Ruth and others are telling us about our kids not being able to wait, you must conclude that these Chinese students were born with more character, more control over their lives and a greater capacity to say no than our young people. I don't believe that. The issue is not what our kids can or cannot do. The issue that makes the difference is the system our kids are raised in – the culture and the media. Saying no is something kids learn to do. In our culture we are not teaching them how to say no and therefore are not expecting them to say no.

Studies show that 90 percent of all Swedish girls have experienced sex before their twentieth birthday. About 65 percent of American girls have had sex by that age. However, only 17 percent of unmarried Japanese girls have lost their virginity before age 20. 1 Are we saying that Japanese girls have more character, more ability and more capacity for saying no than American girls? No. The issue isn't capacity – it is the pressures kids face in our culture and our failure to educate our kids to make proper emotional and ethical choices and to exercise physical control.

♦ Some American Kids Do Say No

Another evidence that our kids are not the helpless victims of their sexual instincts is the simple fact that an average of 35-45 percent of American teenagers are *not* sexually involved. These are kids who could be involved if they wanted to be, but they aren't. The 1987 Survey of High Achievers for *Who's Who Among American High School Students* found that 73 percent of the students had never had sexual intercourse and 61 percent believed that sex should not be a part of a steady romance. 280

Young people are not automatically sexually active. The rates of involvement can decline as well as increase. Dr. Jacqueline Kasun, professor of economics and research analyst at Humboldt State University, makes the following observations about the cultural changes over the past fifteen years:

> When we state that there has been a dramatic increase in teenage sexual activity over the past fifteen years, we also state that historically, sexual promiscuity among teenagers was less common than it is today. Obviously, the desire for sexual activity was the same. The difference is best understood in terms of the greater cultural consensus, the more clearly defined and articulated moral standards, and the greater willingness that once existed of those in authority to actively promote and advocate chastity.
>
> Over the past fifteen years, we have witnessed a degeneration of a moral consensus, and [a growth of] general, moral and ethical confusion along with an unwillingness to state in unequivocal terms that sexual activity outside of marriage is no less than immoral and destructive. Yet even today, the data clearly indicate that teen sex is not inevitable.

Dr. Kasun charts the percentage of never-married women aged 15-19 who have never had intercourse:

Age	1971	1976	1979	1982
15	14.4%	18.6%	22.5%	17.8%
16	20.9	28.9	37.8	28.1
17	26.1	42.9	48.5	41.0
18	39.7	51.4	56.9	61.7
19	46.4	59.5	69.0	61.7

Source: Unpublished tabulations from the NSFG, Cycle III, 1982. Unpublished tabulations from the National Longitudinal Survey of Youth, 1983; Zelnik and Kantner.

The above table indicates that nearly half of all 18-year-old females have never had premarital intercourse. Additionally, according to Zelnik and Kantner, 14.8 percent of all sexually experienced teenagers aged 15-19 have had intercourse only once, and of sexually experienced teenagers aged 15-17, 19.9 percent have had intercourse only once. 380

Kids today can say no to their sexual urges. Even people like Dr. Ruth agree that if a 15-year-old boy wants to have sex with his girlfriend, but his girlfriend doesn't want to have sex with him, he should wait. But wait a minute; that's contradictory! First they say it's unrealistic to wait; the libido is too strong. Then they assert that you can wait if your partner is unwilling. What they are really saying is this: If you and your boyfriend or girlfriend want to have sex, it's *unrealistic* to expect you to wait because "your libido is too strong"; but if you want to have sex and your partner doesn't, it's *realistic* to expect you to wait because "your libido is *not* too strong."

"That's crazy," you say.

You must realize that many of the underlying attitudes and philosophies of secular educators and sex education programs are marked by this kind of double talk, which contradicts standards and belies any personal accountability and responsibility.

♦ Authorities Aren't Saying No

The attitude of so many in positions of authority and influence in our country today doesn't afford our kids a fighting chance to say no to sex. Congressman George Miller says: "We have to stop worrying about whether teenagers are having sex. They are. We have to deal with it from there." 2/1 Miller wants to spend more of our tax dollars on pregnancy-prevention education programs.

Faye Wattleton, president of Planned Parenthood Federation of America (PPFA), believes that sex among teens is "a given. I don't think anyone with a rational mind is going to say that as of a given date there will be no more teenage sexual activity." 3 I'm sure glad Ms. Wattleton isn't in charge of our national anti-drug campaign!

When those in the public eye give up on kids being able to control their sexual instincts, what chance do our kids have of developing a capacity for abstinence?

Let's face it: We will always have some kids who are sexually active, and there will always be unintended teenage pregnancies. But that doesn't mean we should give up on attempts to educate them to the contrary and change their behavior patterns. After all, we will also always have prostitutes, drug addicts, alcoholics, wife abusers, child molesters, rapists, tax evaders and thieves. But we don't stop trying to prevent them from harming themselves and others with their socially unacceptable activities.

Concerning the attitude that more and more kids are going to become sexually active, Dr. Kasun warns that it would be

short-sighted to extrapolate from this that this is an irreversible trend and consequently to abandon our children to sexual promiscuity. The trends can be reversed but only if we are willing to candidly reevaluate existing programs and make the much needed changes. 380

♦ Protection Instead of Prevention

According to PPFA and most other advocates of comprehensive sex education, society's responsibility is to protect teenagers from the unhealthy consequences (e.g., pregnancy and sexually transmitted diseases) of their "given" behavior. Therefore, we should develop school-based health clinics to make contraceptives available and then strongly encourage and educate kids on how to use those contraceptives. Since "they're going to have sex anyway," children must be indoctrinated as to how to have "responsible" sex (i.e., why and how to correctly put on a condom).

If we followed this same line of reasoning in regard to children and drugs, we would immediately abandon the preventative "just say no" campaign in favor of an emphasis on "responsible addiction." Since kids are going to take drugs anyway, we should protect them from the harmful consequences of their actions. We must demonstrate to kids at an early age how to "shoot up" with a clean needle in order to protect themselves from the devastating consequences of AIDS. We must have free syringes readily available at school-based health clinics. And, of course, all these services must be offered to the child without parental notification, let alone consent.

To any complaints about drugs being morally wrong or illegal, the free syringe advocates would respond, "We are not involved in morality. Our programs are value-free and morally neutral. We have such a great teen drug crisis that we can't be concerned about morality." But do we apply this same "morally neutral" approach to that activity or to others where we admit kids are going to do it anyway? Are we morally neutral when kids lie to parents or school authorities, cheat on exams, sexually abuse their brothers or sisters, steal tapes from the local music store or deal drugs? Of course not! Isn't it odd that we only become morally neutral when it comes to teen sexual activity?

"The comparison between drugs and sex is unfounded," the critic may retort, "because the situation is totally different. Drugs are illegal!" So is sex when performed by any man or boy with a girl under 18 years of age. Almost every state in the union has laws on the books forbidding sexual activity under the age of 18. Sex is as much a moral and legal issue as any other teen problem. Why don't we deal with it as such?

The critic may further argue that free syringes are already available in our culture—but they are available only to those who are already addicts. We don't make syringes available to children who have never tried drugs. Yet that's not the same logic used by PPFA and other sex education programs regarding the use of condoms to prevent AIDS and pregnancy. They say condoms must be available and easily accessible to all teenagers. Following that same argument in regard to drugs, you would need to educate all children on why and how to use a clean syringe and make syringes available and easily accessible to all kids.

"But if you make syringes available to all kids," the critic protests, "it would encourage unhealthy experimentation and illegal behavior." Yes it would, and that is exactly what the opponents of comprehensive sex education are saying. **The availability of contraceptives encourages unhealthy, illegal experimentation by children who have never before been sexually involved.**

Why have we adopted a protective instead of a preventive stance with regard to teenage sexuality? Some want us to believe that it's because kids today can't control themselves and so they will be sexually active no matter what we do. That's not true. The Minority Report of the House Select Committee on Children, Youth and Families identified the real reason when it observed: "Progressively over the last twenty-five years, we have, as a nation, decided that it is easier to give children pills than to teach them respect for sex and marriage." 5/386 Young people haven't changed, but the way adults try to help them has.

♦ Fighting Fire With Fire

Bringing in many of the comprehensive sex educators and family planning specialists to help teenagers deal with their sexuality makes as much sense as calling in an arsonist to put out a fire. They don't carry fire extinguishers, they carry flamethrowers! We don't need to throw up our hands in acquiescence, lamenting that kids are going to do it anyway so we'd better protect them—we need to help them learn to say no. *Instead of teaching them about* **birth** *control we should be teaching them about* **self**-*control.* Or in the words of Secretary of Education William Bennett, **"Instead of telling kids, 'Play it safe,' we should be telling them, 'Don't play!' "**

Our culture's bizarre departure from reality in helping teens deal with their sexual instincts was graphically illustrated at the first National Teenage Health Conference sponsored by Emory University in Atlanta, Georgia, on June 19-20, 1978. 381/C-9 The central theme of the conference was guiding teenagers to make their own decisions about sexual activity with due regard to safeguards. About 1,200 students were invited, and many of them attended under the financial sponsorship of family planning groups.

The conference was staffed by counselors who wanted to help teens "feel comfortable" about sexual intercourse. But the *New York Times* reported that the staff members found their task to be more difficult than they expected. One frustrated discussion leader trying to guide her group into accepting the possibility of premarital sex "was repeatedly met with variations of 'you don't need to know about that if you don't mess around.' " The report continued:

> The first frustrated family planner referred to the youngsters' resistance to her ideas as "an extraordinary problem called (by whom, she does not say) the paradox of pregnancy." "These girls just won't admit that they might have a sexual relationship some day," she declared, "and they are precisely the ones who will get pregnant if they do, because they just won't accommodate the possibility of planning on sex by contraception. They feel bound to pretend it was an accident, that they were pushed into sin." She then added: "I sometimes fear that the Judeo-Christian ethic is the greatest contributor to pregnancy that I run into." 381/C-9

This "family planner" urged girls to keep contraceptives in their pockets at all times so that "just in case" they had sex they would be safe. It's the same destructive dog-in-heat mentality toward teen sexual instincts which says, "Look, eventually you're going to do it, so be prepared."

A PPFA leaflet distributed at the conference instructed kids how to help each other put on a condom or apply contraceptive foam as a means of foreplay. Even though they communicated "it's your choice" to the students, only token lip service was given to saying no to sex until marriage. Instead, the nature of the conference said to kids of all ages that it's okay to say yes as long as you play it "safe."

Even though the conference was packed with kids from family planning groups, a large segment of the students were not convinced that sex before marriage is right. A conference survey revealed that 43 percent of the 352 boys in attendance believed that sex should be saved for marriage. One 14-year-old girl "found the whole thing disconcerting and busily looked the other way while a determined counselor sorted through a pile of contraceptive devices, telling how to use each one and where to get them." The 14-year-old's classic comment was: "Well, why do it in the first place?"

♦ Help Instead of Hinder

If our kids are going to succeed at saying no when so much of our culture urges them to say yes, we need to stand beside them. The following letter from a teen echoes this concern:

> *I feel so alone—as if no one cares about what I'm going through. I wish there were someone I could talk to and confide in, someone who's been where I am and could help me through this. I'm so tired of fighting with myself, fighting back my sexual desires, fighting against the sexual desires of my dates. Sometimes I just want to stop fighting. I'm tempted to give up the battle and give in. During those times when I feel so weary,* **I wish I had someone else to encourage me** *and keep me going, someone to fight my battle for me,* **someone to be strong when I am weak** [emphasis added].

Let's give our teens some good news—let's tell them they are not alone!

Young people want to control the sexual area of their lives, and about half of them are showing that it can be done. So instead of undermining our kids with the give-in philosophy of Dr. Ruth and others—"It doesn't matter what you do; kids are going to have sex anyway"—we should respond, "It *does* matter what you do; we're going to help our kids instead of hinder them." **If we don't believe in our kids, how can they believe in themselves? Our kids are not animals, but if we educate them as if they're going to act like animals, we can expect them to act that way.**

♦ Kids Need Stable Standards and Strong Values

How can we help them? Former Surgeon General Koop and Secretary of Education Bennett issued a joint statement saying that "an AIDS education that accepts sexual activity as inevitable and focuses only on 'safe sex' will be at best ineffectual, at worst itself a cause of serious harm." 4/A-3 We must give them more than protection; we must help them with prevention.

Let's not make the same mistakes in Julian which other school districts have made. While I was in Chicago recently, a group of students told me about the "gay rights" speaker who addressed the students at Evanston Township High School. One of his first comments was, "Abstinence is impossible, right guys?"

Sounds to me like this school district was exposing its kids to "a dog in heat" who expected his audience to act the same way.

As long as we have educators, counselors and assembly speakers like this man, the tremendous crisis of teenage sexuality and pregnancies will continue. We are treating our kids like animals **as long as we allow groups like PPFA to say to our kids, "If you're** *not* **supposed to go after a girl for sex,** *what are you supposed to do?*

[emphasis mine]"; 351/17 or, "Don't rob yourself of joy by focusing on old-fashioned ideas about what's 'normal' or 'nice.' " 352/15

Raging hormones, peer pressure, hot movies and suggestive telephone hot lines—there are plenty of influences urging our kids to say yes to sex. We can help our kids by encouraging them that it is okay to say no to sex and yes to moral values. Eunice Kennedy Shriver clearly sees the issue:

> Teenagers want their parents, their teachers, their political leaders to stand up strong for values. And this includes the values of love and sex. . . . We should be repairing the shattered network of family communications whose breakdown is responsible for so much adolescent sexual activity. The young are waiting for challenges, and if we challenge them, they will respond. 10/7

The real problem is not at the physical level—sex organs, unwanted pregnancies, contraception, abortion—but at the emotional level. Our kids are hurting emotionally and crying out for love. They want someone to care for them and guide them through the tough moral choices of adolescence.

In the teen pregnancy program, "A Community of Caring," Eunice Kennedy Shriver said: "Teenagers become sexually active and risk pregnancy, not out of ignorance, but out of lovelessness; not out of an absence of values, not because contraception is unavailable, but because their sexuality has not been given a strong moral context" (November 4, 1988).

The California Educational Code, enacted into law by the State Senate in 1988, rightly states: "Course material and instruction shall emphasize that the pupil has the power to control personal behavior." 79 As school board members, persons who carry the weight of responsibility for the education of our kids, you must uphold this code. I beg you: Don't give in to the false, counterproductive, destructive mentality that the kids are going to do it anyway. Let's give our kids a chance to dream, to think, to choose, to love and to make and act upon right moral decisions. They are not animals; let's not treat them as such.

CHAPTER 3

False Assumption 3

"The Media Tells Teens the Truth About Sex"

NBC recently aired a highly rated special called "Scared Sexless," hosted by NBC anchor Connie Chung. Ms. Chung is a tremendous reporter; I enjoy listening to her—but about halfway through the program she made a comment I could hardly believe. She was being challenged about the media's portrayal of sex. In defense of the media she stated, "The media reflects reality in sexual experience."

Is that the truth? Absolutely not. The media—and I'm talking particularly about the entertainment media—grossly distorts reality in sexual experience. For the most part sex as portrayed on TV, in the movies, in popular music, in the print media and in advertising is fiction, not fact. Unfortunately, our kids have a hard time distinguishing the truth about sex from the media's fantasy.

♦ The Number One Influence on Kids

Most current studies, including a recent Junior Achievement report, show that the media (TV, radio, movies) ranks third behind peers and parents in influencing teen values and behavior. This represents a dramatic shift since 1960 when the media ranked eighth behind such factors as teachers, relatives and religious leaders. 14/4 Our national Why Wait? study showed that kids were influenced by peers first, media second and parents third.

Still, I firmly believe that the entertainment media, not peers, is the number one influence on our kids' sexual beliefs and behavior, on how they determine who they are as sexual beings and on how they treat other people. Why? Because the peers who influence our kids so greatly are also influenced by the media.

What kind of influence is the entertainment media having on our kids today? Former Surgeon General Koop, in a personal interview, explained a report funded by his office:

> In Michigan, in four cities that studied junior high and high school girls, it was found that the girls watch an average of two and a half to three hours of soap operas per day, and that there is one episode of sexual intercourse per hour on those films—almost always between unmarried people. But more surprising to us was that the movies these youngsters wanted to see most were R-rated movies, and we found that 66 to 77 percent of the girls in these four cities had seen the six top R-rated films that year. The fascinating thing to me is that not one of these girls was ever challenged at the box office although all of them were under age, and the movies contained eight instances of sexual intercourse among unmarried people per film. Two of those films had even more than that. One had fourteen. That was so popular with young people that it has now been made into a television series.

I think the media have downgraded morality in this country to the point where kids think if they do what they see, they are behaving according to the norm of society. 31

A study on *The Impact of Media on the Sexual Attitudes of Adolescents* presented at the National Council on Family Relations annual conference concluded that "there appears to be a correlation between the total media time of the students and their premarital sexual attitudes." 672/2

Researchers Anderson and Wright also concluded from their study that there appears to be a strong correlation between the favorite movies of adolescents and their premarital sexual attitudes. When youth selected R- or X-rated movies as their most preferred, the probability that they would have a permissive sexual attitude was extremely high. On the other hand, those who chose PG as most preferred were traditional in their premarital sexual attitudes. 672/6

♦ The Impact of Television

TV—the electronic baby-sitter—has probably done more to shape attitudes of teens than any other single factor of American life, especially with the advent of cable television. Recently the doctors of the American Academy of Pediatrics urged parents to keep their children from watching cable station MTV because of its constant message of sex and violence. According to the Academy's policy statement: "Too many music videos promote sexism, violence, substance abuse, suicides and sexual behavior." 21

The major television networks are feeling the heat from the "freedom of expression" found on cable television. Although network television is still the industry leader, the cable industry is cutting heavily into its market share, and the networks have been forced to do something about it. The fallout is a new low standard for portraying sexual activity on the screen. Art Chapman, president of the Television Critics Association and TV critic for the *Fort Worth Star-Telegram,* said, "In the last year I've become disillusioned; there's been a shift toward more explicit programming." 11/14-21 All the networks except CBS have done away with their departments for program standards, and CBS has reduced its staff in that department.

In a recent *TV Guide* article, "TV's Getting Sexier – How Far Will It Go?" a network executive blasted NBC and its mini-series, *Favorite Son.* He was appalled by the portrayal of sexual bondage, a 60-second strip sequence and a scene where actress Linda Kozlowski *(Crocodile Dundee)* undressed behind a sheer curtain where her nude figure was clearly visible. The executive called it a "quantum leap" in difference from past network programming. 11/14-21

♦ TV's False Message

What does television tell our young people about sex? Mostly lies. Perhaps you think I'm exaggerating to make a point. After all, we all watch television. Is it really communicating lies?

The *Journal of Communication* reports that "television portrays six times more extramarital sex than sex between spouses. Ninety-four percent of the sexual encounters on soap operas are between people not married to each other." 382 What kind of impression does that make on young people, especially when the characters are the "beautiful people" on shows like *Dynasty, Dallas* and *Knots Landing?* Television is telling our kids that most of the sexual activity in the country occurs outside the bounds of marriage. That's a lie.

Roger Simon of the *Los Angeles Times* comments: "In the old days of television, unmarried couples who 'did it' suffered tragically. If a girl had sex out of wedlock, she got pregnant or got hit by a truck or both. And because it was so unreal, it was kind of a joke. It didn't scare kids into not having sex. . . . But TV changed a lot. . . . The *Love Boat* was a good example. On that show, people did it like minks. And no tragedy followed. And no guilt. Sex was as casual as breakfast. But in doing away with guilt, TV also did away with responsibility." 26/6-8

Not everything we see on television is make-believe. Teens see Jerry Hall on television talking about having Mick Jagger's second out-of-wedlock child and saying what a wonderful life she has. A procession of unmarried stars, including Farrah Fawcett and Jessica Lange, have joined Hall in proclaiming on television the "joys" of extramarital pregnancy. Television is telling our kids that premarital and extramarital sex are the norm and that chances of getting pregnant when you don't want to or of contracting a disease are almost nil.

Do kids believe that? Child psychologist Dr. Lee Salk cautions, "A child who has been kept in the dark about sex is going to be highly vulnerable to look upon these scenes as his or her accepted set of values when it comes to sexuality." 20/5 A study by Lou Harris and Associates revealed that 41 percent of teenagers think that television gives a realistic picture of the consequences of sex. What may be even more sobering is that 24 percent of adults believe what they see about sex on TV—one out of four! 27/9

♦ Sex in the Afternoon

What about daytime television—particularly the soap operas—where sex, deception and lack of traditional moral values are so obvious? On the soaps, glamorous women and macho men pass from one sex partner to another like playing musical chairs. According to *Broadcasting* magazine, "Daytime television contained 50 percent more sexual references than prime time . . . 33 instances per hour versus 23. Daytime serials were the chief repository (35 instances per hour) . . . followed by theatricals (30), made-fors (24), sitcoms (24) and prime time serials (21)." 18/121

Here's a letter I received which I believe summarizes the effect of the soaps on many young viewers:

> *When I was a youngster, the soap operas were a part of my daily entertainment. What a mistake to fill the young mind with such thinking! I also purchased sexual-type magazines* (Cosmopolitan, Mademoiselle, *etc.) at a very young age. My mother never monitored what we read (or watched). Thoughts of petting, kissing and sexual intercourse were planted in my mind during a very crucial point in my adolescent life. By the eighth grade I was already acting out, by kissing and petting during recess, what had been planted in my thoughts. This continued during high school. When I moved away from home to college, I began having intercourse.*

Last season on the soap *Another World,* high school senior Thomasina Harding became pregnant. However, her boyfriend quickly married her, got a college scholarship, became the star of the football team and got a good job. "The new baby is beautiful, hardly ever cries and everybody is deliriously happy. It's hard to imagine a less realistic depiction of the experience of adolescent pregnancy." 12/7,17-18 Soap opera sex is a lie.

♦ Sex on the Silver Screen

Picture this real-life scenario: Boy meets girl. Boy and girl find each other attractive and want to get to know each other better, so they set aside an evening to be together. Do they talk? No. They spend $10 (at least) to sit side by side in a movie theater and stare at the screen.

Now picture the on-screen scenario they are watching: Boy meets girl. Boy and girl find each other attractive and want to know each other better, so they set aside an evening to be together. Do they talk? Do they go to a movie? No. They remove their clothes and have sex to the glorious sound of music. The movie has a happy ending.

After the movie the real-life boy and girl still want to get to know each other. Besides, their hormones are roaring after watching a movie which communicated that sex is a great way to get to know someone. Their minds reel (no pun intended!) with visions of skin, strains of beautiful music and the expectation of a happy ending. They look deeply into each other's eyes, fumble with each other's clothes and have sex in the car.

Final real-life scenario: Boy thinks girl is too easy and dumps girl. Girl can't figure out what she did wrong. Both wonder what happened to the happy ending.

Does that sound far-fetched? Read part of a letter I received from a girl in West Virginia who lived it:

> *At age 17 I began dating a boy who had graduated and gotten work with a factory in town. I thought he was cool. Well, one night we went to see the movie* 10. *On the way home we took a detour and had intercourse in the back seat of his mother's car. After five months of dating he broke up with me. I was crushed.*

There seem to be very few movies today portraying positive moral values. Not many movie makers are interested in reality on the screen; the only reality that counts is at the box office. Teen sex films with beautiful music and happy endings keep making money, so movie makers will keep producing them. Sadly, our kids tend to believe that these movies are telling the truth. In reality, most of what the movies portray about sex is false.

♦ Selling With Sex

Sex is a primary ingredient in most advertising. Sex is used to sell everything from automobiles to deodorants. TV commercials, radio spots and magazine display ads suggest that our sex life will improve if we wear designer jeans, drive sporty cars, splash on a certain cologne or brush with the right toothpaste. That's a fantasy.

We are often told that advertising doesn't affect behavior very much. When the public was exerting pressure to remove cigarette ads from TV, the tobacco companies argued that commercials don't change a person's lifestyle, and that media ads would not cause a person to take up smoking. If that is true, why does the tobacco industry spend hundreds of millions of dollars on advertising? **If there is no relationship between TV commercials and viewers' behavior, why do American businesses spend $3 billion annually on advertising for prime time television alone?**

According to *TV Guide,* the number of network commercials run each week in 1981 was 4,079, more than double the figure of 1967. 28/84 In 1983, more than $16 billion was spent on television advertising and more than $5 billion on radio advertising. 29/62-63 And much of the advertising we see is linked with the excitement and allure of sex. Madison Avenue is not telling our kids the truth.

♦ Lying About the Consequences

You may say, "We admit that the excessive examples of sexual activity in the entertainment media and advertising is undoubtedly a bad influence on our young people, but in a society as sexually permissive as ours, where's the lie?"

The media isn't lying about the existence of promiscuity in our society, even though it certainly exaggerates the predominance of premarital and extramarital sex over marital sex and premarital virginity. The lie is that they very seldom portray the negative consequences to promiscuous, uncommitted sex.

Drs. Elster and Hendee of the American Medical Association said of the media lie: **"The behavior has no consequences. People drink alcohol, but don't crash their cars. They smoke, but don't get lung cancer. They have sex, but they don't become pregnant. What kind of message is that?"** 383

For years we have allowed the media to misrepresent casual sex and free love. Young people have been shown that jumping into bed cures everything: personal emptiness and loneliness, and lack of significance, self-esteem or self-fulfillment. Sex is not a cure-all. In fact, sex outside of marriage may be one of society's major "cause-alls." There's no such thing as casual sex or free love without the potential for devastating consequences.

The *Houston Chronicle* reports:

> **Teens . . . lack the life experience that would allow them to view the stories more realistically. . . .** Even news stories on television or in newspapers have an effect. When kids read that teens are more sexually active than ever, they aren't appalled. Rather, they wonder what's wrong with them. 25/18

For the most part, we have allowed our young people to determine their identity as sexual beings on the basis of the misinformation propagated by the mass media. This deception is crucial because our sexuality affects everything we say, hear, think and do. Sexuality is at the core of human existence, and our kids are growing up basing their sexuality on fiction.

♦ The Fantasy of Fiction

When I speak in high schools and universities, I challenge students about their concepts of sexuality. Usually this challenge meets stiff resistance. But when they understand the facts, the students usually nod their heads in agreement.

When I addressed a crowd of 6,000 students at Purdue University in February 1990, I began by saying, "You've been lied to. Your sexuality, how you perceive yourself as a sexual being, and how you treat others sexually is based on fiction." I could feel the crowd tense up. They murmured in disagreement. "I'll prove it to you," I continued. I quoted some of the statistics I shared earlier in this chapter on the number of sex scenes and innuendos American viewers see by age 20.

"The entertainment media has removed almost all the negative consequences of promiscuous, uncommitted sex. That's fiction. How many of you have seen a character on a TV show contract a sexually transmitted disease from their bedroom antics?" About ten hands went up in the audience of 6,000. "You've been lied to; that's fiction. Every day 33,000 Americans get a sexually transmitted disease. 23/53-57 Today, 2.5 million teenagers are afflicted with STDs, 384/10A but chances are you won't see that dramatized, because sex on TV is fiction. **The best thing that could happen for teens today is to see J.R. get VD on TV!** If anyone in real life played around as much as J.R. does on *Dallas,* he would either be dead or paralyzed from the waist down. But you don't see that in the entertainment media because it's fiction."

Then I asked a second question: "How many of you have seen a baby born on TV with a birth defect because of a sexually transmitted disease?" Not one hand went up. "That's fiction. In the past twelve months more babies have been born with birth defects caused by STDs than all the children affected by polio during the entire ten-year epidemic in the '50s. 91/73

By this time the 6,000 students were sober and attentive. I pressed on with my next question: "How many of you have seen a child or teenager in a TV drama or comedy hurting emotionally because his or her parents were divorced?" Not one hand went up. "Amazing," I exclaimed to the crowd, "because hurting children of divorce live in nearly half the houses in this country. But you don't see the hurt on TV. Everyone on TV, even kids whose parents split, lives happily ever after. That's fiction!"

My final question really penetrated: "How many of you have seen someone on TV say no to sex who wasn't in bed after a two-minute commercial?" Again, not one hand went up. "You have been brainwashed. There are countless numbers of people who say no to illicit sex every day. If your sexuality is based on the permissiveness you see on TV, it's based on fiction."

By now the crowd was sitting in stunned silence. They realized that they had bought into the lie about sex which the media so cunningly perpetrates. My experience at Purdue University was no isolated incident. I've seen the same response at hundreds of high schools and universities all over the country—from Stanford to Ohio State, from USC to Florida.

The point is this: **Watching TV to learn how to love makes as much sense as watching a Road Runner cartoon to learn self-defense.** But that's exactly what's happening with our kids. Can you see why a 16-year-old girl who just lost her virginity wrote to me: *"Mr. McDowell, I couldn't compete with television"*?

♦ Distorted Reality

By and large, the secular media does little to reinforce moral values or demonstrate the consequences of irresponsible moral behavior, and thus distorts reality. This distortion cultivates feelings of inadequacy among teens. A tremendous emphasis on the value of a person is placed on the physical. The media displays a constant parade of beautiful women, giving teenage girls an unrealistic standard by which to judge their own attractiveness. What's more, the standard is constantly changing, shifting the focus from breasts to legs to hairstyles to buttocks. It's easy to see how a girl can get a distorted sense of self-worth as she tries to compete on the basis of physical attractiveness. The young male is also affected. He develops totally unrealistic ideas about a woman's true beauty.

Enticing ads, erotic TV and movie scenes and suggestive music lyrics communicate to our teens: "Be sexually active." The focus is on immediate sexual gratification. Yet most concerned parents promote abstinence as the standard for teens. Our teens are getting mixed signals about their sexual behavior; no wonder there is so much confusion. Michelle, a teenager, told me, "Our families and teachers tell us to say no to sex, but often TV, movies and commercials say yes to sex. It's made so glamorous."

Teenagers see, hear and read how others are having sex without any negative consequences and wonder why they are left out. When kids see their favorite actors, actresses, TV heroes or rock stars enjoying sex with no consequences, they will eventually want to emulate them. But their sexual activity will be hollow and unfulfilling because they are basing it on a distortion of reality.

♦ Powerful Influences

What gives the media such power over young people? The amount of time they spend watching, listening to and reading it. The average preschooler spends more time watching television than a university student spends in the classroom earning a bachelor's degree. One study reveals that preschool children watch twenty hours of television a week and grade-school children, twenty-two. "Sleeping is the only activity that commands more of their time. By the age of 18, they will have spent more time in front of the TV set than anywhere else, including school." 33/39

During grades seven to twelve, kids listen to an average total of 10,500 hours of rock music. The total amount of time spent in school over a period of twelve years is just 500 hours more than that. 34/46

As a result of their preoccupation with the media, young people spend less time interacting with real adults. One family magazine states: "The average five-year-old spends only twenty-five minutes a week in close interaction with his father. . . according to one study. That same child spends twenty-five hours a week in close interaction with the TV." 35

Carol Tawarnicky states: "Teenagers are inordinately influenced by the media. They have less interaction with real adults than ever before, so their friends and the 'models' presented in the media have an even greater impact." 25/17-18

While we have been permissively silent, the media in our culture has been telling our children that they will find intimacy by jumping into bed and "getting it on." As a result, most of our kids have developed their concept of sexuality from media fiction without realizing the price tag that comes with free love and casual sex. If we don't wake up and help them see the truth and change their attitudes toward sex, they eventually will pay a high price. One young lady tells of that price:

> *What the movies and soap operas don't tell us about is the devastation and broken hearts that occur due to affairs and premarital sex. I don't make light of the consequences of wrong sexual involvement. Without a doubt, the hardest and most painful thing I've gone through—more than major surgery, tests for cancer, a broken family and numerous job rejections—is getting over a sexual relationship with a married man.*

♦ Changes Are Needed

Either the media or the listening and viewing habits of young people must change if their attitudes about sex are going to change. But would a change in the media have a positive effect on the sexual attitudes of our kids? Media critic Roger Simon thinks so:

> Attitudes about sex . . . won't change without changes on TV. . . . Take a look at what has happened to cigarette smoking on TV. You used to see it on shows all the time. At dramatic moments, romantic moments, fun moments, the hero would light up a cigarette. But think hard about TV today. When was the last time you saw someone light a cigarette? It happens, but not often. And this, more than anything else, has changed the way young people look at smoking. It simply does not have the allure it once did. And that's largely because people on TV don't do it anymore. 26/8

Social commentator Benjamin Stein points out: "Positive images would be more effective—[TV] shows that promote good family life, responsibility and moral choices. If those images were supported by adults in their conversations with teenagers, things might begin to change." 36/14

Before placing all the blame and responsibility on the media, however, I think we must examine what we have done to counteract the situation. Many of us share in the blame because of our permissiveness. How much guidance have we given our children about the kinds of television programs and movies to watch? Have we written to our local television stations when they broadcast something we did not approve of? In most cases I think we have lost the battle without putting up a fight. For years too many of us have been silent about the dangerous effects of the media on our kids. It is time to take seriously the familiar, motivating statement comprised of ten two-letter words:

If it is to be, it is up to me.

If we're going to see a change in our culture's view of sex and a change in our kids' sexual attitudes and actions, we must take the responsibility to see it happen.

CHAPTER 4

➧ A **key section** for busy parents.

False Assumption 4

"Sex Between Consenting Teens Is Nobody Else's Business"

Many people today believe that what happens behind closed doors between two consenting adults (any 15-year-old kid will tell you that he or she is an adult) is private. We're told that the sexual practices of others is none of our business; we can't tell people how to run their sex lives. For example, the government "has no right to enforce laws which affect an individual's private sexual conduct," and schools and churches "should not teach principles to guide or restrict sexual behavior."

The Humanist Manifest II states this position clearly: "In the area of sexuality, we believe that intolerant attitudes, often cultivated by orthodox religions and Puritanical cultures, unduly repress sexual conduct. The right to birth control, abortion and divorce should be recognized. While we do not approve of exploitive, denigration forms of sexual expression, neither do we wish to prohibit, by law or social sanction, sexual behavior between consenting adults." 28/64

Many people will respond, "I guess that's right. Whatever a couple wants to do in private is their business, not mine. After all, if they catch a disease or get pregnant, they will suffer the consequences, not me. Right?"

Wrong! A "private act" of illicit sex can have widespread and horrendous physical, social, political, economical, emotional and moral implications for the society which condones it. Historically, those groups which originated legislation to regulate the sexual activities of a given culture were not primarily religious, such as the Puritans. It was often secular governments who had the common sense to realize that **sex is not only a private act, but also one with potentially appalling public consequences and costs.** Someone always pays for promiscuity—and it's not always the primary participants who pay the most.

♦ Everybody Pays Financially

If sex is merely a private act behind closed doors, why does the government annually pay large sums of money for abortions and welfare? This year, 1.2 million teenagers will get pregnant, most of them unwed participants in a "private act." Do you know that it costs federal and state governments an average of $100,000 in medical and welfare costs for every teen who has a child?

Recently the Associated Press reported:

> Teenage child-bearing cost the nation $16.6 billion last year and the 385,000 babies who were the firstborn to adolescents in 1985 will receive $5 billion in welfare benefits over the next twenty years, according to a study just released. . . . The study estimated that the government spent $16.5 billion last year in welfare costs to support the families started by teenage mothers. This estimate includes payments for AFDC, Medicaid and food stamps as well as the costs of administering these programs. This figure represents minimal public costs in that it does not include other services such as housing, special education, child protection services, foster care, day care and other social services. 83/3

In the next twenty years American taxpayers will pay in excess of $100 billion for the net results of teenage pregnancies. 36/99 *That's an exorbitant public price for a so-called private act.* And you and I are paying it.

The January 10, 1986, issue of the *Journal of the American Medical Association* reported:

> It is estimated that the first 10,000 cases of AIDS in the United States cost $1.6 million in hospital days, $1.4 million in expenditures, 8,387 years of work lost and $4.8 million because of premature death. . . . New York City alone picks up $45 million a year in unpaid hospital bills of AIDS patients. 84/213

It is estimated that the costs for AIDS for just New York will be over $7 billion in the next five years. 99/26

If sex is a private act behind closed doors, why is the U.S. government spending so much money on AIDS research? Why does the U.S. Centers for Disease Control spend so much of its time, at the taxpayers' expense, on sexually transmitted diseases? If AIDS and other STDs are the consequences of private acts between two consenting individuals, why does the public have to pay for them?

The cost of treating the average AIDS victim during the two years it generally takes for the disease to run its fatal course currently averages about $147,000. For many businesses, one or two AIDS cases could trigger a ruinous hike in health insurance premiums. By 1991 it will cost us an estimated $19 billion a year just for AIDS. If we combine that with the costs of other STDs we can expect soon to be paying at least $30 billion a year for the private acts of two people behind closed doors. 386/49 It is estimated that, nationally, "AIDS will be costing between $5-10 billion dollars per annum by the early 1990s." 85

According to health economists Anne Scitovsky of the Palo Alto Medical Foundation and Dorothy Rice of the University of California at San Francisco, "The loss of productivity from these AIDS victims will hit $55,660,000 in 1991 alone—and that is a conservative figure." 86/23 and 87/23

"The estimates of cost of treating projected 400,000 AIDS cases (1986-1992) will cost another $37 billion (about one-third of that under Medicaid)." 90

Health insurance premiums is another cost the public will bear for private sexual activity. A survey by Alexander and Alexander, an employee-benefits consulting firm, showed that "benefits paid out for an employee with AIDS typically exceed $100,000—the average expenditure per afflicted worker consists of $47,702 for health-care costs, $11,285 for long-term disability and $44,363 for death benefits." 88/60

"Acquired Immune Deficiency Syndrome will cost national insurance companies over $100 billion in life, health and disability claims by the year 2000, shows a recent study by the Society of Actuaries." 89

If sex is a private act between two people behind closed doors, and if the government, the school and the church have nothing to say about what happens there, why are PPFA and various pressure groups demanding millions upon million of dollars for public school sex education beginning in the third grade? Ironically, many groups which pressure for public funding of abortions and care for victims of sexually transmitted diseases also defend their "right" to the private sexual freedom which is causing these great social problems. Their position is a gross philosophical contradiction.

Sex is not a private act when persons who practice casual sex come out from behind closed doors and demand that the government spend billions of our dollars to combat and cure their STDs. Sex is not a private act when teenagers become pregnant behind closed doors and then pass the costs of those children on to taxpayers.

♦ Some Pay With Their Health

The rapid and widespread growth of sexually transmitted diseases, with all the terrible suffering they bring, is another way society pays for private promiscuity. Twenty years ago there were only a handful of sexually transmitted diseases. Today there are fifty-one. 387 Approximately every nine months a new one is discovered. Every day 33,000 Americans will contract an STD. That's 12 million this year! 23/53

A newcomer in the past few years to the list of sexually transmitted diseases is the dreaded AIDS virus. Almost every day there are more articles and TV reports about the enormity of this disease. It is estimated that in the next three years hundreds of thousands of babies will be born with this deadly AIDS virus.

An honest answer from a sex partner about a sexually transmitted disease is no guarantee that a person is safe. Even while dormant in one person, an STD can be transmitted to another. Dr. Edward Wiesmeier, director of the UCLA Student Health Center, warns students that "one chance encounter can infect a person with as many as five different diseases." 23/56

A young married man urged me, "Please keep telling people about the price of casual sex." When I asked him why, he said, "I've had a real loose lifestyle with a lot of free love and plenty of casual relationships. When herpes came onto the scene, it didn't really change my lifestyle even though I knew you can never get rid of it. Fortunately, I never got it.

"Now a whole new strain of herpes has hit nationwide," he continued. "You won't hear much about it; it's asymptomatic. You don't even know you have it. You don't have blisters, but you can still pass it on. The one way you know for sure you have it is if you have a child born with a birth defect. But that didn't change my lifestyle either.

"Then AIDS came on the scene. That got my attention. It's fatal. So, I decided, okay, that's it. I'm going to change my lifestyle, fall in love, settle down and have children. That's exactly what I did. Then my wife gave me herpes."

Last fall, over a period of fifty days, twenty-four women spoke to me who were each carrying three to six sexually transmitted diseases they had contracted from their husbands. Many of the diseases were incurable and/or cancer-producing. Several of the women said that their doctors strongly admonished them to be tested for cancer every six months—for the rest of their lives. When their husbands played around sexually, some before marriage and some after, they weren't just participating in innocent, private affairs. Their so-called private acts will affect their wives and children for as long as any of them live.

Several months ago a woman drove eight hours to talk with me at a conference. As soon as she arrived she fell apart emotionally. Ten years earlier her husband of twenty-three years left her and their two teenage girls and ran off with another woman. Just that week the woman's doctor told her that she was carrying three STDs from her husband – one of them incurable – which had been dormant in her for all those ten years. She wanted to kill her husband. She would be reminded every day, for the rest of her life, that sex behind closed doors is not a private act.

A 35-year-old woman drove to my home to ask for help. At the age of 32 she had married a man who told her he was a virgin like she was. The morning she came to see me her doctor had just told her that she had contracted three STDs – two incurable and one cancer-producing. Talk about a woman being crushed. She is carrying in her body three diseases from her deceptive husband. *Try telling this woman that her husband's private acts have no consequences on her personal life.*

Except within the commitment of a monogamous marriage relationship, there is always a price to be paid for engaging in sex. Medical authorities say you must now consider not only your current sex partner, but also all of your partner's other sexual involvements during the past ten years. 225; 31 It is possible for a person to be carrier of an STD like AIDS for ten years without knowing it.

Think about sex as a private act between two individuals in light of the following medical nightmare involving one 16-year-old girl who was responsible for 218 cases of gonorrhea and more than 300 cases of syphilis. "The girl had sex with sixteen men. Those men had sex with other people who had sex with other people. The number of contacts finally added up to 1,660. . . . What if the girl had had AIDS instead of gonorrhea or syphilis? You probably would have had 1,000 dead people by now." 92/A12

A recent bulletin from the U.S. Centers for Disease Control declares that **the only certain way to avoid sexually transmitted disease is for a monogamous man to enter into a monogamous relationship with a monogamous woman. There is no other positive way.** If everyone practiced monogamy, STDs would soon be nonexistent.

♦ Some People Pay Emotionally

Perhaps the most difficult cost society bears from private, casual sex is the emotional toll. Guilt, suspicion and fear always are associated with unwanted pregnancy, abortion and STDs. Now, with the threat of a nationwide AIDS epidemic, the greatest emotional weight is on those who fear that their private sexual activity with another person will result in their contracting AIDS.

Almost every state has a task force to combat the spread of AIDS among heterosexuals. A great fear today in the hearts of promiscuous heterosexuals is that of receiving a phone call from an AIDS task force worker: "Hello, are you alone? Your name has been given to us. Can we talk?" Imagine how you would feel getting a call like that.

After a meeting with a group of high school students in Orlando, Florida, I was approached by a big, husky, handsome young man. Tears were streaming down his cheeks as he told me how he'd spent his entire life striving for his father's love. "I've done everything I can to get my father to put his arms around me, to hug me, to tell me, 'I love you.' He never did. So about six months ago I joined the Marines. I got so lonely that when I met this girl I went to bed with her. I'm a Christian. It's the only time in my life I've done something like that. She gave me herpes."

Then the tears really began to flow. "Josh," he asked, "will anyone ever love me?" He will be paying emotionally for his one private act for a long time.

After a speaking engagement I was approached by a woman who was nearly hysterical. "For God's sake help me, please!" she sobbed. "I was married for four years. My husband had never been in the hospital a day in his life. Then last January they told us he had AIDS, and twelve days later he was dead. They traced the disease back to an affair he had six years ago."

Her husband's death was only part of the tragedy. She continued, "Do you know what they told me I have to do every three months for the next several years? I have to go into the clinic to be tested to see if I'm going to live for another three months. Mr. McDowell, do you know what that's like? I go to bed at night, but I can't sleep. I have nightmares. I wake up in the morning and I go to work, but I can't concentrate. All I think about after leaving the clinic is that I have to go back in a matter of weeks or days to see if I'm going to live another three months." What a price this woman is paying for her husband's private act!

I talk to people like this three to five times a week. Another woman came to me just broken-hearted. She was about 23 years old, and she was crying. She said, "I've been married three months. Last week my husband came down with an acute case of gonorrhea. They traced it back to an affair he had four years ago."

Would you want to try to rebuild trust in that relationship? Do you know what it's going to take for them to work through their emotional crisis? It will take years—if they don't give it up.

Dr. Lawrence Laycob says that "when you're casual about sex, chances are the person you're casual with has been casual with someone else. So there's a third, fourth or twenty-fifth party out there that you have no knowledge of." 33/56

Former Surgeon General Koop soberly stated,

> It is a very frightening thing. Today if you have sexual intercourse with a woman, you are not only having sexual intercourse with her but with every person that woman might have had intercourse with for the last ten years and all of the people they had intercourse with. 31

In an appearance on Tom Brokaw's AIDS documentary, Dr. Theresa Crenshaw, past president of the American Association of Sex Educators, Counselors and Therapists, commented, "If you have sex with one person, you are having sex with everyone that person ever had sex with before you." 225

A husband goes out and cheats on his wife by having sex with a prostitute; it happens all the time. The average prostitute in the United States has had sex with 2,000 men. That man didn't just have a private act of sex with a prostitute. He had sex with the prostitute, plus her 2,000 partners, plus all of their partners for the past ten years—up to 12,000 people. Then that man has the audacity to go home and have sex with his wife! His wife didn't have a private act in bed with her husband. She had sex with her husband, plus the prostitute, plus her 2,000 partners, plus all their partners for the last ten years. That's a lot to handle as a wife.

Think of the emotional implications within a marriage if the husband has an extramarital affair. Even if he repents and goes back to his wife, she could become frigid because of a legitimate fear: "If I have sex with my husband now, it's as if I'm having sex with the other woman and everyone she's had sex with." The price is awesome.

This is hard to say, but it's true: **It's a medical fact that you're bringing every sexual partner you've ever had, and all their partners, into your marriage bed every night.** That's quite an emotional price to pay for a night of sexual pleasure.

♦ Children Often Pay

Even our children are paying a huge price for the private sexual activities of their parents.

Because of the sexual practices of others, we who are parents are faced with a solemn task. We must explain to our children that they cannot have peace of mind on their wedding night (or afterward) unless they know the detailed sexual history of their mate and all their mate's partners for the past ten years. It won't be easy telling that to my three daughters and one son. But I've got to tell them, and they will have to bear that emotional burden because that's what private, casual sex is going to cost them.

I recently read a report released by the U.S. Centers for Disease Control. It was heartbreaking. The report told about the rising number of pregnant woman who will require birth by Caesarean section because of sexually transmitted diseases. If their babies were delivered normally, most would be born blind and with other side effects from passing through a birth canal contaminated by STDs.

In New York, HIV-infected mothers are having between 500 and 1,000 infected babies per year. 93 A study of Massachusetts women who gave birth found that one in 500 was infected with the AIDS virus. 94

Dr. Daren Hein, director of a program in New York sponsored by the American Academy of Pediatrics that serves and studies teens with AIDS, says: "One in a hundred 19-year-old women giving birth statewide is infected with the AIDS virus, as are one in 1,000 15-year-olds. Half of the city's [New York] teenage girls with AIDS say they got [AIDS] by having sex with males." 97/D1

European researchers followed 219 infants of mothers with AIDS for up to two years. "It appears that 25 to 30 percent of the babies will themselves be infected with the virus." 95 A study by Dr. Sheldon Landesman and others at the State University of New York in Brooklyn found "an infection rate of at least 40 percent in newborns of mothers with AIDS." 95

AIDS Prevention reports: "Since 1981, more than 1,100 children in the United States have been diagnosed with AIDS, mostly as a result of being born to an HIV-infected mother. It is believed that two to three times as many children, aged one minute through 12 years, may be infected with the AIDS virus, but are not yet showing symptoms. One hospital reported that lifetime care costs for children with AIDS average $90,437 per child." 96

Children are paying the price, not only in the United States, but also around the world. The USSR's communist newspaper *Pravda* reported "a tragic incident in which at least twenty-seven babies and four mothers became infected with the AIDS virus at a children's hospital facility. Possibly many more were infected, and some 3,000 children are being tested in an effort to determine more precisely the extent of the problem." 100/5 The children were given blood transfusions, and the blood was tainted with the AIDS virus.

A great price for private sex will be paid by the orphans and foster children left behind by AIDS victims. *USA Today* reports: "Within the next few years, New York will have 10,000 orphans whose parents have died of AIDS." 98/2D

In New York,

> More than 30,000 single mothers with AIDS, who have an average of two children, will die in the 1990s, leaving the city to cope with 60,000 foster children–tripling today's load. Imagine placing 60,000 kids whose mothers have died of AIDS and who may themselves be at risk. The human cost is tragic. 99/26

In our society even unborn human beings frequently pay for their parents' sexual irresponsibility by dying as a result of abortion. I don't know about you, but that makes my heart ache. When we ignore God's loving, protective commandments, someone always pays the price. No sexual encounter is free or private when others have to pay for it.

No longer can anyone say that sex is a private act between two individuals behind closed doors. Each individual takes into his act of sex every person he or she has ever had sex with. That can be terrifying for a lot of people, especially for those who have more than one partner.

At a student gathering, I was asked, *"Isn't abstinence unrealistic?"*

"No, it's not," I replied. "Fifty percent of you here have never been sexually involved. Statistics show it; half of you have never had sexual intercourse."

Some said, "Yeah, but what if we have?"

"I don't care what your background is," I answered. "I strongly encourage you, no matter how many experiences you've had, that you start right now to practice abstinence. Because if you don't, and you keep adding partners, you're playing a game worse than Russian roulette. The medical statistics prove it."

CHAPTER 5

➧ A **key section** for busy parents.

False Assumption 5

"Safe Sex Is Really Safe"

The cry of our generation is, "Safer sex!" "Use a condom; no glove, no love!" PPFA, Dr. Ruth, proponents of school-based clinics, and comprehensive sex educators urge us, "Never leave home without one."

The phrases "safe sex" and "safer sex" can easily cause confusion. The advocates of comprehensive sex education coined the term "safe sex" for encouraging condom use, and the universities sustained the false concept by sponsoring "Safe Sex Week" programs. Then, after strong opposition based on medical research into the failure rate of condoms and other methods of contraception, they changed the phrase to "safer sex." One can wonder how long it will be before they change that phrase to something else.

An organization which is deeply involved in AIDS education and information in the homosexual community advises: "Have all the hot sex you want. Just be sure to make it safer. . . . Always use a condom. . . . Be creative and enjoy SAFER SEX! [emphasis theirs]" 229

A full-page ad placed in the *New York Times* by a large city health department urges: "Don't die of embarrassment. . . . If you decide to have sex, using a condom is your best protection. It's as simple as that. . . . So start carrying condoms, and tell your partner to use them." 230

Another poster distributed by the same city health department proclaims to women: "DON'T GO OUT WITHOUT YOUR RUBBERS. You just can't be sure who has the AIDS virus. So, if you choose to have sex, protect yourself [emphasis theirs]."

"The country has become involved in 'condom-mania,'" former Surgeon General Koop confessed. "I don't feel particularly happy about the role I've played in that. Condoms are a last resort." 268

The term safe sex is tragically misleading. The word *safe* means "free from damage; secure; escaping injury unharmed." Accordingly, safe sex should refer to sexual activity which is free from personal injury or harm (unwanted pregnancy, disease, etc.). But the statistical evidence is quite clear that the highly touted condom cannot guarantee safety. At best all that those who use them can hope for is sex that is a little "safer." Dr. Gerald Bernstein of the University of Southern California summed it up: "Using condoms is not really what people are talking about when they say 'safe sex.' It may be safer sex, but I think it's a misnomer to say condoms are 'safe sex.' " 123/6,28

The only 100-percent safe way to prevent pregnancy is abstinence. The only really safe way to avoid STDs is a monogamous man and a monogamous woman in a monogamous marriage. **Apart from abstinence or monogamy, safer sex is a fantasy.**

♦ Do You Know the Facts?

Recently I was invited to give the concluding talk during "Safe Sex Week" at the University of North Dakota. The auditorium was jammed to capacity—about 3,000 students. As I often do in an opportunity such as this, I opened my talk with a statement which sent a rumble of discomfort through the crowd: "You've been brainwashed!"

When the students settled down I continued. "You've had an entire week of 'safer sex' indoctrination: speakers, experts, videos, films, classes and symposiums. You've been challenged, motivated, encouraged, indoctrinated and pressured about using condoms to ensure safe sex. To top it all off, you were given a 'safer sex packet.' But you've been lied to."

At this point the crowd was becoming a little indignant with me. Then I lowered the boom with one question: "After all the information on 'safer sex' you have received this week, how many of you know the statistical failure rate of the condom?" *Not one hand went up!* Suddenly the auditorium was as quiet as a cemetery. They looked at each other with expressions of astonishment. They realized they hadn't been told the whole truth about safer sex.

I have received the same response from students of more than twenty universities in the past few months. It happened at the University of Michigan with 2,500 students and at Auburn University with almost 8,000 students. Northwestern University in Evanston, Illinois, was in the midst of a push for on-campus condom machines just before I came to speak. There were newspaper articles, editorials, symposiums and debates. Even Dr. Ruth had spoken there. But when I posed the question about knowing the statistical failure rate of condoms, not one student in the crowd of 1,400 raised his hand.

I want to share with you the facts about condoms and the two greatest problems facing the proponents of free love and casual sex: unwanted pregnancies and sexually transmitted diseases. I believe the data will convince you that condoms and safe sex are mutually exclusive.

♦ Condoms and Pregnancy

Does use of a condom guarantee safety from unwanted pregnancy? No. That's a false assumption. Planned Parenthood's research—reported in their own journal, *Family Planning Perspectives*—revealed sobering facts about birth control methods in 1986. The chart below identifies some percentages of unplanned pregnancies for single women. Notice: None of the methods, including the condom, were totally reliable:

Percentage of Unplanned Pregnancies Within the First Year of Contraceptive Use

Age	Pill	IUD	Rhythm	Condom	Diaphragm	Spermicides	Other Methods	No Method
Under 18	11.0%	10.5%	33.9%	18.4%	31.6%	34.0%	21.1%	62.9%
18-19	9.6	9.3	30.6	16.3	28.3	34.0	18.7	62.9
20-24	7.2	6.9	23.9	12.3	21.7	23.5	14.2	7.6
25-29	5.0	4.8	17.4	8.6	15.6	17.0	10.0	36.3
30-44	1.9	1.8	7.0	3.3	6.2	6.8	3.9	15.7
All	5.7	5.4	23.0	10.8	23.3	19.4	15.4	44.7

122/204 (See also 239/H121,122.)

There are many reasons for such a high failure rate (18.4 percent) of condoms with teenagers. One basic reason is that young people are susceptible to impaired judgment from alcohol, drugs, sexual excitement, etc., which interferes with the proper use of condoms, making failure more likely. 225

The 1989 facts on birth control and pregnancy are even more sobering:

> The failure of birth control methods results in unplanned pregnancy about 30 percent more than previously believed. . . . Depending on the method, between 6 percent and 26 percent of couples using birth control experience an unplanned pregnancy. . . . The failure rate was:

6% for the pill
14% for the condom
16% for the diaphragm and rhythm
26% for spermicides . . .

About 43 percent of the nearly 3.3 million unplanned pregnancies occurring each year happen to people using some method of birth control. . . . Half of the pregnancies end in abortion. 124/18

Though statistically more reliable than some other methods, the condom is far from being fail-safe in preventing pregnancy. Researcher Dr. George Grant points out:

When first-year failure rates are extrapolated, i.e., estimated, over extended intervals using the binomial probability formula, the following chances for pregnancy are found:

- A fourteen-year-old girl faithfully using the pill has a 44% chance of getting pregnant at least once before she finishes high school.
- She has a 69% chance of getting pregnant at least once before she finishes college.
- She has a 30% chance of getting pregnant two or more times.
- Using condoms, the likelihood of unwanted pregnancy while she is in school rises to nearly 87%. 666/30

♦ The Pill, Pregnancy and STDs

Notice from the chart above that the pill (oral contraceptives) appears to be one of the most effective methods for preventing pregnancy. Yet while the pill has enjoyed great success on one front of the sexual revolution, it has produced devastating results on another front. Common sense dictates, and medical history of the past fifteen years confirms, that *the pill does not prevent sexually transmitted diseases.*

Dr. Robert Hatcher, in *Contraceptive Technology,* warns:

Unlike condoms or diaphragms, oral contraceptives (OCs) provide no physical barrier to the transmission of sexually transmitted diseases (STDs). OCs have, in fact, been linked by some to increasing STD rates by (1) causing abandonment of barrier methods, and (2) leading to increased sexual activity. 278/139

During the '60s everyone hailed the pill as the "messiah" of birth control and sexual liberation. Women proclaimed their freedom from the fear of pregnancy. Promiscuous sex became "safe"; it was "legitimized." Barriers came down and sexual activity went up.

Were the medical profession, women's groups, PPFA, family planners, health teachers and university professors who were hailing the pill short-sighted? **They didn't realize that a non-barrier contraceptive** (the pill) **would usher in one of the most devastating**

epidemics of sexually transmitted diseases in history. Their enthusiasm blinded them to the total-person experience of the act of sex. Reveling in safety from pregnancy, they ignored the long-term health consequences of promiscuous sex with or without the pill.

We are repeating the same mistake with condoms. **Are sexual decisions still being based on short-term desires instead of long-term consequences?** We won't have to wait twenty years to see the devastating failure of the condom as we did with the pill. It may only take another five years. The tragedy is that again we are going through on-the-job training at the expense of our young people.

♦ The Case of the Leaky Condom

One of the main reasons condoms cannot guarantee safety against pregnancies or STDs is that some of them leak. The Department of Health and Human Services reports: "One of every five batches of condoms tested in a government inspection program over the last four months failed to meet minimum standards for leaks." 123/6,28 Present FDA standards allow up to four condoms per thousand to leak water in lots acceptable for sale to the public. 267

FDA inspectors "checked more than 150,000 samples from lots representing 120 million condoms. The agents had to reject about one lot in ten of domestic condoms because too many leaked. Imports turned out to be worse—one in five lots was rejected." 130

♦ Condoms and AIDS, HIV, and Other STDs

Pregnancy isn't the greatest danger posed by condom failure. An AIDS virus is 450 times smaller than a sperm.

Consumer Reports notes that scanning the membranes of skin condoms under an electron microscope reveals:

> layers of fibers crisscrossing in various patterns. That latticework endows the skins with strength but also makes for an occasional pore, sometimes up to 1.5 microns wide. That's smaller than a sperm, a white blood cell or even some gonorrhea bacteria. But it's more than 10 times the size of the AIDS virus, and more than 25 times the size of the hepatitis-B virus."119

"To keep AIDS from spreading," states a Department of Education position paper, **"a condom must work ten times better [than for birth control]. A woman is fertile roughly 36 days a year, but someone with AIDS can transmit it 365 days a year."** 225 Furthermore, consider the following facts:

- Only the female can get pregnant, but the AIDS virus (and other STDs) can infect male and female.

- Pregnancy can occur only from semen entering the vagina, but the AIDS virus can infect other parts of the body through exposure to contaminated blood or body fluids even when the condom is used correctly. 225
- Condom failure in pregnancy prevention produces a new life, but condom failure in AIDS prevention produces death.

Even if "safer sex" reduces other sexually transmitted diseases, it doesn't necessarily reduce the prevalence of HIV infection. 225 The cases of HIV infection almost tripled among San Francisco homosexuals between 1980 and 1984 (from 24 percent to 68 percent) even though safe sex techniques resulted in a 73-percent reduction of rectal gonorrhea cases in men attending San Francisco city clinics during the same period. 266 One reason for the HIV increase could be that it was latent or dormant.

A study titled "Incidence and Risk Factors for Female to Male Transmission of HIV," conducted by an international group of scientists, found that "the incidence of female to male transmission of HIV after *a single sexual exposure* was 8 percent [emphasis mine]." 116

In another study, thirty female prostitutes and sixteen persons from a hospital staff each tested ten latex condoms in vaginal intercourse. Six people dropped out. Condom rupture occurred at least once for seven of the remaining forty persons. Overall condom rupture rate was 5 percent. The study concluded: "Truly safe sex with an HIV-positive partner using condoms is a dangerous illusion." 114

A Department of Health and Human Services task force concluded that "there are no clinical (human trial) data supporting the value of condoms" in preventing the spread of a range of diseases, including syphilis, herpes, hepatitis-B and HIV. 123/6,28

Dr. Nicholas Fiumara, director of the Massachusetts Department of Public Health, writing in the *New England Journal of Medicine,* warned that condoms are "useless" against gonorrhea and syphilis:

> The current epidemic of gonorrhea in the United States and in Massachusetts has prompted many physicians to ask us about the effectiveness of the condom as a prophylactic against this disease. The answer to this question is theoretically yes, but the effectiveness of the condom is such as to make it completely useless as a prophylactic.
>
> The condom is effective against gonorrhea provided there is no preliminary sex play, the condom is intact before use, the condom is put on correctly and the condom is taken off correctly. However, the male population has never been able to fulfill the very first requisite.
>
> Even if all these [four] conditions are fulfilled, a condom incompletely protects against syphilis because it protects only the part it covers . . . It does not cover . . . the areas that are bathed with the secretion of the female during the sex act.

> In summary, then, its effectiveness makes the condom useless as a prophylactic against gonorrhea, and even under ideal conditions against syphilis. 243/972

♦ Condoms and Anal Sex

Former Surgeon General Koop warned that condoms fail at "extraordinarily high" rates in anal sex. According to Koop:

> The rectum was not made for intercourse. It's at the wrong angle; it's the wrong size; it doesn't have the same kind of tough lining that the vagina does. It has its blood supply directly under the mucosa. Therefore, you would expect a great many more failures of condoms in rectal intercourse than you would in vaginal intercourse. 247

In a Pittsburgh study, 8 percent of gay/bisexual men reported condom breakage, and 5 percent reported condom slippage. 245 In a 1987 study of seventeen homosexual couples engaging in 200 acts of anal intercourse with condoms "especially designed for the study, 15 percent of the condoms slipped off and 11 percent ruptured. . . . Even assuming a low risk of HIV transmission of 1 percent at each intercourse, the probability that a partner of an HIV-positive person will become infected within a year with intercourse three times weekly will be 8 percent and within three years 21 percent." 114 The researchers concluded: "Since [complete satisfaction] can never be guaranteed, [condoms] should be used with restraint. Changes in sexual behavior remain the goal." 244

In more emphatic language than federal health officials have used previously, a U.S. Public Health Service task force recently warned that "the risk of condom failure in anal intercourse is so high that the practice should be avoided entirely—with condoms or without." 271

♦ A Deadly Choice

The condom is not a safe sex choice; it is dangerous and potentially fatal. Dr. Harold Jaffee, chief of epidemiology for the Centers for Disease Control, states: **"You just can't tell people it's all right to do whatever you want so long as you wear a condom.** It's just too dangerous a disease to say that." 250

Dr. Theresa Crenshaw, past president of the American Association of Sex Educators, Counselors and Therapists, and member of the Presidential AIDS commission, says that "if the wrong information [about condoms] is given, the effort will fail. It will cause death rather than prevent it. . . . **To say that use of condoms is 'safe sex' is in fact playing Russian roulette.** A lot of people will die in this dangerous game." 252/2

Dr. Malcolm Potts, president of Family Health International and one of the inventors of condoms lubricated with spermicides, admits: "We cannot tell people how much protection condoms give. . . . **Telling a person who engages in high-risk behavior to use a condom is like telling someone who is driving drunk to use a seat belt."** 253 and 254

Dr. Victor Cline, professor of psychology at the University of Utah, emphasizes that the condoms-equals-safe-sex message is offering kids a deadly false sense of security:

> If kids buy the notion that if they just use condoms they will be safe from AIDS or any other sexually transmitted disease whenever they have sex, they are being seriously misled. They should be correctly informed that having sex with any partner having the AIDS virus is life-threatening, condoms or no condoms. It would be analogous to playing Russian roulette with two bullets in your six chambers. Using condoms removes only one of the bullets. The gun still remains deadly with the potential of lethal outcome. 126

Dr. Michael Wilder, an AIDS expert on the staff of the Kaiser Permanente Hospitals of California, called me recently to talk about the deadly AIDS crisis. After only twenty minutes on the phone with him, I was scared. I said, "Sir, if you knew your partner had AIDS, would you commit yourself to having sex with that person using a condom only 1/100 of an inch thick?"

He said, "Mr. McDowell, not only would I not commit myself to such an unreliable method, but I don't know one medical expert in the world who would–certainly none of my colleagues."

♦ Risk Reduction/Risk Elimination

Richard Smith, a specialist in AIDS and sexually transmitted diseases, has worked for 20 years in the field of public health. At present he is involved in monitoring and coordinating AIDS counseling test sites. After years of researching the threat of AIDS and STDs in light of the "safer sex" crusade, he rightly discerns the fatal mentality of those who propagate *risk reduction,* as contrasted to *risk elimination.*

Smith advises:

> Present policy regarding prevention of sexually transmitted diseases and pregnancy is divided into two fundamental messages: (1) those which eliminate risk; and (2) those which reduce risk. The rationale is that since not all people will choose to change behavior sufficiently to assure risk elimination, we, therefore, should also provide information that will reduce risk but not eliminate it. However, careful examination of the facts, human nature and our public mandate compel us to both restructure and refine the premise.

For example, introduction of the fatal and incurable Human Immune Virus (HIV) into our society has caused a sobering re-examination of past rationale which apparently has been relatively ineffective in halting the spread of AIDS. First, we should understand that just because choices are given does not mean that all choices are of equal merit. Second, since some of those choices are more factual than others, they are *de facto* more objective, therefore less subjective, and consequently deserve more emphasis. Liken this fundamental principle to balancing two objects of unequal weight where you must place the *heavier* object *closer* to the fulcrum in order to achieve the balance.

Accordingly, we must then persistently encourage risk elimination as opposed to risk reduction in the face of this deadly, incurable virus. In fact, as Dr. Goedert said in the *New England Journal of Medicine,* "Reducing risky sex rather than eliminating it is like incompletely immunizing a population—there is little benefit to the individual or the community." 671/1339

Furthermore, as public officials, we have the moral and legal responsibility to emphasize and encourage that which is most effective because the failed result is death.

Particularly in this crisis climate, the current disproportionate emphasis on risk reduction is irresponsible and perhaps even legally liable. For example, as prevention against AIDS this so-called safe sex or risk reduction by definition accepts a certain index of death, doesn't it? In fact, it could be argued that the over-reliance upon such a flawed message essentially encourages a death index because it presumes and endorses the philosophy of acceptable losses. Both as a parent and public health professional that has a chilling and haunting effect upon my conscience. What does it do for yours? Yet, abstinence by definition does not include death, does it?" 670/2

♦ Knowledge Alone Is Not Enough

Possessing information about the risks of pregnancy and STDs does not necessarily translate into modifying sexual behavior. In their massive condoms campaign, the National Education Associa-tion's guide for teachers, *The Facts About AIDS,* states: **"Health education that relies only on the transmission of information is ineffective.** Behavioral change results only when information is supported by shared community values that are powerfully conveyed." 257/16

Will the knowledge imparted in safer sex education effectively combat AIDS? According to one study, apparently not. Knowledge of so-called safer sex techniques did not prevent most men who practiced anal sex from engaging in unprotected sex.

Of those engaging in anal sex within the last six months

- 65% possessed knowledge of safe sex;
- 90% agreed that condoms can "reduce the spread of AIDS"; and

- 91% identified anal sex as the highest-risk sexual behavior regarding AIDS transmission.

Yet most still practiced that high-risk behavior. Within the past half year, 65 percent engaged in anal sex. Of those,

- 62% "never" or "hardly ever" used condoms during anal intercourse;
- 64% said their partners "never" or "hardly ever" did;
- 72% reported multiple sexual partners within the past six months; and
- 24% reported half or more of their sexual partners were anonymous. 245

A National Institute of Health study of 4,955 gay and bisexual men found:

- 51% still practiced receptive anal sex (though that proportion not practicing it increased).
- More than two-thirds did not use condoms with anal sex (although condom use doubled).
- Almost half (44%) still used nitrate inhalants.
- Although the study found a "marked" decrease in dangerous sexual behavior, the reductions weren't sufficient when measured against the dangers of risky behavior. The authors stated that "further reductions are clearly warranted." 264/213

As a result of a 1987 survey of University of Maryland students, the researchers stated, "We found that knowledge is reasonably high, yet there is little personalization of risk or behavior change due to AIDS." 258

- 95% of students know about AIDS prevention, but most don't change their behavior.
- Of students practicing anal sex, 68% said they made no change, and only 27% said they practiced it less frequently.
- Of students having sex with prostitutes, 56% made no change, and only 37% did so less frequently.
- Of students sharing needles, 76% made no change, and only 14% did so less frequently.

A review of four studies conducted at U.S. universities concluded:

> The collective results revealed that the majority of students are reasonably knowledgeable about the transmission of AIDS virus and proper preventive measures. Unfortunately, only a minority are translating their knowledge into behavioral change. . . . Students tend to see AIDS as "someone else's problem." 259

The chairman of the American College Health Association's task force on AIDS, Dr. Richard Keeling, acknowledges that some people are not reachable through education:

> There is a despairing theory in health education that says until there is some horrible baseline number of people who have died, the disease doesn't become personal enough to the rest of the community for it to take fundamental changes in behavior seriously." 260/3

The *Journal of Family and Marriage* reports: "Our findings suggest that knowledge and sex education courses [are] not successful in reducing the chances of out-of-wedlock childbearing." 662/250

The study, "The Role of Responsibility and Knowledge in Reducing Teenage Out-of-Wedlock Childbearing," concluded: "Although sex education is often promoted as a way to reduce the incidence of early pregnancy, our results suggest that simply requiring more students to take more sex education, as it is currently provided, is not the answer." 662/251

In spite of education, powerful denial mechanisms often inhibit behavioral changes. "Even those who are educated about safer sex practices sometimes resist making changes. There's a tremendous difference between education and behavioral change," said Dr. Neil Schram, former chairman of the Los Angeles City-County AIDS Task Force. "Look at cigarette smoking or seat-belt use or drunk driving. People are educated about the dangers of all those things. They just never think it will happen to them. The key word is denial." 265

Some infected people intentionally continue unprotected sex despite education about AIDS and counseling to change their behavior. "Patient Zero" ignored repeated warnings about his infectious status and deliberately exposed hundreds of his sexual partners to AIDS infection before he died in 1984. 261

Comprehensive sex educators are pressing for more knowledge and availability of birth control devices for teens. Both state and federal legislatures are passing bills to allocate millions of dollars based on the claims of PPFA and others that education is the answer. Yet PPFA's own Lou Harris poll shows that most teens do not use birth control because:

(1) they prefer not to (30%);
(2) there is no time to use it (30%);
(3) they lack knowledge of or access to birth control (14%).
138/6,28

Only 14 percent lacked knowledge or access to contraceptives.

By 1976, "Only 3 percent of teenagers who did not use birth control said it was because they did not know how or where to obtain it." Zelnik and Kantner, 1979, quoted in 145/154

A *New York Times* writer began her story by relating a personal experience:

> I was sitting at a table with half a dozen 16-year-old girls, listening with some amazement as they showed off their knowledge of human sexuality. They knew how long sperm lived inside the body and how many women out of 100 using a diaphragm were statistically likely to get pregnant. One girl recited the steps of the ovulation cycle from day one to day twenty-eight. There was just one problem with this performance: Every one of the girls was pregnant.

This would be a good story to keep in mind as we get closer to making a decision on whether more (and earlier) sex education in the schools and giving contraceptives to teenagers is the answer to our teen sex problem. As one person laments: "One listens in vain for any of them to advocate, 'Just say no!' Oh, they would say, they are not averse to telling young people to abstain from sex. In reality, though, **they are like parents who would tell their children it's best not to cheat, but then go on to say, 'If you have to cheat, however, let me tell you how to keep from getting caught.' "** 147

♦ Abstinence and Monogamy

We must realize that sex was designed as a total-person experience for a monogamous man and a monogamous woman in a monogamous relationship. We had better listen to warnings like the one published in the *New England Journal of Medicine:*

> It is clear that the use of condoms will not eliminate the risk of transmission [of HIV] and must be viewed as a secondary strategy. On the basis of current data, only celibacy and masturbation [in the light of HIV and various STDs, this is now being questioned] can be considered truly safe. 131/1240,1341.

Dr. Art Ulene, family physician on the *Today Show,* writes:

> In an educational video designed for junior high and high school students, youngsters were told that the best they could do to protect themselves against AIDS was to "know their partner" (whatever that means to a teenager), wear a condom during intercourse, avoid anal intercourse and not make sexual decisions while using drugs or alcohol. . . . I'm sorry, but that's not the best they can do. [The video] forgot to mention abstinence, which is the only behavior that carries a 100-percent guarantee of safety. 226 and 225

The *Journal of the American Medical Society,* based on reports by the Center for Devices and Radiological Health, the Food and Drug Administration, the Division of Sexually Transmitted Diseases, the Center for Preventions Services: AIDS Program, the Center for Infectious Diseases, and the Centers for Disease Control, proposes:

> Abstinence and sexual intercourse with one mutually faithful uninfected partner are the only totally effective prevention strategies. Proper use of condoms with each act of sexual intercourse can reduce, but not eliminate, risk of STD. Individuals likely to become infected or known to be infected with the human immunodeficiency virus (HIV) should be aware that condom use cannot completely eliminate the risk of transmission to themselves or to others. Condoms are not always effective in preventing STD. Recommendations for prevention of STD, including HIV infection, should emphasize that risk of infection is most effectively reduced through abstinence or with a mutually faithful uninfected partner. 133/1925-27

An article on AIDS and blacks concludes: "abstinence is the best way to prevent sexual transmission, mutual monogamy is the second best way and wearing a condom is a poor third." 120 Let me put it this way: **When it comes to our kids' sexuality, if you want to fool Mother Nature, use margarine on their toast instead of butter, not condoms and the pill in place of abstinence.** Remember: It's not only "not nice" to fool Mother Nature, but it's also not very smart.

Dr. Victor Cline warns that he would "anticipate the very real possibility in the future of lawsuits initiated by some infected teenagers or college-age adults against those educational institutions or organizations promoting this kind of inaccurate information and the false sense of security it promotes among sexually active young people." 126

Who is liable when a school-based clinic or sex educator propounds condoms and safe sex to his students, and then one or more of them gets pregnant, contracts herpes or worse—gets AIDS? "That's a very serious point," an Illinois attorney told me once. "Call the school board, the school superintendent and the people who are running the clinics. You will find that they are ducking; they don't know. Try calling the school's insurance company, and everybody will say, 'Not me, boss, not me.' And yet you know that when the children start getting herpes or AIDS or abortions, we're going to have some juicy lawsuits."

It's an issue school board members should seriously consider.

If one of my children were given a condom by the school health teacher or a school-based health clinic, or were encouraged to go to a PPFA office to get one, and then got pregnant or contracted a sexually transmitted disease, *believe me: I would sue the school board, the school and the teacher for everything they had!*

CHAPTER 6

False Assumption 6

"Teens Don't Need Parental Involvement in Sexual Decisions"

A number of states now have laws on the books which require parental consent for a teenager to receive contraceptives or to have an abortion. Family planning groups would have us believe that restricting access to contraception and abortion by requiring parental involvement will result in more teenage pregnancies. They argue that comprehensive sex education apart from parental involvement, including easy, confidential access to contraceptives and abortions, will reduce pregnancies.

However, when you look carefully at the statistics, you will see that the exact opposite is usually true. When parents are not involved in their children's sexual decisions, pregnancies increase. Dr. Jacqueline Kasun, professor of economics at Humboldt State University in Arcata, California, concludes from her extensive research, "If the intent is to reduce premarital sex activity and pregnancy among teenagers, there is no evidence that sex education will help." [134] In fact, there is considerable evidence that limiting access to contraception and abortion through parental consent can actually reduce pregnancy.

♦ State Statistics

Consider the case of Minnesota: "The state law, which became effective in August 1981, requires doctors to notify parents of minors who get abortions. Exceptions are allowed if a girl gets a court order saying that she is mature enough to make her own decision or that notification isn't in her best interest." 224 The law resulted in Minnesota girls under the age of 18 having fewer abortions and fewer babies in 1982 than they did in 1980. The House Select Committee on Children, Youth and Families found that within 18 months of the law going into effect the abortion rate was down 40 percent, the birthrate was down 23.4 percent and the pregnancy rate down 32 percent. "It would appear that women under 18 are reducing their risk of pregnancy," said Paul Gunderson, the health department's chief of statistics. 224

Minnesota health officials confirmed:

> The number of abortions reported for Minnesotans in this age group had dropped from 2,327 in 1980 to 1,564 in 1982. Some experts speculated then that this would mean a sharp increase in births. But figures . . . show that the number of babies born to Minnesotans age 17 and younger decreased from 2,035 in 1980 to 1,778 in 1982. The surprise finding raises new questions about the effect of a parental notification law that went into effect between those two years. It also raises the possibility of some changes in adolescent sexual patterns [as a result of parental notification]. 135

Critics of the consent law in Minnesota immediately claimed that the girls were going out of state for abortions. Yet the *Star Tribune* reported: "The number of Minnesota minors involved going out of state would be much too small to explain the large decrease in abortions for girls under age 18 in Minnesota." 135

Other states had similar results with parental consent laws:

> *Rhode Island:* Between 1981 and 1983, following enactment of a parental consent law for 12- to 17-year-olds in 1982, the birthrate declined 2 percent, abortion rate dropped 44 percent and pregnancies fell 30 percent. 390
>
> *Massachusetts:* Between 1980 and 1982, following enactment of a parental consent for 12- to 17-year-olds in 1981, the teen pregnancy rate decreased 15 percent. 391
>
> *North Dakota:* No sex education is required by the state, and teens can obtain contraceptives only with parental permission. North Dakota has the lowest rate of teen pregnancy in the United States.
>
> *Utah:* In 1980 the state passed a law requiring parental consent for minors to be given birth control, and rates of pregnancy and abortion among girls 15-17 fell. 136

In contrast, look at the state of Virginia. In cities which recently instituted comprehensive sex education, the *increase* in teen pregnancy was as great as 58 percent in some cities and averaged 20 percent in all the cities combined. In Virginia cities without compulsory sex education, the *decrease* over the same period of time was as great as 42 percent in some cities and averaged about 16 percent in all the cities combined. 392

Similar results have been recorded in parts of Europe. Teen abortions declined in England following a 1984 court ruling which prohibited giving prescription contraceptives to girls under 16. 137

♦ A Case for Barriers

There are three major barriers which cause many teens to question premarital sexual involvement. A Planned Parenthood poll shows that teens who avoid sex do so because of worry about diseases (65 percent), fear of pregnancy (62 percent) and worry over parents' reactions (50 percent). 138/6,28 Our national Why Wait? study revealed the same **barriers to sexual promiscuity: fear of pregnancy, fear of sexually transmitted diseases and fear of their parents finding out**.

Planned Parenthood vigorously campaigns for legislation and for community and education programs which will eliminate all three of these barriers. At the same time the pitch to kids is five-fold:

1. *Since you're going to do it anyway, we can keep you from getting pregnant by giving you contraceptives.*

   The fact that contraceptives cannot prevent all pregnancies is well-established, but the kids are usually not told that.

2. *We can keep you from getting a sexually transmitted disease by giving you condoms.*

   That's not true either, but the kids don't know it.

3. *We can provide an abortion for you if you do get pregnant.*

   Sadly, that is true.

4. *We can do all of the above without ever telling your parents or asking their permission. And if they ask for your file, we will remove whatever you don't want them to know.*

   One of the primary components of most school-based clinics is confidentiality from parents. A clinic staff member in New Mexico explains how they keep parents in the dark: "We keep a separate page (in the child's records) for each type of service provided to the student. The ones relating to family planning or other services that kids don't want their parents to know about are flagged. Then, if they (the parents) ask to see the file, we just remove the flagged pages." 139/5 This infuriates me as a parent.

5. *All of these services are provided free.*

   Free to the students, but their parents, who may oppose such services and from whom knowledge of these services is often deliberately concealed, will pay for them with their tax dollars.

Dr. Jacqueline Kasun, who has written extensively about the influences on teenage sexual behavior, 443; 444 objects to the abolition of these barriers which serve to protect teens against the dangerous consequences of casual sex.

Referring to the studies by Marsiglio, Mott and Deborah Anne Dawson reported in the PPFA journal, Kasun points out:

> The authors have omitted what is probably the most important determinant of differences among young people in levels of premarital sex activity and pregnancy. Like good market analysts (though they are sociologists) they have carefully measured and reported the influence of race, religion, education, and family stability, but they omitted the key determinant of demand–the price. What is the "price" of premarital sex activity for a teenager? It is, like any other price, the terms on which it is available. A youngster who is given free contraceptives by her school birth control clinic without her parents' knowledge and with the promise of a free and confidential abortion in case of pregnancy, faces a low price for premarital sex activity. She can be expected to consume more of it than a girl with less easy access to contraceptives and abortion. Though sociologists may not admit it, it is an established fact well understood by most people that human beings–and teenagers are human beings–do respond to incentives and disincentives. 134

PPFA and other family planners want to remove the three barriers–fear of pregnancy, fear of STDs and fear of parental knowledge–to decrease the consequences of teenage sexual activity. In reality, lowering the "price" increases the activity and raises the probability of negative consequences among our kids.

♦ Parents as Heroes

Teenagers not only need parental involvement in the sexual decisions, but the majority of them also want to seek and heed their parents' advice. Kids want their parents' love and understanding, and they want a relationship with their parents so they can talk with them. They want to be able to come to their parents in good times as well as bad. They want to look to their parents as their heroes.

While I was visiting the University of Wisconsin, a professor shared with me a study they conducted to find out who teenagers claim are their heroes today. Of all women, mothers were the heroes of teenage boys and girls by greater than a 6-to-1 margin over any other women. Of all men, fathers came out ahead by better than a 2-to-1 margin with no close seconds.

But as is so often the case with teens, these statistics are ideal; this is the way our kids *want* it to be. They desperately want their parents to be their heroes. In some ways they are, but often teens act in ways which deny that they revere their parents as heroes. Why? One reason is that teens follow many other heroes and have many other role models in their lives, especially as they move from dependence on their parents to the independence of adulthood.

There is also another reason, a more important reason. Rebellious teen behavior in many cases is a cry for the attention of their parents. Kids want their parents to care, to function as the heroes they want them to be.

As mothers and fathers we have an incredibly vital position of influence with our kids. It is a serious and sobering responsibility. "Parenting is now much more demanding," says Michael Carrera, professor of health sciences at Hunter College in New York and former president of the American Association of Sex Educators, Counselors and Therapists. "But parents must be attentive and involved, particularly in the early years. . . . **In shaping the values of young people, parents are more powerful than any clinic, any teacher, any peer."** 142/68

♦ Closer Family Ties

Studies show that 86 percent of teens today desire closer family ties. Of teens from divorced homes a full 74 percent said their parents did not try hard enough to make their marriages work. The same number felt that it was too easy to get a divorce in this country. 73

A recent Gallup Poll finds virtually unanimous public support among teenagers for more emphasis on traditional family ties: 144

	1978	1981	1988
More family ties	91%	92%	94%
More respect for authority	89	89	89
More sexual freedom	29	25	22
More marijuana acceptance	20	13	8

While I was speaking at a youth conference in Dallas, forty-two junior and senior high school students made counseling appointments with me. Their number one question was, "Josh, what can I do about my dad?" When I asked what they meant, they gave answers like, "He never has time for me"; "He never takes me anywhere"; "He never talks to me"; "He never does anything with me." I asked all forty-two of them, "Can you talk with your father?" Only one said yes.

I asked all the girls, "If you got pregnant, could you go to your father and share your problem with him?" Most of them didn't feel they could. That's heartbreaking, isn't it? If there ever is a time when a young woman ought to be able to go to her father and talk to him, it's in a situation like that.

The Why Wait? survey, "Teen Sex Survey in the Evangelical Church," showed that in homes where the children did not feel loved by their parents, twice the number participated in sexual intercourse—an increase from 19 percent to 35 percent—as those in homes where they did feel loved. Parental inattentiveness creates a "love famine" that affects both parents and children. It also can create a vicious self-perpetuating cycle in which parents who are starved for love raise children who are even hungrier for love. The results can be devastating.

♦ Sex Education Begins at Home

Whether parents are aware of it or not, sex education of children begins at home. And children want it this way. The Why Wait? study, which has been confirmed by other studies, shows that teens want to learn about sex from their moms and dads. Kids chose their parents first overwhelmingly in this survey—and there was no close second. 393 Parents are the child's earliest role models of love, affection, authority and values, including sexual values.

In one study kids rated parents as being the most influential in their sex education: "55 percent noted them as having a 'great deal of influence.' Only 26 percent noted siblings as having had this much influence, whereas over one-third of the respondents rated church and close friends as being that influential." 197

In the same study, "parents were rated highest in terms of influence, [however] friends were rated higher as sources of sex information—84.6 percent of the respondents said "parents" as compared to 46.2 percent who said "friends." Siblings were cited even less often as a source of sex education (21.5 percent), and the church was rarely mentioned (10.8 percent). Other major sources of sex education included school (78.5 percent) and books (80 percent)." 197

What is the relationship between the sexual attitudes and behavior of parents and their children's sexual attitudes and behavior? Students who responded to a questionnaire indicated that their attitudes were similar to their perception of their mothers' attitudes. Students' attitudes toward premarital sexual permissiveness for males "were significantly related to their perceptions of their mothers' attitudes." 197 It was also discovered that young people's "attitudes toward sexual permissiveness for females were highly correlated to their perception of their mothers' attitudes toward sexual permissiveness for females." 197

Parents were rated as more influential when family strengths were higher in these areas:

(1) "shows affection toward me"
(2) "stands behind me when times are rough"
(3) "expresses appreciation to me"
(4) "is available to talk to me when I need him/her." 197

♦ Talking About Sex With Parents

Parents have a powerful influence on their children's sexual values through what they say and model. In fact, parents and children just being together, whether or not they say or do anything, has a profound effect on a child's sexual behavior. The National Survey of Family Growth (1982) showed that both "maternal education of twelve or more years and presence of both parents in the home at age 14 reduce the odds [of sexual promiscuity] at ages 14-16." 141/162-63,166

A study on teenage sex-related values and behavior was conducted by sociologist Brent Miller of Utah State University, and it was reported in "The Family's Role in Adolescent Sexual Behavior." Miller discovered that the more openly parents discussed their own sex-related values and beliefs with teens, the less their children displayed either negative sexual attitudes or promiscuous behavior. He also showed that teens who learned sexual facts from parents were significantly less likely to be sexually active than those who first heard about sex from their friends. 394/73-130

Researcher Terri Fisher, associate professor of psychology at the Ohio State University branch in Mansfield, discovered that

> children who readily discuss sex with parents have values more similar to the parents than do those who have little family communication on the subject. . . . Children and parents have vastly different views on whether there is a lot or little discussion of sex; parents say they talk a lot about it, and children say they talk little about it. . . . It's easier to get mothers to talk about sex than to get fathers to do so. 143

Another study provides more interesting data on the subject of sex communication in the home: "Girls are more likely to have had discussions with their parents than are boys. Whites and blacks are more likely than Hispanic teenagers. And those whose parents are college graduates are more likely to have talked about sex with their parents, but they are no more likely to have talked about birth control." 27/40

Two-thirds of all teenagers have at some time "talked to their parents about sex and how pregnancy is caused."

42% of teenagers say they would be nervous or afraid to bring up the subject.

50% say they would not be nervous or afraid to bring up the subject.

Older teenagers are more likely than younger ones to report discussions with parents about birth control. Among 16- and 17-year-olds:

46% have had such a discussion.

31% have not talked with their parents about either sex or birth control. 27/39

The most heartbreaking statistic from this study revealed that "28 percent of [teens] have had no talk of any kind with their parents about sex." 27/39

Another study investigated the influence of family variables on the sexual attitudes and knowledge of sixty-five college students:

> *Parents were rated highest in terms of influence* on sexual opinions, beliefs, and attitudes, but were rated lower than friends, schools, and books as sources of information. Specific family strengths as perceived by the students were related to amount of parental influence, parents' past reaction to sex education, and sexual permissiveness of parents. Sexual knowledge was not related to any of the family variables.

However, what was lacking was "parental involvement in educating children about sexuality. Only about 15 percent of young persons said they were satisfied with their parents' discussions about sex." 197 (See also 395.) On the other hand, when parents do discuss sexuality with their children, "It appears to have a positive effect in terms of sexual responsibility." 396/231-45

In discussing formal versus family influences on sexuality, Keeney and Orr say that ultimately "the family will continue to play a far more pivotal role than any school or outside agency in setting an example and establishing values for young people and in providing them with the information they need in order to behave wisely." 397/491-96 (Cited in 197.)

When students were asked who ought to teach kids about sex and sexual behavior, 96.9 percent thought that sex education should come from parents, but only 55.4 percent thought that their parents agreed. In actual behavior, respondents rated their parents' reaction toward sexual issues/education as follows:

(1) 43.1% avoided discussion.
(2) 21.5% gave information but discussions were uncomfortable.

(3) 24.6% gave basic information and were comfortable.
(4) 10.8% were comfortable discussing any aspect of sexuality.

More than half the respondents claimed that their parents had discussed sexual development (58.5 percent) and moral issues (65.9 percent), but the majority had not discussed:

sexual intercourse (69.2%);
sexually transmitted diseases (87.7%);
pregnancy (52.3%);
birth control (.7%);
(had not discussed) any topics (23%). 197

Whether or not sex educators will admit it, teens need their parents to help them develop a positive sexual awareness in the midst of an often negative atmosphere. Our kids may not always admit their need for parental assistance and guidance, but studies have shown that they respond well when parents provide a positive model of sexuality and foster positive communication on all topics of sexual awareness.

If we sincerely want to help kids work through their sexuality, we must help their parents. As we work to equip the parent for his nurturing role during his or her child's adolescence, we will strengthen the bond between parent and child and thus help heal our society of its moral woes.

Part Two

Six Myths About Comprehensive Sex Education

Comprehensive Sex Education (CSE)

Definition and brief explanation

CSE is a reference to sex education programs and curricula that go beyond treating the sexual area through biological or physiological and reproductive instruction all the way to teaching (and most often advocating) birth control, a sexually active lifestyle, and abortion for adolescents.

Often in CSE programs there is a direct teaching on birth control, and it indirectly advocates abortion. CSE curricula very seldom mention abstinence. If they do, it is not presented as the healthy choice nor supported vigorously. You will notice also that a CSE program makes little, if any, mention of heterosexual marriage or the traditional family unit.

Comprehensive means "all inclusive." The goal is to teach everything on an equal footing, whether it be sexual deviancy, heterosexual marriages, gay marriages, etc.

Comprehensive sex education has been defined by some, i.e., the Planned Parenthood-commissioned Lou Harris Poll of 1986, as including at least four of the following six topics:

(1) biological facts of reproduction;
(2) coping with sexual development;
(3) different kinds of birth control;
(4) information about where to get contraceptives;
(5) information about preventing sexual abuse; and
(6) facts about abortion.

It is also very important to realize that CSE programs often redefine certain terms used in their curricula. For example, some programs redifine *monogamy* to mean you are only having sex with one person at that time. They redefine the word *abstinence* to mean that maybe you'd had sex before but you are waiting at that moment. You must examine carefully the way they use both *abstinence* and *monogamy*.

CHAPTER 7

➧ A **key section** for busy parents.

Myth 1

"Comprehensive Sex Education Is Value-Free and Morally Neutral"

WARNING: Sections of this chapter will be extremely offensive to you—and they should be. However, we felt these sections need to be included to alert you. We want you to gain a true picture of the information, especially some of its language and instructions, being disseminated among our children in the name of "value-free, morally neutral sex education."

In the past twenty-five years it has become generally accepted that any teaching about sex in the public schools should be free of moral judgments. "A moralistic education," says Sol Gordon, "seeks to influence children to accept a particular religious or idiosyncratic point of view." 5 According to many people, the present generation has no business imposing its views on the next generation. We're told that our kids have minds of their own and must be allowed to use them. The teacher must act only as a neutral catalyst for discussion to help students discover their own values.

It has become moralistic, and therefore unacceptable, to tell public school students that certain sexual activities are wrong while others are right. "We must be value-free and morally neutral and let students make their own choices." "Sex education should present all the options for sexual expression without explicitly encouraging or discouraging teen sexual activity." Former Secretary of Education Bennett summarizes this position (which he opposes): "While students are told it is okay to say no to sex, they are not told they ought to say no." 38/4

Perhaps the greatest deception perpetrated on the parents of teens in this country is the myth of value-free, morally neutral sex education. I have never met anyone, let alone a teacher, who can act as a neutral catalyst on any subject, let alone sex. Whenever a kid is around an adult, the adult's values will be communicated either verbally or nonverbally. For example, a ninth-grade teacher told her class that she and her boyfriend were going away together over Christmas vacation. One of the boys brashly asked, "Are you going to get laid?"

The teacher responded with a gleam in her eyes, "Now, I can't tell you that, can I?"

Was this teacher's relationship with her class value-free and morally neutral on the topic of sex? No!

There is no such thing as value-free, morally neutral sex education. Mary Lee Tatum is a board member of SIECUS (Sex Information and Education Council of the United States), a prominent sex educator, adjunct faculty member at the University of Virginia and a co-laborer with PPFA. Tatum acknowledges that "no one is value-free." What an acknowledgment of truth! Teachers must deal with that fact. 428/139

Anne Marie Morgan, formerly an educator and psychology teacher and now a parent, observes:

> Despite its claims of being "neutral," comprehensive sex-ed is not truly value-free. Listing certain options gives value to them, with the endorsement of the authority of the State and the school behind those options. If, for example, a parent has taught his child that abortion is wrong, and the school says that it is not, but merely one of many options, this undermines the parent's attempt at inculcating that value. For years, liberals have used this as an argument against school prayer, saying that the very presence of the prayer at school lends the credibility and authority of the school and State to that prayer; it would then possibly undermine what a parent was trying to teach—even if the child did not participate. Equal, comparable choices are not taught by the school for other activities; for instance, stealing is wrong, not an option. Therefore, the child may be hearing confusing messages from his authority figures, subverting values generally taught at home or, at the very least, traditional American mores. 198

It's not a question of whether or not sex education teaches values or morals; it's a question of whose values and which moral code is best or right. The claim that comprehensive sex education is value-free and morally neutral is a myth.

♦ The Case Against Moral Neutrality

Comprehensive sex educators and Planned Parenthood argue that we live in a pluralistic society of many different faiths and beliefs and that our Constitution forbids us from including those beliefs in our teaching. Therefore, they say, we must be accepting of all views and take a value-free approach, just giving the facts and not siding with any position. The curriculum guides prepared by these groups are loaded with devices to help students explore the options, evaluate the choices involved, identify alternative actions and examine their own values. They provide facts, definitions and lots of options about sex for the students, but that's all; no instruction about what's right or wrong.

What's wrong with this kind of teaching? Former Secretary of Education Bennett exclaims:

> It is a very odd kind of teaching—very odd because it does not teach. . . . It displays a conscious aversion to making moral distinctions. . . . The words of morality, of a rational, mature morality, seem to have been banished from this sort of sex education.

To do what is being done in these classes is tantamount to throwing up our hands and saying to our young people, "We give up. We give up. We give up teaching right and wrong to you. Here, take these facts, take this information, and take your feelings, your options, and try to make the best decisions you can. But you're on your own. We can say no more!" It is ironic that, in the part of our children's lives where they may most need adult guidance, and where indeed I believe they most want it, too often the young find instead an abdication of responsible moral authority. . . . When adults maintain a studiously value-neutral stance, the impression likely to be left is that, in the words of one twelfth-grader, "No one says not to do it, and by default they're condoning it." And a sex education curriculum that simply provides options, and condones by default, is not what the American people want—nor is it what our children deserve. 37

Coleen Mast, a health educator and consultant, knows the frustration that teachers face in teaching sex education. She tells of a high school teacher who was assigned the task of teaching freshman sex education. He was troubled that the materials focused on the biology of intercourse and the use of contraceptives without teaching moral values. He wanted to know how much he could teach about the morality of sex before he would be offending parents and violating legal education guidelines.

Mast explains:

> As a public health educator, I was familiar with the uncertainties that this teacher was expressing. Educators have become confused about what values, if any, they may present in their classes. . . . Since there seems to be

> no moral consensus, who is the teacher to think he or she can determine what values his students should be taught? And who is the teacher to show disapproval of sexual behaviors that are, to the modern mind, simply other options from which his students may choose? Who is the teacher to define what constitutes "normal" sexuality, "pornography," or "immorality"? It would appear that there is little else left to teach other than the impersonal facts. As for values, the students must decide for themselves what constitutes the most "comfortable" choice. 202/543-44

Perhaps the strongest case against the concept of moral neutrality in education is found in the confession of Dr. W. R. Coulson, co-founder and research director of a project to test what has come to be known as "affective" or "value-free" education. The late Carl Rogers was the principal investigator in the project which operated out of the Western Behavioral Sciences Institute in La Jolla, California, and was funded through a foundation governed by the R. J. Reynolds family, owners of the nation's second largest tobacco company.

Rogers and Coulson began the experiment in 1967 in a college, two high schools and fifty-seven elementary schools operated by the sisters of the Immaculate Heart order. Their admitted purpose in the project was to suspend the standard of reason and replace it with the standard of feelings. Dr. Coulson writes:

> Carl Rogers confessed our intention: It had been our plan early on, and years later was still the hope of Rogers as the most determined member of the team, to invert the relative importance of ideas and emotions in classrooms all over the world. He told the interviewer, "I think the stress on the rational mind is greatly misplaced. To isolate his thinking apparatus as though that was the man, I think that just disregards an enormous amount of his feelings, his physiological reaction, his genetic makeup, etc." 39/20-21

By 1968, the second year of the project, some of the staff members were beginning to pick up on the totalitarian potential of the project's philosophy, and they became uneasy. One staff member expressed the suspicion that he and his colleagues "hadn't been playing fair." Dr. Coulson relates his comments:

> We didn't think rationality and argumentation deserved the emphasis academics usually give them; we thought the exploration of feelings is a more complete process and inherently more democratic. Everybody has feelings. No one can say you don't feel what you know you do feel. But they can say your ideas are wrong. So we wanted the schools to focus more on feelings, and we didn't want to get into an argument about it; arguing was what we thought had been overdone. 39/20-21

The faculty was a little slower at perceiving the disastrous impact the project would have on their students, their career and their schools. Coulson continues:

> School personnel who later became opponents of the new, affective, value-free movement in education—our own version being called the "person-centered" approach—were not yet aware that the project proposed to cancel the very profession they'd trained for. They didn't know just how irrelevant we held the work of "professing" to be. Many had entered education for a time-honored purpose, to initiate youth in the life of the mind. They didn't realize that our philosophy questioned those very notions, initiation and mind. Traditionally, educators have believed that responsible adults possess necessary knowledge. Young people who fail to listen, who fail to receive and appreciate this knowledge, become vulnerable to exploitation and finally lose their freedom. But our person-centered vision of classrooms characterized by facilitative, nonjudgmental, value-free and therapeutic commitments held no brief for traditional educational ideals. 39/20-21

Eventually the Immaculate Heart school system, which had co-operated with the project, collapsed. Coulson and Rogers gave up their revolutionary idea as pre-emptive and unworkable. But by that time affective, value-free, morally neutral education had gained a significant foothold in the educational community and the business world, which it still enjoys. Coulson states that R. J. Reynolds "continues to participate through Tobacco Institute sponsorship." 39/21

After Carl Rogers died, Coulson wrote these sobering words:

> He [Rogers] and I and our project teammates owe the nation's parents an apology, for we alerted industry leaders to the potential for profit that lies in affective education. The surgeon general has pointed out that a healthy tobacco industry depends on getting kids to experiment with cigarettes: millions of replacements are needed each year for smokers who die or quit, and adults are no longer willing to start. Affective education turns kids into starters. The research is clear and consistent on this, with numerous studies yielding the same result: **getting facilitation instead of teaching causes students to become more interested in making decisions than in doing what's right: Right becomes whatever they decide** [emphasis mine].
>
> The bad effects don't end with smoking. Youthful experimentation with sex, alcohol, marijuana and a variety of other drugs—whatever's popular at the time—has been shown to follow affective, value-free education quite predictably; we now know that after these classes, students become more prone to give in to temptation than if they'd never been enrolled.
>
> One cause lies in an educational philosophy that calls on students and teachers alike to disbelieve in the concept of temptation. Moral absolutes are routed in affective education in favor of a psychotherapeutic imperative called "running the risks of personal growth," and this turns out to be identical with what dealers in dangerous substances and ideologies applaud. The idea of free choice for children suits them fine. So it turns out to be a deadly scheme we hatched those twenty years ago. 39/20-21

It is time for all who hold to traditional values to take a stand in opposition to this kind of sex education. The two principal reasons are:

First, there is *no such thing* as morally neutral sex education. It is a myth! And **second,** morally neutral sex education–even when it advocates and dispenses contraceptives–*does not reduce teen sexual activity or unwanted premarital pregnancies*. (See Myths 2, 3, 4 and 5.)

♦ The Myth of Moral Neutrality

Is it possible to teach sex education from a neutral point of view that does not reflect the world view presuppositions of those who design or teach the materials? I don't think so. Telling children that their sexual behavior is a personal choice is not being morally neutral. Barrett Mosbacker observes:

> It is philosophically and intellectually impossible to be morally neutral. To claim either actively or passively that there are no moral absolutes is to embrace moral relativism and situational ethics. This is a moral frame of reference. Either sexual activity is presented as having moral parameters, or as having no parameters, but both are equally moral statements. 6/24

Dr. Sigfried Ernst, M.D., of Germany states that "there is no value-free human sexuality because its basic sense is the creation of new human life and human life is never value-free." 40

"It is impossible to teach knowledge without values," says Nathan Quinones, chancellor of New York City's schools. "The question is: whose values?" 9/92

The subject of sex, except for the topic of human biology, can never be taught without communicating values. The real question is what kind of values do we want taught? Drs. Alexandra and Vernon Mark contend:

> Most of the proponents of permissive sex education pride themselves on the fact that they do not make value judgments; they studiously avoid preaching. That is what they say. It might even be what they think. But that doesn't make it true. What they are doing is systematically and relentlessly imposing their own value judgments on our society, and they are indeed preaching–their personal brand of sexual religion. 44

Planned Parenthood and their research arm, the Alan Guttmacher Institute, along with numerous sex clinics and sex education programs, argue they are value-neutral. They also boast that neutrality is a "good" thing. But "good" is a value word! How can they claim to be value-free and morally neutral while making such a value judgment on their programs? It's a contradiction.

Educators may have good intentions about helping teens discover their sexual values. But it is not neutral to tell kids, "It's okay to say no to sex and it's okay to say yes to sex. Whichever one you feel right about is okay." That's a moral statement offering two contradictory moral choices, and that communicates pluralism which says that ultimately *everything* is okay. But even pluralism is a value-oriented, morally based posture. No matter how they cut it, the comprehensive sex educators' position on sex education is not morally neutral.

One of the great ironies, which also reveals the sheer insanity of the argument for moral neutrality, is that the proponents of morally neutral sex education often demand that parents, churches, etc., not impose their morality—particularly sexual abstinence—on their own kids and other teens. How bold, how ludicrous, how moral-oriented, how value-oriented! **I can't believe the gall of anyone insisting that parents encourage their own teens to turn against parental values in order to follow a view which is the exact opposite.** Such a demand is anything but morally neutral.

♦ Presuppositions of Moral Neutrality

There are two basic views of sex education. The traditional view says that sex education is for the purpose of preparing young people to enjoy to the maximum the marvelous gift of sex within the context of marriage and to the betterment of society. In contrast, those who promote morally neutral sex education believe that young people primarily need to be trained to use contraceptives and make choices. Comprehensive sex education is seen as a means for reducing the number of unwanted teenage pregnancies and slowing the spread of sexually transmitted diseases.

Behind these two diverse purposes are radically different moral presuppositions. Advocates of value-free, morally neutral sex education see man as the product of a long evolutionary process. He is a sexual animal who is not necessarily monogamous or heterosexual. Sex has no meaning beyond pleasure and the propagation of the species. There is no reason to exercise control over one's sexual behavior. In fact, any restriction or prohibition of sexual behavior is seen as harmful.

Current sexual theorists of this persuasion believe that sexual dysfunction (which, by the way, is widespread today) is the result of Puritanical or Victorian repression perpetuated by religion. The Marks comment:

> At the heart of present-day theories on sexuality in America is the notion that "an inadequate, impaired or distorted sexual life is a cause of mental or emotional disease." This thought is not unique. It has been around for hundreds of years. Its corollary, the idea that all normal and abnormal mental functions are sexually motivated, is not new either. Both notions are founded on the concept that "appetite determines behavior." 44/1

Is this a morally neutral view? No!

Compare the so-called morally neutral view to the Judeo-Christian world view which sees man as created in the image of God with dignity, worth and potential. Sex is an expression of love, not the satisfaction of lust. Man has the ability to make moral choices and control his sexual behavior. Within the commitment of a monogamous marriage relationship, sexual intercourse is a beautiful and profoundly meaningful act—the primary form of interpersonal communion between two persons who are uniquely different and yet complementary to each other.

Because of the supreme value placed upon marriage and the family in this view, premarital and extramarital sex must be prohibited. Furthermore, the exploitation or perversion of any sexual relationship is not only counter-productive, but degrading and damaging to anyone involved. According to this view, some forms of sexual behavior are very right, while other forms are very wrong.

Obviously, this view of sexuality is not morally neutral, but it doesn't claim to be. Those who claim moral neutrality are in fact hiding behind a clever facade which "gives the impression of being neutral and objective. . . . As they write and as they teach, their moral—or immoral—presuppositions or assumptions will come through." 6/24

What I don't understand is, why do advocates of moral neutrality seem to limit their interest to sexual behavior? Why don't they take this approach with other kinds of behavior? Mosbacker shares my concern: **"No responsible teacher, parent, school superintendent or counselor would take a [value-free, morally] 'neutral approach' to stealing, lying, cheating on exams or violence. Yet, this is precisely what is being done in the area of sexual activity."** 6/4

It makes no sense to me why we seem to have this curious double standard when it comes to teaching about sex. Tottie Ellis writes:

> Just imagine if a teacher, in a unit on alcohol, were to describe in full detail the methods of getting drunk, or spend time talking about drunk driving without offering any moral judgment as to whether driving while intoxicated was right or wrong, but says, "If you decide to drive and drink, here are some ways to avoid detection: This is 85-percent safe, this one is 92-percent." We would think the teacher incompetent. 45/8A

♦ The Perils of Moral Neutrality

Isn't this "pseudo-neutral" approach harmful to students? Of course it is. Former teacher Anne Marie Morgan agonized about how supposedly value-free, morally neutral comprehensive sex education can be overwhelming and counterproductive for teens. She states:

> Sex educators do not acknowledge that adolescents are immature and not adults, and therefore should not be expected to consistently make

adult-level decisions. Our laws recognize the immaturity of teenagers in restricting minor access to alcohol and tobacco products, as well as other areas, such as marriage-licensing, consenting for medical care, and entering into contracts. Yet, sexuality educators expect adolescents to make adult-level decisions in areas of sex, family planning, and abortion, when frankly, even adults don't always make the most appropriate choices at times. . . . In addition, developmentalists, such as Piaget, have emphasized that most minors are not abstract, but concrete thinkers who are easily confused and unable to rationalize the future implications of present actions. This is not referring to intelligence, but to the level of cognitive decision-making skills in their development. Even when given information and the choices, an adolescent will often choose the concrete (immediate gratification) rather than avoiding the abstract (some problem which is vague and hard to conceptualize). Comprehensive sex-ed does not recognize the immaturity of adolescent decision-making. Teens need fewer choices and consistent, firm messages conveyed by all authority figures. 198

CBS Morning News featured the University of Michigan on their program in February 1989. They chose the University of Michigan because of the alleged racism on campus. (Racism and rape are rampant on university campuses all over the country.)

Kathleen Sullivan, the former morning news co-host, asked several students to appear on the program to state what they would like the American people to know about them as students. The first student was a black woman who spoke about the subtleties of racism on campus. The next young man looked straight into the camera and said, "What I would like most for the American people to know about students is that we need moral guidance. We need to know what is right and wrong."

At that point, Ms. Sullivan interrupted him and retorted from what appeared to me to be an attitude of arrogance, "If you want religion, there are private schools you can go to."

The student explained, "Ms. Sullivan, I'm not talking about religion. I'm talking about moral guidance—what's right and wrong."

To that she replied, "Well, you don't come to a public university for that," and then cut him off and went on to the next student.

I don't know if I was mad or simply hurt that a major network spokesperson would make such a statement. What are young people supposed to do: go to a private school for moral guidance and to learn what's right and wrong, then transfer to the University of Michigan? One thing is sure: If Ms. Sullivan had a daughter attending the University of Michigan who had been raped several times, she would angrily attack the faculty and administration for their inability to educate their students that rape is wrong—but she already stated that you don't go to a public school to get moral guidance to know what's right and wrong. Let's face it: Not everyone can go to a private school to learn moral behavior and what's right and wrong.

Here's the irony. Several months later, CBS anchor Dan Rather presented an editorial commentary on radio concerning the brutal rape of a female jogger in Central Park. His comments centered on how the brutality of the teens who attacked the girl reflected what was happening in our country. He concluded that we need to get back to teaching morality to our kids–what's right and wrong.

I sat in my car amazed. A CBS morning news person says we shouldn't teach right and wrong, and the evening news anchor says we must. If CBS had a noon news program, would they recommend that all young people enroll in a private school for two years? (The above account of Sullivan and Rather is from my memory and notes, since CBS would not provide a transcript, or a video or audio tape or even confirm my recollections. I trust I have been accurate in my account.)

Another peril of "morally neutral" sex education is that it actually promotes sexual activity. Mosbacher states: "Unfortunately . . . once it is accepted that teenage sexual activity is not a moral issue that can be addressed in sex education programs, there is an inevitable slide into open acceptance of such activity." 6/4

Dr. Edgar J. Woody, M.D., in his editorial, "Teenage Morality–Another Look," in the *Journal of the Medical Association of Georgia*, points out:

> True feelings of security, love and purpose in life seem rather remote to many . . . teenagers. Is it any wonder that, when they achieve some measure of freedom from their parents, they should seek gratification in early sexual encounters, without much thought of the consequences? To expect them to grasp the significance of the consequences is absurd. Peer pressure from other similarly deprived youngsters effectively fans the flames of their passion. The illogical conclusion becomes, "Why should I deny myself pleasure when all of my friends are enjoying themselves?" 46

How can we guard our kids against the perilous effects of morally neutral sex education? Dr. Woody has some good ideas:

> That sexually active teenagers be educated about the reproductive capacity of their bodies is a good thing. But without concomitant education in the spiritual/moral sphere, this education by itself is almost self-defeating. *Consider this analogy*: Give a person a loaded gun, educate him regarding its use, and lose him in a crowded park without an appreciation for the value of human life. Without the instilling of a moral code you have a potentially dangerous person who can wreak havoc on his own as well as other lives. But, you say, one must teach a person about the gun and how to use it correctly; otherwise that person may, through ignorance and negligence, hurt himself or others. This is true. But can you not see how in the absence of a moral code in which human life is valued, he is still dangerous? . . . I contend that unless and until teenage pregnancy prevention programs

reinforce moral values, they will continue to fail in their efforts to effect a significant reduction in teenage pregnancy [emphasis mine]. 46

♦ Values and Character

What so many sex educators overlook today is that sex is a social act involving at least two people. As a social act, the way partners treat each other is not determined by the physical or biological aspect of sex: how the penis enters the vagina, how a condom is rolled on, etc. Rather the relationship is determined by the character of the individuals. And character is based on values. **We dare not teach sex to young people without teaching character, and we cannot teach character without teaching values.** If we surrender the responsibility for developing morality, values and character to our children alone, then we must be ready for the devastating physical and social consequences they will suffer.

In a "value-free, morally neutral" comprehensive sex education class, educators, teachers, therapists and counselors strongly urge men and women to ask each other about their past sexual experiences and whether they have been infected or exposed to a sexually transmitted disease. This is their message to young people to ensure safe sex. However, June Reinisch, director of the Kinsey Institute for Research in Sex, Gender and Reproduction, warns that "in the dating situation, you can't believe and act upon information that comes from your partner." 47/1D Why? Because people without character and values lie, especially about their sexual activities. Asking a potential partner about his or her sexual history won't keep you from getting AIDS, new research suggests. "It's a risky technique, particularly for women, since it appears that men will more frequently be dishonest," says psychologist Susan Cochran of California State University, Northridge. 47/1D

How safe is sex without character?

The *San Diego Union* printed the results of the study published in the *New England Journal of Medicine* (conducted by Drs. Susan Cochran of California State University in Northridge and Vickie Mays of UCLA). The headline of the *Union* article read, "Lies and sex make dishonest bedfellows." In the study,

> 34 percent of male respondents and 10 percent of women admitted they had "told a lie in order to have sex." Even more said they would lie if a situation arose where it would be to their advantage.
>
> "The implications of our findings are clear," they wrote in today's *New England Journal of Medicine.* "Patients should be cautioned that safe-sex strategies are always advisable, despite arguments to the contrary from partners."

The survey, which gave no margin of error, was based on questionnaires filled out by 196 men and 226 women at colleges in Southern California. . . . In the survey, 47 percent of the men and 60 percent of the women believed they had been lied to for purposes of sex.

"One can probably assume that their reports of their own dishonesty underestimate rather than overestimate the problem," the researchers added.

The 422 people the researchers questioned were heterosexuals aged 18 to 25. Asked if they would disclose the existence of another sex partner to a new one, 22 percent of the men and 10 percent of the women answered, "Never." On the flip side, 29 percent of the women, but only 10 percent of the men, said yes. The rest said they would "after a while" or "if asked."

"Women will lie in order to achieve a relationship, while men will lie for both sex and relationships," she said. 359/C-4

The *New England Journal of Medicine* reports that "young people are advised to select potential sexual partners from groups at lower risk for HIV in part by asking about partners' risk histories. Unfortunately, this advice overlooks the possibility that people may lie about their risk history. 663/774

The study found that

sizable percentages of the 196 men and 226 women who were sexually experienced reported having told a lie in order to have sex. Men reported telling lies significantly more frequently than women. Women more often reported that they had been lied to by a dating partner. When asked what they would do in hypothetical situations, both men and women frequently reported that they would actively or passively deceive a dating partner. Though again, men were significantly more likely than women to indicate a willingness to do so. 663/774

Drs. Cochran and Mays, in a letter to the editor of the *New England Journal of Medicine,* share the results of their research regarding both men and women and their dishonesty in sexual relationships:

Dishonesty in Dating

	Percent	
	Men	Women
History of disclosure		
Has told a lie in order to have sex	34	10
Lied about ejaculatory control	38	
or likelihood of pregnancy		14
Sexually involved with more than one person	32	23
Partner did not know	68	59

Experience of being lied to		
Has been lied to for purposes of sex	47	60
Partner lied about ejaculatory control		46
or likelihood of pregnancy	34	
Willingness to deceive		
Would lie about HIV-antibody test	20	4
Would lie about ejaculatory control	29	
or likelihood of pregnancy		2
Would understate number of previous partners	47	42
Would disclose existence of other partner to new partner		
Never	22	10
After a while, when safe to do so	34	28
Only if asked	31	33
Yes	13	29
Would disclose a single episode of sexual infidelity		
Never	43	34
After a while, when safe to do so	21	20
Only if asked	14	11
Yes	22	35

663/774

Cochran and Mays concluded:

> The implications of our findings are clear. In counseling patients, particularly young adults, physicians need to consider realistically the patients' capacity for assessing the risk of HIV in sexual partners through questioning them. 663/774

How safe is sex without character? In light of the research which shows that people constantly lie about their past sexual experience, the following, by Sally Ann Stewart in an article in *USA Today,* seems ludicrous: "William Staytone, professor of human sexuality at the University of Pennsylvania, says the direct approach is best. I think the person can be open about it by saying, 'You may be as concerned as I am about this. I want to assure you that I'm free of any disease, and I hope you can assure me of the same,' Staytone says. Carol Ellison, a sex therapist in Oakland, California, agrees, 'I think you have to be clear what your own values are.' " 49/5D

The Norfolk (Virginia) Department of Public Health put out a pamphlet titled "Safer Sex" which counseled: "It is best to know your sexual partners. Make it a habit to exchange names and phone numbers in order to protect each other. Avoid all types of anonymous sex including 'one-night stands' and 'pick-ups.' " 398

But we must realize that often both partners will lie through their teeth. We had better make sure that vulnerable men and women, people with character, values and morals will not be coaxed into a potentially dangerous liaison. **Crude though it may sound, when it comes to many men, "an erect penis has no conscience"–or morals or values, we might add.**

♦ Examples of "Morally Neutral" Sex Education

In this section I want to share with you a number of examples of the material which I found shocking and offensive, but which is being distributed in public schools around our country in the name of value-free, morally neutral sex education.

Be aware that sex education in our public schools varies greatly from state to state and even from school district to school district. I recommend that you examine carefully the sex education materials being used by school districts in your area.

Consider the way one school district deals with the subject of homosexuality: "The sex-curriculum guide for elementary schools in my city specifies that children will 'develop an understanding of homosexuality,' 'learn the vocabulary and social fads' relating to it, 'study the theories concerning it,' view films and engage in role playing about homosexuality, and take tests on it." 50/1 Morally neutral?

Not only do many "morally neutral" public school curriculums advocate that "our society must strive to sanction and support various forms of intimacy between members of the same sex," but masturbation also is championed as an excellent way to relieve sexual tension, especially for women: "In a 'sexuality' course for teachers, given recently by my county health department, I heard the instructor deplore the fact that so many otherwise well-informed girls and women 'have never been told anything about masturbation' and 'don't even know they have a clitoris.' " 50/1

The PPFA promotes and distributes a number of pamphlets to sex education classes. Two of these pamphlets were given to a coed class of eighth-graders in a Norfolk, Virginia, middle school in March 1988. One is titled "Proper Use of Condoms," which explains their use. The other pamphlet is titled "Safer Sex," which advocates creativity in sexual activity and describes safe sex techniques such as mutual masturbation, showering together, visual fantasies, using your own sex toys, anal intercourse with condom and oral sex with urine contact. In both of these pamphlets, information was provided for help or counseling. The recommended resources included the National Gay Task Force, the Gay Men's Health Crisis and the Virginia AIDS Hotline. This information was provided by the Norfolk Department of Public Health. Value-free? Morally neutral?

In another eighth-grade sex education class in Virginia, a quiz was given asking for the definition of more than fifty terms used in what we would call the basest kind of street language. Pejorative terms for women abounded in the quiz.

I was given a copy of that list of terms, and, frankly, it left me stunned! We may have heard some of these words in a locker room, but when I began my research, I certainly did not expect to see them in a "morally neutral" eighth-grade sex education course. I had listed a dozen or so of the terms in this chapter, but my publishers and I, after much discussion, decided to remove them, though they undeniably would have verified our more general statements about sex education.

In the widely used book, *Finding My Way: Student Guide,* recommended by the Virginia Department of Education for their Family Life Education (FLE) program, the following are explained and quizzed: oral sex, incomplete orgasm, fetishism, bestiality, the moral rightness of homosexual relations between a young boy and a man, voyeurism, masochism, sadism, incest and rape. Value-free? Morally neutral? What do you think?

A teenaged girl and her boyfriend walked into the Planned Parenthood office in Escondido, California. She said she had just turned 15 and wanted to know about sex. They gave her two of the books quoted below: *Changing Bodies, Changing Lives* and *The New Our Bodies, Ourselves.* As of May 1987, these two books were recommended by Planned Parenthood for 13- to 19-year-olds.

As you read these excerpts, imagine a school-based clinic or sex education class giving these books and/or teaching these concepts to your 13-year-old child or grandchild without your knowledge or permission. (I couldn't imagine it even *with* your permission!) Then visualize your tax dollars paying for this sexual indoctrination. Too horrible to think about? Tragically, it's happening all over our country.

- *Boys and Sex,* recommended and distributed by PPFA:

> Premarital intercourse does have its definite values as a training ground for marriage or some other committed relationship. . . . It's like taking a car out on a test run before you buy it. 51/117
>
> [Specific instructions on how to masturbate. These include several techniques that go way beyond what most of us would consider normal.] 51/49
>
> It's better to have a good deal of petting . . . [explicit advice on the procedure] before the first intercourse takes place. 51/125
>
> There are many possible positions. [Vivid descriptions are given for three specific positions for intercourse.] 51/127
>
> Any of the farm animals may become a sexual object—ponies, calves, sheep, pigs, even chickens or ducks. Dogs are also commonly used, but cats rarely. . . . If this kind of sexual behavior should ever happen to you, you

would be best to keep knowledge of it from other people. . . . Feel secure in your self-knowledge that you are not a monster, no matter what society may say. 51/171-172

- *Girls and Sex,* recommended and distributed by PPFA:

When she's old enough and ready to be aroused, excitement will make her lips go soft and open, so that the next step inevitably occurs – tongue-kissing. From there petting proceeds, [graphic descriptions of heavy petting, hand-to-genital stimulation and oral-genital stimulation]. 52/74-75

There are many girls who regret after marriage that they didn't have premarital intercourse, because they've come to realize what a long, slow learning process it can often be after marriage. 52/96

- *Changing Bodies, Changing Lives,* recommended and distributed by PPFA:

If your parents or other adults who play a parental role in your life have talked to you about sex, their voice may be saying, "You're too young to be in the back seat of a car with a girl!" If you feel your parents are over-protective, their message may not be helpful. If they seem to fear your sexuality, or if they don't want you to be sexual at all until some distant time, you may feel you have to tune out their voice entirely. Or it may be strong enough only to make you feel guilty. But if your parents seem to trust your judgment and basically just want you to take care of yourself, their voice of carefulness can help you make decisions you will be glad about. 53/87

For some couples, petting includes touching each other's genitals. [The statement that follows in this material is a boy's explicit description of mutual masturbation with a girlfriend. The account concludes with the boy's saying] "It was great." 53/96

In some ways, oral sex is the most intimate kind of lovemaking. [Oral sex and its "benefits" are described in detail here.] 53/97

[Specific techniques for oral sex described here.] It is a kind of love-making that many people find very pleasurable and exciting (and it doesn't risk pregnancy). Many others don't feel comfortable with it at all. . . . What you do should feel right for you. 53/96

[The emotions and physical feelings involved in oral sex are described in provocative, first-person dialog here, much like a "love story."] 53/97

When both are ready for intercourse, [full particulars of physical changes that take place in preparation for intercourse appear here, and the paragraph continues with a clear description of movements and techniques that can lead to orgasm.] 53/101

Parents who react against their child's "coming out" [as a homosexual] are often thinking of the stereotypes of what gay people are. They may need to learn more before they can open their minds. 53/120

Gay and bisexual teenagers need to meet other people like them for friendship and support, but this can be difficult. Call a local hot line, or possibly a local service agency. Gay bars often are among the only places to find openly gay people. Many teens find their way into gay bars despite being under the drinking age. Bars have been a lifeline for lesbian and gay people. 53/121-122

Lesbians make love in lots of ways. [Description of various woman-to-woman sexual techniques.] 53/122

Gay men, too, have many ways of making love. [Description of various man-to-man sexual techniques.] 53/122

- *The New Our Bodies, Ourselves,* recommended and distributed by PPFA:

The question of whether or not to sell ourselves to men [in prostitution] is a false one: The real question is how to sell ourselves in the way that is least destructive to ourselves and our sisters. That is not a decision any one of us can make for any of the others. 54/113-114

[Again, first-person dialog is used, this time to portray the "turn-on" of anal sex.] 54/178

Did you find the preceding paragraphs offensive? I hope so! As a parent I found them extremely offensive. I have in my files additional, even more explicit samples which illustrate the extremes that some sex educators will go to in order to promote teen sexuality. Many school administrators believe that as long as they avoid that level of explicitness, the program is okay. The problem is, *almost all* comprehensive sex education programs open the door for that degree of extreme explicitness.

- "You've Changed the Combination," a pamphlet published and distributed by Rocky Mountain Planned Parenthood, Denver, Colorado:

(The title refers to a broken relationship in high school where one of the former sexual partners has changed the combination on his/her locker. This pamphlet is frequently distributed to adolescent boys in the San Diego Planned Parenthood Clinics. The instruction contained is as far removed from value-free and morally neutral as you can get.)

Sex is best between friends. Not quickest, just best. Ask anyone who knows. . . . There are only two basic kinds of sex: sex with victims and sex without. Sex with victims is always wrong. Sex without is always right. . . . One way to avoid having victims is, of course, to have sexual relationships only with your friends. If you can't manage that, at least try to observe the ground rules. . . . Be honest about your intentions: If this is a one-nighter, and you don't intend to be around, say so. If you're just lonely and down, say so. If this is a girl you've just met and she agrees, you're in the clear, provided that she's old enough to have some sense. 55/10-12

Sexual sickies grow up in homes in which sex is taboo [emphasis added]. 55/14

Decide honestly what you want from your relationships with women. Do you want a convenient warm body? Buy one. That's right. There are women who have freely chosen the business. Buy one. Do you want a virgin to marry? Buy one. There are girls in that business too. Marriage is the price you'll pay, and you'll get the virgin. Very temporarily. 55/18

- *One Teenager in Ten: Writings by Gay and Lesbian Youth,* promoted and sold by PPFA:

(This book is a part of "Project 10," which began in 1984 at Fairfax High School in Los Angeles. It is currently being implemented at secondary schools throughout the Los Angeles Unified School District. Project 10 was prepared by the Office of Counseling and Guidance Services Branch, Los Angeles Unified School Districts, 6520 Newcastle Avenue, Reseda, CA 91335; telephone (818) 997-2485. This material has not only been sent to me by numbers of concerned teachers and principals, but last week I also received a resource flyer from PPFA itself, promoting *One Teenager in Ten.* The following "testimony" is by a 16-year-old named Amy.)

> I had known my dance teacher for three years. . . . We became lovers the weekend I was asked to give a special dance presentation. . . . She was 23. She said, "Let me help you take this off." I cooperated with her so my arms could be freed, leaving the costume hanging at the waist, with my breasts bare. Placing her hands . . . [a graphic, sensuous description of how the dance teacher "made love" to the girl follows]. 399/52-54

- In Virginia, one of the books advocated for sex education was *The Dynamics of Relationships: Alternative Sexual Lifestyles.* In this book, homosexuality is not treated as value-neutral. Homosexuality is said not to be a sign of maladjustment under any circumstances; in fact, those opposed to homosexuality may be the maladjusted ones. 400

In a sex educators' workshop, the instructor insisted that the prevailing theme of sex education is that "children from the sixth grade on must come to accept [homosexuality] as normal. . . . [A workshop participant suggested that a good experience is to have two ten-year-old girls 'role-play' two male lovers.] . . . Parents who quote Scriptures against homosexuality are 'irrational'; their minds are perverted."

We can't expect kids to practice abstinence if the adult authority figures in their lives promote promiscuity. For example, PPFA, as part of its program for Valentine's Day activities, distributed Valentine cards with bright red condoms attached and a printed message, "Love Carefully." This level of taste was also expressed in "Love Carefully" T-shirts, buttons, etc. For other examples of sex-enhancing materials, see *True to Life,* Planned Parenthood publication #1558. PPFA claims its publications are "useful in secondary schools reading courses." 57/4

"Condomania" is sweeping the country, and PPFA and other sex educators resort to all kinds of "educational methods" to get kids to wear condoms. 201/489-90 Their methods include having kids role-play teens who have been sexually active "for a long time." 358/256 Kids are often required to attend a "safer sex dance party," where they dance to "hot music with sexual messages." The music and games are used to instruct and help kids feel comfortable when they "roll condoms down the penis." 356 They use cucumbers as penises so kids can practice fitting condoms. 357

"Creative ideas for encouraging condom use among teens" are suggested by an influential national organization, The Center for Population Options, which has played a leading role in the movement to place health clinics in schools. These ideas include:

- Encouraging teens to carry one for a friend. If all teenagers carried condoms, they would be prepared for situations where "it just happened." They also could help their friends out.
- Homework assignments. Leaders can develop an optional assignment for teens to purchase a packet of condoms. This helps a student develop skills for purchasing personal products at a pharmacy. . . . *In some schools, students can't pass their health class without buying a condom!*
- Condom couplet contest. Ask students to develop two-line rhymes promoting condoms to sexually active teens.
- Role plays. Girls can be asked to develop answers for boys who say, "But it's like taking a shower with a raincoat on." Boys can develop responses to girls who say, "But I'm on the pill"; or, "Do you have a disease or something?" 228/10,16,17

Remember: Many sex educators would like to bring all the above material into *Julian's junior and senior high schools.* They would like our kids to wear their T-shirts and play their condom games.

If you have any remaining doubts as to whether teaching and providing students with birth control techniques is morally neutral, consider the Dartmouth College "safe sex kit." Gregory Fossedal, a "media fellow" at the Hoover Institute and former editorial writer for the *Wall Street Journal,* researched the safe sex kit and writes:

> Students arriving at Dartmouth College this winter received . . . free of charge what Dartmouth is pleased to call the "safe sex kit." One enclosure is the brochure . . . which describes options for "enjoying sex to the fullest without giving or getting sexual diseases." Similar kits, health experts say, are available at many colleges—and some high schools—around the country.
>
> Dartmouth's sex kit included two free condoms, plus a lubricant and "rubber dam" recommended for love acts between two men. . . . Women students . . . may receive the controversial morning-after pill.
>
> Dr. John Turco of Dartmouth's health service denies that the sex kit "promotes promiscuity." Dartmouth, he says, is not condoning anything, but rather, seat-belt-like, serving to "protect those who already drive." (Sure, and if Dartmouth handed out needles, marijuana bongs, cocaine spoons, and a handbook on the do's and don'ts of freebasing, you would not be promoting drug usage, just a safe trip.)
>
> In fact, Dartmouth is condoning a certain view of human sexuality rather explicitly. When one student phoned the college health office to ex-

> press doubts about the safety and morality of the morning-after pill, she was told: "Well, it's a #*@* of a lot better than pregnancy, isn't it?" A student who asked whether anal sex is "kind of dangerous" was eventually told: "It's an individual preference, of course. Whatever's comfortable and feels natural to you."
>
> How does one react to such events? Are they silly? Sad? Outrageous? If you're unsure, consider this. Imagine—just imagine—that instead of the safe sex kit, Dartmouth or Yale or Stanford or Ohio State were passing out copies of the Bible. Picture it: the faculty resolutions, *New York Times* headlines, the lawsuits, the protest, the gnashing of teeth.
>
> The tragedy . . . is, it is near impossible to conceive of such an event. Yet the "safe sex kit"—at Dartmouth and perhaps your alma mater—is not only imaginable, not possible, but fact. 58/B7

Few instructional programs, if any, are or even come close to being value-free or morally neutral. **I know that I could never honestly teach sex without revealing my own convictions**. Do we really care what happens to our own children, to all children? I think the teen promiscuity which is so prevalent today is largely the result of a new morality which claims to be value-free and morally neutral but isn't. It's about time that concerned parents and leaders make the content of the sex education programs in their local schools a matter of personal concern. What have we done in this area to help our children in Julian?

♦ The Violent Side of Moral Neutrality

One more important issue must be discussed here: Rape, the violent side of "value-free, morally neutral" sex education. Teaching about the physical and biological aspects of sex while avoiding the issues of values, morals and character leaves young people with unclear boundaries concerning rape, especially date rape. I firmly believe that value-free, morally neutral sex education is largely responsible for the sobering statistics on rape in our country.

According to FBI statistics,

> Rape is committed in this country every six minutes. Nationally, the number of reported rapes has increased more than 20 percent from 1978 to 1987, with more than 91,000 forcible rapes documented in 1987, the most recent year in which figures are available. . . . According to yearly crime totals compiled by the Dallas Police Department, rape has steadily increased in the last five years: There were 568 cases in 1984, 620 in 1985, 669 in 1986, 771 in 1987 and 1,260 in 1988. 61/D11

Between 1977 and 1986, rape increased by 42 percent, making it the most rapidly growing major crime in the United States. 61/D11 The number of rapes in the United States increased 526 percent between 1960 and 1986. 62

More than 50 percent of college women are sexual victims. Administrators concerned about sexual aggression on campus should be interested in a new 210-page manual, *The Prevention of Rape and Sexual Assault on Campus.* The cost is $35 plus $2.50 handling. Contact: Campus Crime Prevention Programs, P.O. Box 204, Goshen, KY 40026.

A national study of 1,700 sixth- to ninth-grade students, presented at the 1988 National Symposium of Child Victimization in Anaheim, California, revealed:

65% of today's students state it is acceptable for a man to rape a girl if they've been dating for more than six months.
25% said it was acceptable to rape a girl if a guy spends money on her.
87% said it is acceptable for a husband to rape his wife.
31% said it is acceptable for a guy to rape a girl if she had been sexually active before.

Morally neutral sex education has nothing to say about rape being wrong. Such a judgment would be "value-oriented and morally based." No wonder the incidence of rape in our country is so staggering. Kids who are taught to do what feels good cannot discern where their own sexual freedom violates that of another.

Rape is considered the most under-reported felony, and accurate figures are difficult to compile. The Center for the Prevention and Control of Rape teamed with *Ms.* magazine and Mary P. Koss, Ph.D., then a psychology professor at Kent State University, and conducted an enlightening study. Over a three-year period, 6,100 undergraduates were surveyed on thirty-two college campuses with these results:

25% of those women were victims of rape or attempted rape.
84% of those raped knew their attackers.
57% of the rapes happened on dates.

In one year 3,187 women reported suffering:

328 rapes (as defined by law);
534 attempted rapes (as defined by law);
837 episodes of sexual coercion (sexual intercourse obtained through continual arguments or pressure);
2,024 experiences of unwanted sexual contact (fondling, kissing or petting committed against the woman's will).

The average age when a rape incident occurred (either as perpetrator or victim) was 18.5 years for both men and women.

27% of the women whose sexual assault met the legal definition of rape thought of themselves as rape victims.

75% of the men and 55% of the women involved in date rapes had been drinking or taking drugs just before the attack.

Of the 3,187 female college students questioned:

15.3% had been raped.
11.8% were victims of attempted rape.
11.2% had experienced sexual coercion.
14.5% had been touched sexually against their will.
42% of the rape victims told no one about the attack.
5% reported their rapes to the police or sought help at a rape-crisis center.
55% of the men who raped said they had sex again with their victims.
41% of the raped women said they expect to be raped again;
30% of the women identified in the study as rape victims contemplated suicide after the incident.
31% sought psychotherapy.
22% took self-defense courses.
82% said the experience had permanently changed them.

In the year prior to the survey, 2,971 college men reported that they had committed:

187 rapes;
157 attempted rapes;
327 episodes of sexual coercion;
854 incidents of unwanted sexual contact.
16% of the male students committed rape.
84% of the men who committed rape said what they did definitely was not rape.
10% of those who attempted a rape took part in episodes involving more than one attacker.
38% of the women who had been raped were 14, 15, 16 or 17 years old at the time of their assaults.

In a landmark survey financed by the National Institute of Mental Health, 7,000 students at thirty-five colleges and universities across the country were interviewed. Psychologists surveyed more than 400 students at Washington State University. Five percent of those women and 19 percent of the men did not define forcible sex or the man's coercion as unacceptable behavior. Rather, they felt that under certain conditions it might be acceptable for a man to force sex on his companion. These conditions included if the couple had been dating for a long time, if she had let him fondle her, if she wasn't a virgin or if she had "led him on." 60

Read the following letter from a rapist in light of the moral neutrality perpetrated by comprehensive sex education today:

I had a belief system set up so that I could rape. It went like this: Most women secretly want to be raped; most women will not report being raped; if it is reported, it will not go to trial; if it is taken to trial, the rapist will be found not guilty; if he is found guilty, he will not get much time.

I now realize that all these are lies. Lies I had to tell myself in order to allow myself to rape.

After the first rape, I began to use other justifications for raping: The women I raped were all giving it away anyway, so why not get some myself? It is not like we were doing anything that these women had not done before. If they knew me, which they did not, they would have given it to me.

You can see how all of these things worked together to let me rape. They were all necessary, but where did they come from? This is where it gets sticky. I had my first rape fantasy after watching the TV movie, A Case of Rape, *starring Elizabeth Montgomery. In this movie, a man she meets gets into her apartment to use the phone while her husband is out of town. He rapes her. Although she starts to, she does not report it. Later on, she is raped by the same man again. This time, she does report it and it goes to trial. You guessed it, he is found not guilty.* 62 and 64/9A

♦ A Moral Dilemma

When those who are in authority over adolescents do not promote and model moral character, virtue, self-control, fidelity and abstinence, they in fact surrender the teen's moral and character development to the media, Hollywood and peer pressure. Mosbacker points out that this "neutral" or "objective" approach, "provides no moral framework or foundation for decision-making that leads the students directly away from sexual activity, which should be the goal of any sex education counseling program. Instead, this approach effectively sets students adrift upon a sea of cultural chaos and sexual exploitation without compass or rudder." 6/23-24

I think this excerpt from a recent Minority Report of the House Select Committee on Children, Youth and Families is an insightful summary of our predicament:

> Every generation has inherited the difficult job of bringing children to adulthood, and the same problems have presented themselves. . . . Why does the problem seem so much more difficult in this generation? Have we really failed in our efforts to prevent pregnancies to unmarried teens? Or is it truer to say that we have abandoned them? **Progressively, we have, as a nation, decided that it is easier to give children pills than to teach them respect for sex and marriage.** 66/386

Nationally syndicated columnist William Raspberry, echoing former Secretary of Education William Bennett, wrote:

> Birth control clinics in school may prevent some births. That I won't deny. The question is, what does it teach? What lessons does it teach? What attitudes does it encourage? What behaviors does it foster? I believe there are certain kinds of surrender that adults may not declare in the presence of the young. One such surrender is the abdication of moral authority. Schools are the last place that that should happen. [67]

♦ The Moral Solution

Raspberry goes on to say that when it comes to sex education, the best and really the only acceptable instruction adults can offer to adolescents is abstinence: Don't do it. [67] If we are going to help our kids, we must give them positive, value-oriented, morally-based principles. Even most teens know that!

Researchers report that mere factual "knowledge alone has little impact and that even peer pressure is less powerful" than what they call "the student's internalized beliefs and values." In a recent national poll, 70 percent of the adults surveyed said they thought sex education programs should teach moral values, and about the same percentage believe the programs should urge students not to have sexual intercourse. Believe it or not, teens agree. According to a recent survey, seventh- and eighth-graders who have chosen not to engage in intercourse say that the greatest influence on their decision is the fact that "it is against my values for me to have sex while I am a teenager." [68]

I do not believe that "morally neutral education" can ever provide an adequate basis for saying no to premarital sex. It certainly does nothing to build a young person's understanding of the concepts of family or character. Sex education without traditional values is not only pointless, but it is also harmful to young minds.

Some responses to this chapter:

This chapter, as originally written, contained a number of word-for-word excerpts from the explicit material some of our kids are receiving in school. However, as the work on the book progressed, my associates and I struggled with whether it would be too offensive to you, and we realized we could not publish it as it was. Therefore, we revised it, removing some of the most offensive terms and phraseology, and we sent copies of the original chapter and the revision to several well-known educators and community leaders, asking for their reactions and recommendations. All agreed the original version was too offensive. Regarding the revision, the replies were markedly varied. One said, "You should take out [even from the revision] anything that is at all graphic. It is not appropriate for a book by Josh or from the publisher."

Another said, "I'd say, *print it.* Those who miss the point and get mad at you probably won't be very effective in the battle anyway. Those who can be stirred to sustained action by the frankness will be the warriors who will stay the course. Isn't that the real reason you're writing/publishing this book?"

One said, "Normally I would ask my wife to give her opinion on something like this. However, I would never expose her to prurient language such as that contained in the report. . . . I was shocked at some of the descriptive language employed." He went on to say, "I understand Josh's desire to have readers slam their fists on the table in disgust against the public school system and their sordid sex education program. I fear that [if you print it] more will slam their fists on the table in disgust with Josh McDowell and Here's Life Publishers."

A pastor said, "I feel the material was handled very well and see no problem with it at all." An institute leader said, "I hope you can retain at least a measure of the quotes in the book so as to communicate to the readers the reality of what is going on. My concern is that you will be able to find the fine line where people will take offense at the material—but not at Josh or at the publisher for revealing it."

One thoughtful respondent said, "If someone buys this book, it is because he is interested in the subject. He has already qualified himself to be willing to receive what is in it. I don't see any problem with it."

As a result of all these responses, and some others, I felt it the better part of wisdom to take out of the chapter some of the most explicit and graphic material. It has been replaced with bracketed explanations. At the same time, I want to be sure you do get the impact of the lewd and pornographic language our kids are getting in the name of "sex education." I hope that has been accomplished.

You may have need for the exact material for use in your organization or in your own efforts to stem this tide of comprehensive sex education. If so, write me, explaining your need, and I will be happy to send you copies of the appropriate text. You will be shocked and alarmed at what is there.

Write to me at: P. O. Box 391, Julian, CA 92036.

CHAPTER 8

Myth 2

"Comprehensive Sex Education Increases Responsible Teen Contraception"

Proponents of school-based health clinics, seeing that many teenagers don't consistently employ various methods of birth control, strongly advocate that clinics be placed in or near every middle, junior high and senior high school. They believe that greater accessibility to contraceptives will encourage more sexually active students to use them.

Those who oppose school-based health clinics in or around our schools see them as a threat to the morality of the students for several reasons:

(1) Accessibility to clinics and contraceptives creates a climate of legitimacy or acceptability to illicit sexual activity.

(2) They communicate values about premarital sex that is at variance with the values and attitudes of many of their parents.

(3) They eventually increase teen premarital sexual activity, abortions and unwanted births.

I want to share with you three case studies illustrating the impact of school-based health clinics, and the contraceptives they offer, on the schools they served. I believe you will agree with me that the sex education which is available in these clinics does not increase responsible contraception.

1. Chicago, Illinois

DuSable High School received nationwide attention and a lot of media coverage for its "successful" experience involving a contraceptive-dispensing school-based clinic. School administrators decried the fact that during the 1984-85 school year, prior to establishing a school-based health clinic, 300 of their 1,000 female students got pregnant. After the clinic was opened, they proudly heralded that only thirty-five girls got pregnant in the first half of the 1985-86 school year.

But when all the facts finally came to light about the program, what little corroborative evidence existed told a different story. The analysis of the DuSable program was so unscientific and unverifiable that only a couple of observations are necessary to discredit their so-called success.

First, school officials admitted they kept no records of the numbers of pregnancies before the operation of the clinic. Laura Devon, the information officer for "Ounce of Prevention," one of the clinic's funding sources, admitted that "300 pregnant girls" was an estimate based on casual sources and interviews with school officials.

Second, school officials could not produce the statistics for the number of abortions girls received as a result of clinic exposure. There was no data to show how abortions reduced the teenage births at the school during the clinic's operation.

2. St. Paul, Minnesota

Another highly acclaimed study is the St. Paul, Minnesota, clinic's evaluation of its success at encouraging responsible teen contraception in two schools. The study showed a reduction in the number of teen births. Planned Parenthood reported in 1980 that the number of pregnancies in the two schools declined each year between 1976 and 1979 (see Table A on the next page). Also, the percentage of female students who obtained contraceptives at the clinic rose from 7.1 percent in 1977 to 16.4 percent in 1978 to 25.0 percent in 1979. 402 The study also showed a 23-percent decline in births.

On the surface the clinic appears to be successful. However, as Table A suggests, there are some serious flaws in the study which discredit the clinic's boast at developing responsible contraception in its participating students.

To begin with, a school administrator admitted that the schools could not document the decrease in pregnancies. 109 Furthermore, the report did not show the correlation between the reduction of births and the decline of female students enrolled in the schools.

Table A
St. Paul M.I.C. Adolescent Program
Progress Report September 1982—June 1983

Number of Active Clients:	Site 1	Site 2	Site 3	Site 4	Total
Total pregnant adolescents registered*	12	27	9	8	56
Pregnant adolescents followed medically**	1	6	7	1	15

* The number of pregnant adolescents registered represents all patients registered in the clinic as prenatal.

** The number of pregnant adolescents followed medically represents all patients receiving their prenatal care through the clinic. **The difference between the two numbers equals those registered patients who either miscarried, terminated the pregnancy or went elsewhere for care after their registration** [emphasis mine]. 403

Michael Schwartz, in "Lies, Damned Lies, and Statistics," explains, "We are not told what the total female enrollment in the two schools was in each year, but by matching the percentage with the hard figures we reach the totals: 1267, 1018 and 948." 216/4 The relationship in the decrease of births (23 percent) and the decrease (25 percent) of student enrollment shows there was actually an increase in births.

Next, the school did not have a means for determining *all* the teen births which occurred. The Support Center for School-Based Clinics admitted that "most of the evidence for the success of that program (St. Paul) is based upon the clinics' own records and the staffs' knowledge of births among students. Thus the data undoubtedly do not include all births." 217/14

It is possible that abortions were the reason births declined. Family planners are emphatic on promoting abortions for birth control. For example, in the spring of 1984 the King County (Seattle) Planned Parenthood executive director's annual report boasted that during the previous year "we made fourteen adoption referrals and 2,695 abortion referrals." There is no evidence that the same policy wasn't in effect in the St. Paul clinic.

Another flaw in the St. Paul study is that it didn't note the correlation between the decrease of births and the increase of abortions, showing the former but omitting the latter.

Also, as Table A explains, the difference in the number of pregnant teenagers who were registered in the clinics and those who were followed through on is remarkably different. This large discrepancy is one of the major reasons a reduction in births is apparent. There is no means of verifying clinic data. Those who have vested interest in the success of the clinics are also responsible for reporting their effectiveness. This clearly represents a conflict of interest and causes all unverifiable data to be suspect.

It is important to realize, as Mosbacker points out, that "the St. Paul study showed a drop in the teen birth rate rather than the teen pregnancy rate. Accordingly, it is quite likely that the reduction in the fertility rate was due at least in part to an increase in the number of abortions." 193/4 Schwartz explains, "We still do not know whether the rate and/or number of pregnancies changed or how many students submitted to abortions." 216/5

Finally, the St. Paul study failed because it was not replicable and did not control outside factors. Marie Dietz, a research analyst, states:

> Since its comparisons were done in a cross-sectional way between the school before and after clinic presence, other variables affecting birth rates could have been affecting all school populations. The suggested approach to show whether this occurred or not is to compare the clinic school with other schools or a school which is similar in the school demographics (number of students, race of students, and socio-economic status of students) and to see if there is a significant difference between the birth/fertility rates of the school with a clinic and without a clinic. This was not done. Therefore, the widely publicized findings of the teenage contraceptive clinic which supposedly showed a drop in the birth rate are simply not supported by the data presented in the research report. 218

The St. Paul study does not supply sufficient grounds for any kind of a policy decision on school-based health clinics by the government or by individual school districts.

3. Baltimore, Maryland

A school-based clinic program was instituted at two junior and senior high schools in Baltimore, Maryland. Researchers from Johns Hopkins University evaluated the program and reported their findings in the PPFA journal, *Family Planning Perspectives:* 404/119-26

1. Students in the experimental schools displayed a greater knowledge of sexuality than students in the control schools.
2. Students in the experimental schools displayed a greater tendency to use effective forms of contraception than students in the control schools.
3. The average age at which experimental-school students became sexually active rose from 15 years and 7 months to 16 years and 2 months.

4. Over a 56-month period, the adolescent pregnancy rate among students in grades nine through twelve in the experimental school dropped 30.1 percent, while in the control school the pregnancy rate increased 57.6 percent. 219/124

Again, the statistics look impressive at first glance. But on closer scrutiny there are a number of significant flaws "in the research design which prevents one from being able to verify the conclusions of the Johns Hopkins study." 220/7

Research analyst Dr. Jacqueline Kasun and sociologist Dr. Tobin Demsko each evaluated the Baltimore program extensively. Excerpts from their evaluations reveal the weakness of the Baltimore study in determining the success of the school-based clinics. In her paper, "The Baltimore School Birth Control Study: A Comment," Dr. Kasun writes:

> The most conspicuous failing of this study of the Baltimore school birth control clinic program is that it does not take account of girls dropping out of school due to pregnancy. . . . Since only 10 to 20 percent of pregnant students at the schools in question entered the pregnant minor program . . . and since it is estimated that as many as one-half of such drop-outs may be due to pregnancy . . . the omission of these girls represents a major loss of information and casts serious doubts on the study's conclusion that the clinic program reduced sex activity and pregnancy.
>
> Secondly, in estimating pregnancy rates, the authors calculate pregnancy rates as percentages of the sexually active only, rather than among all the girls exposed to the clinic program. This means that even if pregnancy rose as a result of the clinic program, if it rose less rapidly than sex activity, it would appear as a reduction. Thus two failures could be made to appear as a success. . . .
>
> In addition to these serious problems with the Baltimore study, there are others as well. The authors' failure to give numbers, rather than percentages or percent changes, in any of the categories studied, conceals the fact that the numbers are very small in many cases. . . . Similarly, in attempting to measure changes in sexual behavior, the declines in enrollment and attendance as well as the need to exclude students who were already sexually active when the study began, greatly reduced the numbers available for observation. In addition, response errors are often as high as 40 percent on questionnaires regarding private behavior and experience.
>
> It must be concluded therefore that the Baltimore study has failed to demonstrate that birth control clinics in schools reduce sex activity or pregnancy. 405

A second in-depth analysis was done by Dr. Demsko in "School-Based Health Clinics: An Analysis of the Johns Hopkins Study" (The Family Research Council, Washington, D.C.):

1. Johns Hopkins researchers did not specifically state whether the study was cross-sectional or longitudinal. From the information available, it seems clear that the study was cross-sectional

because it utilized anonymous questionnaires at both the control and experimental schools . . . making it impossible, therefore, to track individual students over time. 219/5

2. Accordingly, the study did not control for student mobility (transfers, drop-outs, etc.) in and out of the control experimental schools. . . . The sample size of female students at the experimental school dropped more than 30 percent between the first and last measurements. This decline was approximately three times larger than the corresponding drop at the control schools. They did not explain why the decrease was so much larger (drop-out seems to be because of pregnancies)—especially among girls—at the experimental schools.

3. Since the students at the control school were measured on four different occasions, it is difficult to compare the questionnaire results from the experimental and control schools. Among other things, this discrepancy prevents one from knowing how great a role, if any, a "testing" effect played in influencing student questionnaire responses.

4. The study contains no raw figures or percentages for a number of standard demographic variables such as marital status, academic achievement, or family characteristics. Thus, there is little for one to work with in assessing the initial comparability of the experimental and control school populations, and there is no information to aid an assessment of the change in demographic characteristics over time. Since such factors could affect pregnancy rates, this omission makes it impossible to verify the researchers' assertion that school-based clinics were responsible for the reported decline in pregnancy rates at the experimental schools.

5. The experimental senior high school served as a magnet school which attracted some highly motivated young people. . . . Research has shown that students motivated by academic achievement are more inclined to develop the behaviors necessary to delay pregnancy.

6. Another discrepancy between the two groups of students concerns pregnancy rates prior to the implementation of the clinic program. According to the JHU researchers, the pregnancy rate at the senior high experimental school was "considerably lower" than that at the senior high control school. 219/6

Unfortunately, the Johns Hopkins researchers did not explore the possible reasons for this discrepancy nor did they account for its potential influence on their study's final outcome.

7. The absence of other information hinders critical review of the Johns Hopkins study even further. While the JHU researchers noted that three years after the start of the experimental program "92 percent of female students age 15 and older had attended a professional facility," 219/122 they did not distinguish between students who attended the clinic for family planning services and those who did not. 219/124 Moreover, the researchers apparently did not measure changes in the frequency of sexual activity—a factor which has a bearing on pregnancy rates even when contraception is used regularly.

The pregnancy percentage rate declined in the Baltimore study, but the actual pregnancy rate increased. Note that when the increase in the number of sexually active students is more than the increase in the number of pregnancies, the percentage of pregnancies appears as a decrease—but that is misleading.

♦ No Measurable Impact!

Faith placed in school-based health clinics to increase responsible contraception and reduce pregnancy is, for the most part, unfounded. The Muskegon, Michigan, area Planned Parenthood and the Muskegon Heights Public Schools Health Clinics reported that, in their programs, "There was no significant change in the pregnancy rate." 221/2

A study of ten cities in four states concluded:

> The comprehensive model assumes that timely interventions of health, educational, and social service agencies will help young women to make informed decisions about the resolution of their pregnancies (abortion, adoption or parenthood). . . . The scant evidence available on program effectiveness shows these to be optimistic goals. 222/77

Douglas Kirby is the former research director for the Center for Population Options which is committed to comprehensive sex education and school-based health clinics. In 1988 he released the results of their study on the effectiveness of school-based clinics:

> We have been engaged in a research project for several years on the impact of school-based clinics. . . . We find basically that **there is no measurable impact** upon the use of birth control, nor upon pregnancy rates or birth rates [emphasis mine]. 223

In light of failures like those above and others, Dr. Kasun asks:

> Does sex instruction in classrooms and school clinics have no effect at all? . . . There has been a measurable impact, but not a positive one. For one thing, the researchers (other than Kirby) have consistently concluded that sex education leads to increased use of contraceptives, even though this effect is offset, or more than offset, by the increase in sex activity. This

increased demand is good for the contraceptive business and may help to explain why the pharmaceutical industry has supported the drive for sex education and school clinics. 201/497-8

I personally believe that comprehensive sex education, school-based health clinics and the promotion of contraceptives will eventually become counterproductive to the teen sex dilemma because they will not reduce teen pregnancy, abortion or sexual activity.

CHAPTER 9

Myth 3

"Comprehensive Sex Education Does Not Increase Teen Promiscuity"

Family planning groups insist that comprehensive sex education and easy access to contraceptives does not encourage an increase in teenage sexual promiscuity. That's a myth. Numerous studies show that family planning endeavors do encourage both sexually active and inactive teens toward increased promiscuity.

♦ Classes Provoke Sexual Activity

Planned Parenthood's own study, conducted by Lou Harris and Associates, clearly shows that "comprehensive sex education programs significantly increase the percentage of teens becoming sexually active, while limited sex education, and especially those with no sex education classes, discourage kids from becoming sexually active." According to the Harris study of teenagers who have had sexual intercourse, 46 percent had comprehensive sex education and 42 percent had no sex education. 138/53

Planned Parenthood's journal, *Family Planning Perspectives,* reports the findings of researchers Marsiglio and Mott in their study,

"The Impact of Sex Education on Sexual Activity, Contraceptive Use and Premarital Pregnancy Among American Teenagers":

> These models suggest that, even when factors that might be associated with both the likelihood of taking a course and the outcome variables are controlled, prior exposure to a sex education course is positively and significantly associated with the initiation of sexual activity at ages 15 and 16. 140/151-60

The National Research Council, in a report titled, "Risking the Future," points out that the increased rate of sexual activity in teens "is directly related to birth control information and provision to adolescents." 186/165 Sociologist Philip Cutright of Indiana University adds that in the sex education programs he studied "venereal disease is actually found to increase. . . . The reason for negative results is that the programs stimulate much higher rates of sexual activity." 187

In Planned Parenthood's *Family Planning Perspectives,* Dr. Deborah Anne Dawson, a survey research consultant, concluded: **"Prior contraceptive education increases the odds of starting intercourse [at the age of 14] by a factor of 1.5."** 141/166, 168-9 A factor of 1.5 might not seem like much, but in actuality it is a staggering 50-percent increase!

Lou Harris and Associates conducted a poll for PPFA titled, "The Relationship Between Sexual Activity and Sex Education: Analysis of the Results of the 1986 Harris Survey." (Study 864012) The study, as analyzed by Dr. Jacqueline Kasun, showed:

> Young people aged 12 to 17 who had had sex education had higher rates of sex activity than their peers without sex education. . . . These figures showed that 64 percent of 17-year-olds who had had "comprehensive" sex education (i.e., including information about contraception) had had intercourse. The rate was higher than the corresponding percentage for the group that had no sex education (57 percent) and also higher than the percentage for the group that had some but not "comprehensive" sex education (51 percent). 201/494

But the Harris group went on to claim that the higher level of sexual activity associated with sex education in their study is the result of age differences. Dr. Kasun argues that

> differences in age affect all of their results—that is, older youngsters have a higher probability of having had sex education, and they have a higher probability of engaging in sex as well as a higher probability of using contraceptives. The age factor did not deter Harris from concluding that sex education increases the use of contraceptives, but the agency cried foul when the equally obvious tendency to increase sex activity was pointed out. 201/495

Dr. Kasun continues:

> A problem with the Harris survey was that it apparently did not determine whether respondents had received sex education before or after initiating sex activity. The poll showed, however, that 75 percent of young people who receive sex education do so before the end of eighth grade, but only 30 percent of those who are sexually active initiate sex before age 14. This suggests that the majority of sexually active youngsters have received prior sex education. [Dr. Deborah Anne] Dawson estimated that 57-65 percent of all teenagers receive formal contraceptive education before they first have intercourse. 201/494

It's no wonder that Trish Knightly, Planned Parenthood's National Director of Education, confessed to Nancy Firor of the *Cincinnati Enquirer* in a telephone interview that PPFA's Harris Poll "has been very much of an Achilles' heel for us." 314 /E1-E2

♦ Contraceptives Provoke Sexual Activity

The claim that the availability of contraceptives does not affect teenagers' involvement in promiscuity is also a myth. Dr. Robert Kistner of the Harvard Medical School, one of the developers of the pill, admitted to the American College of Surgeons in 1977, **"About ten years ago I declared that the pill would not lead to promiscuity. Well, I was wrong."** 182 Dr. Kistner's confession was confirmed by another developer of the pill, Dr. Min Chueh Chang: "It's made them more permissive." 183/A16 (Cf. 109.)

Dr. Reichelt, studying teenage clinic patients in Detroit, discovered: "After issuing oral contraceptives there was a 50-percent increase in sexual activity after one year. Having intercourse went from 4.3 times a month before visiting the clinic to 6.8 times afterward." 184/57

A random survey of 400 family physicians and psychiatrists has shown that "81 percent believed there was an increase of sexual involvement among teenagers due to increased availability of contraceptives." 188/147 The following bar graph reflects the results of the inquiry:

Has increased availability of contraceptives led to increased sexual activity among teenagers?

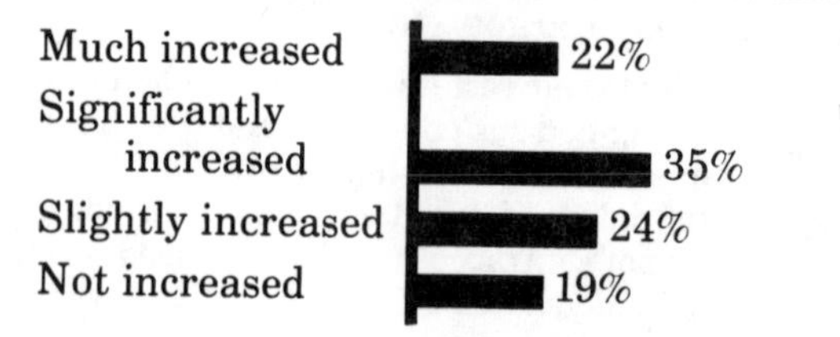

Dr. S. DuBose Ravenal, a pediatrician, admits in the *North Carolina Medical Journal* that he is "very concerned about the increased teenage sexual activity following the providing of contraceptives." 189/606 His concern is well-founded in light of the frightening parallel increase in pregnancies, abortions and sexually transmitted diseases in sexually active teenagers.

Dr. Kasun warns: "Of the young people who have had 'comprehensive' sex education, 11 percent engage in sex without using contraceptives, thus risking disease or pregnancy. Of those without the instruction, the proportion is 9 percent. It is true, as the Harris staff says, that youngsters who have had sex education do use more contraceptives, but they also engage in more sex, and this is the stronger effect." 201/495

♦ Promiscuity Is Illegal

In most states, comprehensive sex education as it is now taught encourages sexual activity between minors, which is illegal. For that reason, the California State Senate mandates in its sex education guidelines that "course material and instruction shall advise pupils that it is unlawful for males of any age to have sexual relations with females under the age of 18 to whom they are not married, pursuant to Section 261.5 of the Penal Code." The State of California recognizes something that many sex educators don't: Kids must be protected from the dangers of promiscuity, not by wearing condoms, but by teaching them to abstain from illegal sexual activity.

♦ Sex: A Basic Survival Need?

I believe that the increase in sexual activity among teenagers is due in part to the sex education premise that sex is a basic human survival need which must be satisfied. For example, the proposed eighth-grade sex education curriculum for Dickinson County Schools in Virginia specifies that "the primary factor to be presented is the development of one's own sexual identity and *the importance of satisfying basic needs* [emphasis mine]." (If you think the Dickinson County example is an isolated case, be aware that Virginia is only one of fifteen states targeted by Planned Parenthood for the implementation of Family Life Education curriculum.)

Calling sex a basic human need puts it in a category with food and water. That's like mixing apples with oranges. Strand a man and a woman in the desert without food and water, and I'll guarantee you that their survival need after five days will not be for sex. They won't be crawling across the sand in search of a condom-dispensing machine. Sex will be the farthest thought from their minds, even if they are both naked and have a copy of *Playboy* and a PPFA brochure on safe sex.

And after a few more days they will both be dead, but it won't be from lack of sex.

However, strand the same couple on a lush tropical island with all the food and water they need, and even if they never have sexual intercourse, they will survive indefinitely. Sex educators seem to infer that this couple will die if they don't satisfy their "need" for sex. Sex may be a strong drive, but it's not a basic survival need. We can't live without food and water, but we can live without sex.

Furthermore, what if the man feels the "need" for sex and the woman doesn't? If he buys into the idea that sex is a basic need which must be satisfied, he's not too far from justifying the rape of his not-so-needy companion. Similarly, if we convince our kids that sex is a need which must be satisfied, what will keep them from sexual abuse of others, date rape or more serious sex crimes?

Family planning advocates may object, "This is outrageous! Without birth control, this couple will 'be fruitful and multiply,' overpopulate the island and eventually die because they exhausted their supply of fresh water and food with so many mouths to feed. The same thing will happen to our country if we listen to these pro-abstinence, anti-family planning, anti-condom fanatics!"

Please note: **Advocates of pre-marital abstinence are not all against family planning within marriage, but they are against advocating and promoting contraceptives among teenagers.**

If a couple which is committed to a life-long monogamous relationship asks me what they should do about precautions against pregnancy, I would not say, as many school and family planners do with our kids, "Here's a flyer from the Norfolk, Virginia, Health Department on condoms. Study it carefully." Nor would I send them to a PPFA counselor for advice. Instead, I would encourage them to talk with their gynecologist. Ask him or her about the pros and cons of contraceptives—their risk rate and failure rate.

Contrary to what comprehensive sex education communicates, sex is not a need to be satisfied, but a desire to be controlled through abstinence until it can be properly and safely fulfilled within a monogamous marriage.

♦ Sexual Behavior: My Right?

There is another facet to the myth that sex education does not encourage teen sexual activity. Family planners believe that kids are autonomous and have the right to determine their own sexual behavior. For example, Dickinson County's proposed Family Life Education curriculum states: "The first step in learning to set limits for yourself is recognizing that *you have the right* to decide on the sexual behavior that is *best for you. The right is yours* . . . whether it means not having intercourse, or not wanting to hold hands, or even not wanting to discuss sexual matters, *only you can decide* what your sexual conduct will be" (emphasis mine). In their *Insider* magazine (May 1988), Planned Parenthood took much of the credit for seeing that FLE curriculum was implemented in Virginia.

I believe it's dangerous even to mention FLE's directive to kids, let alone make it mandatory for schools to teach it as Dickinson County suggested. Let's analyze the directive and you'll see why.

First, if our kids have the right to decide what's best for them, where did they get this right—from educators, the FLE authors, Planned Parenthood or the Virginia legislature? Is it an "inalienable right" guaranteed by the constitution? Is it a right granted by God, parents or the school board?

Second, if we have the right to decide what's best for us, what about everybody else? Do we ever think about them and their rights? It's obvious that sex is a social act involving two or more people. Does our right to this social act condone rape, date rape, sex abuse, incest or lying to a partner about sexually transmitted diseases in order to do what we feel is best for us or to satisfy our needs? Try talking about rights with a victim of one of these crimes.

Third, when we say, "Only you can decide," what are we saying about responsibility to parents, society, government, school, church and God? Do we offer kids the same right to decide what's best for them concerning drugs, alcohol, cheating, stealing, murder, etc.? At what age does this inalienable right to decide about sexual behavior begin—10, 12, 13, 15, 17?

These questions scare the living daylights out of me as a concerned parent of four children. I don't want my children dating someone who has been indoctrinated with the right to decide his or her own sexual conduct. Can you imagine your child marrying someone who has been conditioned to do what's best for him or her? What a heartbreak! If you don't believe me, ask a woman whose husband raped her, sexually abused her or coerced her into committing distasteful sex acts in the name of what was right for him. Ask a mother whose eight-year-old girl was sexually molested by her father because he had the right to decide what was best for him.

Apply this approach to a rape case at the university where I recently spoke. According to the female student (I'll use the name Cindy), a male student (we'll call him Tom) raped her in his fraternity house. Cindy brought charges against Tom. According to the campus newspaper interview, Tom's defense was, "Cindy wanted it just as much as I did." Whether she wanted sex as much as he did is not the issue; *Cindy did not want it from Tom!* Then Tom had the audacity to say, "I can't believe she didn't appreciate what I was doing"!

Imagine that Tom was a product of the Virginia sex education program cited above. Could he base his legal defense on the fact that he was taught–in a mandatory sex education class in a public school funded by taxpayers' money–to meet his sexual needs in a way that was right for him? "I not only had to memorize the material," Tom argues from the witness stand, "I was also tested on it. If I had not agreed with the teacher, I would have been penalized in my final grade for the class. And I needed an *A* to graduate and get into college. So I learned it."

Imagine also that Tom had been exposed to other sources which promoted the values of comprehensive sex education:

- As a 15-year-old he got a book from Planned Parenthood, written by Dr. Pomeroy, which informed him that there were many benefits to premarital sex.
- He read the Human Manifesto II which assured him that he had the right to determine his sexual conduct.
- He attended a seminar given by a comprehensive sex educator who warned him not to listen to his parents.

In his closing argument, Tom says, "I was taught the benefits of premarital sex, so I decided to share those benefits with Cindy. I was also taught to meet my sexual needs in a way that was best for me. I enjoy sex more when it is forced. When a girl resists, it turns me on. Cindy decided not to have sex with me, but my sex education taught me my decision was more important. And I decided to have sex with her. Besides, almost every time a girl says no on TV she really means yes. Why am I being punished for doing what I was taught to do?"

Now imagine that you're the jury. Would you have difficulty bringing a verdict of guilty against Tom for acting out in society the very values society inculcated in him?

This example is fictitious and extreme, but the comprehensive sex education curriculum cited and the values it teaches are fact. Teens exposed to these programs are becoming sexually active at an alarming rate. Perhaps only a fraction of them will become rapists, date rapists, sexual abusers, etc. Still, the grief other promiscuous teens will bring to themselves and others through unwanted pregnancies, abortions and STDs which accompany their sexual "rights" is horrendous.

This section can best be summed up by the comments of Dr. W. R. Coulson, one of the co-founders of values clarification: **"We know that after [sex education] classes, students become more prone to give in to temptation than if they'd never enrolled."** 39/21

Comprehensive sex education **does** increase teen promiscuity.

CHAPTER 10

Myth 4

"Comprehensive Sex Education Reduces Teen Pregnancies"

Family planners have contended for years that comprehensive sex education, including easy access to contraceptives and free abortions, will solve the problem of teen pregnancy in this country. This myth is the heartbeat of Planned Parenthood and of advocates for school-based clinics. It is their major thrust for raising funds, implementing curriculum and pacifying concerned parents and legislators.

As you shall see, though, the evidence shows this belief to be nothing more than a fantasy. In fact, just the opposite is true. Numerous studies reveal that family planning methods and comprehensive sex education produce a dramatic *increase* in teenage pregnancy.

♦ Discerning an Important Difference

There is a significant difference between the pregnancy rate of teen girls and the birth rate. The birth rate of pregnant teenage girls in 1982 was only 47 percent. The chart on the next page reveals the pregnancy rates, abortion rates, miscarriage rates and birth rates for women aged 15-19 over a ten-year span. Though the pregnancy rate skyrocketed from the 1960s to the 1970s, the rate has increased only slightly since the early 1970s. Notice that the abortion rate represents a real "epidemic" among teenagers, which accounts for a gradual decline in the birth rate for teenagers over the past decade. 111

Adolescent Pregnancy Rate and Outcomes, 1970–1982

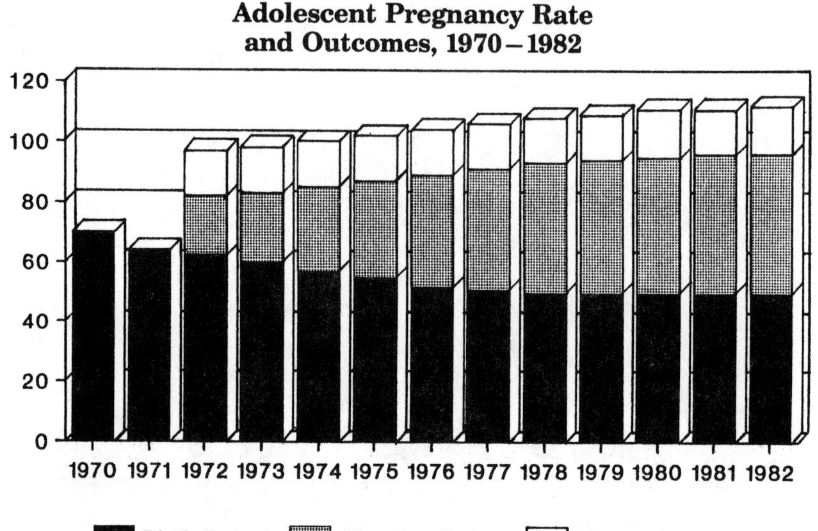

The House Select Committee on Children, Youth, and Families warns policymakers to be cautious when hearing the phrases "pregnancy rate" and "birth rate" used interchangeably. As the Committee points out, "Many groups cite high 'pregnancy rates' when describing the need for implementation of certain family planning programs, but when showing the effectiveness of the proposals, the groups frequently cite a decrease in 'birth rates,' leading the public to believe that family planning, rather than abortion, has reduced the problem of teenage births." 109/2

The above observations are not made to indicate a lessening of the seriousness of the teenage sexual situation but rather to get public officials and educators to see the real crux of the problem. Perhaps this will help all of us make decisions affecting our kids based upon fact and not media hype. Greater attention needs to be given to the causes of teenagers becoming sexually active. Remember the axiom: A problem well defined is a problem half solved.

♦ Curbing Births, Not Pregnancies

Drs. Joseph A. Olsen and Stan E. Weed are researchers with the non-profit Institute for Research and Evaluation. Their study, "Effects of Family-Planning Programs for Teenagers on Adolescent Birth and

Pregnancy Rates" was completed under a contract with the Brigham Young University Law School as part of an ongoing research project dealing with legal, social and public policy issues concerning children, youth and families. The study was reported in the *Family Perspective Journal* (which is not PPFA's journal). 145/152-170

Olsen and Weed concluded,

> A reduction in teenage fertility [births] due to greater adolescent participation in family planning programs similar to that reported by a number of other researchers has been replicated and confirmed. Although the lower fertility may be due to easier access to abortion, the findings of our study and other studies indicate quite clearly that greater teenage involvement in family planning leads to decreased childbearing among adolescents. 145/167

However, they discovered something other studies had overlooked or hidden: Although births to teens decreased, pregnancies increased.

> Greater teenage involvement in family planning programs appears to be associated with higher, rather than lower, teenage pregnancy rates. The observed effect is dramatically different from one hypothesized on the basis of the expected reduction in adolescent pregnancies due to improvements in contraceptive practice among teenagers attending organized family planning clinics. 145/167

In a *Wall Street Journal* interview, "Curbing Births, Not Pregnancies," Dr. Weed related that their interest in the research "was prompted by the rising trends in teenage pregnancy rates, despite large federal expenditures to help fund family planning clinics and extend contraceptive services to teenagers." Weed's findings are summarized in the following charts: 146

	1971	1981
National expenditure for clinics (in millions of dollars)	$ 11	$442
Number of teenage clients	300,000	1,500,000

	1972	1981
Pregnancy rate for 15-19-year-olds (per thousand)	95	113
Teenage abortions	180,000	430,000

Noting that the overall size of the teen population was unchanged over the ten-year period, Weed concluded:

> One must reconcile the rise in teen pregnancies with major program efforts that saw a five-fold increase in teenage clients and a twenty-fold constant-dollar increase in funding. . . . As the number and proportion of

teenage family planning clients increased, we observed a corresponding increase in the teenage pregnancy and abortion rates: 50 to 120 more pregnancies per thousand clients, rather than the 200 to 300 fewer pregnancies as estimated by researchers at the Alan Guttmacher Institute (formerly the research arm of the Planned Parenthood Federation). We did find that greater teenage participation in such clinics led to lower teen birthrates. However, the impact on the abortion and total pregnancy rates was exactly opposite the stated intentions of the program. The original problems appear to have grown worse. 146

Weed and Olsen conducted a second study to double-check the findings of the first. The second study's conclusions

were very similar to those from the first study: lower teenage birth rates, higher abortion rates, no reduction in teenage pregnancy rates. . . . *Apparently the programs are more effective at convincing teens to avoid birth than to avoid pregnancy.* Birth avoidance can certainly be accomplished by resorting to abortion. Unfortunately, that is not what the effort was set up to do nor the basis on which it was funded [emphasis mine]. 146

The following graph illustrates the findings of Weed and Olsen's second study. The clear bars depict the projected reductions (1981) of teenage births, abortions and pregnancies based on implementation of family planning programs. This projected reduction was a major reason the federal government and many state legislators decided to fund family planning. The black bars are the observed effects by Weed and Olsen five years later (1986). 146 and 196

Impact of Teenage Family Planning Programs Projected Versus Observed Changes in Births, Abortions and Total Pregnancies (per 1,000 teen clients, 1980)

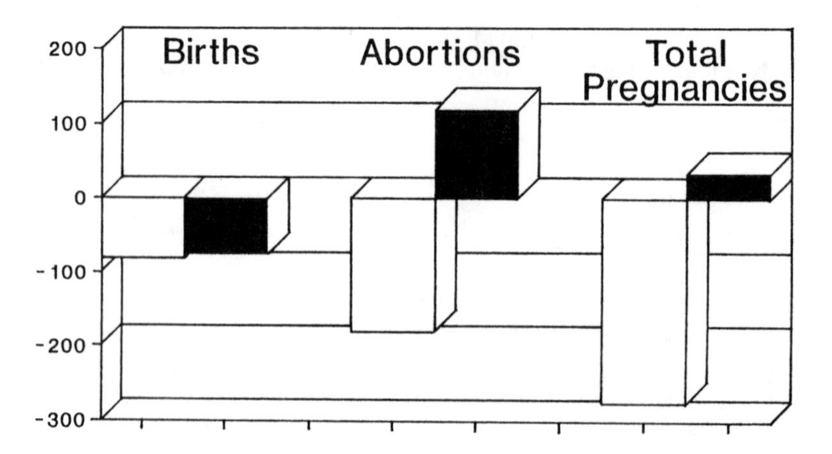

- These statistics represent the remaining effects after accounting for race, poverty, urbanization and residential stability.
- Total pregnancy includes miscarriages, which are estimated to be 20 percent of births and 10 percent of abortions. 406, 146 and 196

A similar study by Weed and Olsen concluded:

> A regression analysis of interstate variation in 1978 birth and pregnancy rates shows about thirty fewer births to adolescents for every 1,000 teenage clients served by organized family planning programs, an effect similar to that reported in a number of previous studies. However, instead of the expected reduction in teenage pregnancies, greater adolescent involvement in family planning programs was associated with significantly higher teenage pregnancy rates. 196/153

It is too late to reverse these heartbreaking results of so-called family planning. However, we can learn from past mistakes not to duplicate the shortsighted errors of others. For our kids' sake and for the future of our families and country, I hope we have learned a lesson.

♦ Contraceptives and Pregnancy

If comprehensive sex education and easy availability of contraceptives really solved the problem of teenage pregnancy, you would anticipate a correlation between contraceptive availability and decrease in pregnancies. However, even studies reported in Planned Parenthood's *Family Planning Perspectives* demonstrate that the exact opposite is true. The following chart illustrates the point: 153 (Also cited in 190.)

Contraceptive Use and Pregnancy

	1976	1979	Increase
Premaritally sexually active women			
Aged 15-19 who always used contraceptives	28.7%	34.2%	19.2%
Pregnancy rate among always users	9.9%	13.5%	36.4%

In their drive for federal, state and local funds, family planning proponents plead that comprehensive sex education, especially the use of contraceptives by teens, will produce a dramatic reduction in teenage pregnancy. They would like every teenage girl in America to carry condoms in her purse and use them to prevent pregnancy "just in case" she decides to have sex. But here are the facts:

- There are 10 million teenage girls in the United States. Last year one million pregnancies were reported in that group. A million pregnant teenagers is totally unacceptable to family planning proponents. They want to provide comprehensive sex education, including free condoms, to these 10 million girls.

- Comprehensive sex education and easy access to contraceptives does not discourage sexual activity, it encourages it. Giving free condoms to 10 million teenage girls will encourage sexual activity in 10 million teenage girls.
- The documented failure rate of condoms used by teenage girls to prevent pregnancy, confirmed by Planned Parenthood, is 18.4 percent. 122/204 (See also 239/H121,122.)
- Therefore, if all 10 million teenage girls became sexually active, and every one of them used condoms, the result would be 1.8 million pregnant teenagers. In other words, if family planning adherents were given all the money they wanted to implement their program, and every teenage girl was given free condoms, there would be a positive net increase of 800,000 pregnant teenagers.

If one million pregnant teenagers is totally unacceptable to family planners, how much more unacceptable is 1.8 million pregnancies? Yet family planning groups continue to seek funding for comprehensive sex education to "reduce" pregnancies!

An excellent case in point is the state of Virginia. Statistics show that in every school district which taught comprehensive sex education–with only one exception–the number of teen pregnancies went up. The average increase was 17.3 percent, but in some districts the increase was as high as 50 percent. At the same time, in the school districts that were *not* teaching comprehensive sex education, all but one had a decrease in pregnancies (all school districts were selected at random). The average decrease was 15.8 percent, with some decreases reaching 42 percent! (For a comprehensive look at Virginia's Family Life Education program, see chapter 20–Part Four, Resource #1.)

♦ Contraceptive Failure in Teens

> The reality of contraceptive failure lies mainly in the lack of reliability in practice. For example, three of five married couples contracepting will have unplanned pregnancies over a five-year period. Adolescents will have four to five times that failure rate. Why the contraceptive failure? [Because] adolescents are typically risk-taking, and impulsive. They deny reality. In the final analysis, increased sexual activity with contraceptive failure results in an increase of illegitimate pregnancies. 148/1

As you consider your approach to teenage sexual behavior, consider that "even among teens who use oral contraceptives regularly and follow the ideal pattern prescribed by Planned Parenthood, the pregnancy rate is 5.8 percent." 149 "Planned Parenthood has been aware of the high failure rate for teens since the early 1970s. In *Family Planning Perspectives,* Norman Ryder published a study showing that the ineffectiveness rate for young women using oral contraceptives was four to five times that for older women." 150 In light of the high failure rate, why does Planned Parenthood insist that their programs are effective?

In 1980, Planned Parenthood's own journal admitted that teenage contraception was not stemming the increasing tide of pregnancies: **"More teenagers are using contraceptives and using them more consistently than ever before. Yet the number and rate of premarital pregnancies continues to rise."** 154/229

There are several ethical issues associated with contraception endorsement for teenagers. For example, Dr. James Ford, M.D., says, "It is dangerously misleading to tell a girl that she won't get pregnant if she takes the pill." 151 The Human Life Center adds, "It is perhaps one of the cruelest myths to lead children to believe that pregnancy cannot occur if contraception is used." 152

♦ Ineffectiveness of Family Planning Programs

What about the recently established school-based health clinics which freely dispense contraceptives to teens? Have they been effective in reducing teen pregnancies?

Between 1970 and 1975 the number of teenagers nationally involved in organized family planning programs quadrupled. In that same period abortion became legal and widely available to teenagers, and instruction in the use of contraceptives became part of the sex education curriculum through much of the country. Did these factors, as claimed, reduce teen pregnancies during this period? No. According to the findings of Kantner and Zelnick, premarital pregnancy during that period increased 45 percent. Premarital intercourse increased 41 percent. In their study on sexual activity of teenagers, Kantner and Zelnick found that the pregnancy rates for sexually active females between the ages of 15 and 19 actually increased when their sexual activity increased—even when contraceptives were used regularly. 153

Susan Roylance compared fifteen states with similar social demographics and rates of teenage pregnancy in 1970. Testifying before the U.S. Senate Committee on Labor and Human Resources (March 31, 1981), she reported that **states with the highest rate of governmental expenditures on birth control also had the greatest increases in abortion and illegitimate births between 1970 and 1979.** 190

After carefully reviewing the sex education programs which were initiated in California public schools in the 1960s, Dr. Jacqueline Kasun, wrote:

> California has provided and promoted sex education at all grade levels; it has sent pregnancy counselors into schools and has provided and promoted contraceptives and abortions to teenagers at public expense without parental knowledge. In the process, California has consistently spent twice as much as the national average on government-funded birth control. And what are the results? By 1981 California's teenage pregnancy rate rose to a level 30 percent above the national level, and the teenage abortion rate more than tripled. . . . After years of extremely high expenditures and effort in this area, we have the highest rate of teen pregnancy in the entire nation . . . and the highest rate of teen abortion. 176

Dr. Kasun wrote to me personally about an even greater failure in her own community:

> *In Humboldt County, where we have several "model" programs and government family planning, expenditures per person have been much higher than in the nation, and adolescent pregnancy has increased ten times as much as in the nation. The reason this increase in pregnancy has not resulted in an increase in births is that Humboldt County has had a greater than 1,000-percent increase in teenage abortions during the past decade, more than fifteen times the rest of the nation.*

Dr. Kasun found that

> states which spend most heavily to provide free contraceptives and abortions have the highest rates of premarital teenage pregnancy. The rate of premarital teenage pregnancy is more than twice as high in California as in Idaho or South Dakota; and California spends more than four times as much per capita as the other two states on free birth control. *The notion that teenagers can be deterred from becoming pregnant by more and easier access to contraceptives and abortions is like expecting people who are given free gasoline to reduce their driving* [emphasis mine]. 134

Here are a number of other reports from authorities in the field which clearly show the ineffectiveness of comprehensive sex education to reduce teen pregnancies:

- Richard Weatherby, *Family Planning Perspectives* (PPFA): "Comprehensive programs . . . are not the magic bullet that will solve the problems associated with unintended teenage pregnancy and parenthood. Nor should they be expected to do so." 157/77
- Deborah Ann Dawson: "Prior contraceptive education increases the odds of starting intercourse at [the age of] 14 . . . by 50 percent." 141
- Senate subcommittee report: "With more than 5,000 'family planning clinics' operating in the United States, many of them with the help of federal funds, and sex education courses in many public schools, it is

clear that contraceptive information alone is not the solution to the unwanted consequences of sexual activity." 158

- Congressional budget office report: "Since Title X federal funding for family planning programs began in 1971, the number of teenage girls in subsidized birth control programs increased 397 percent; who used contraceptives but became pregnant increased 266 percent; who had abortions increased 107 percent; who contracted an STD increased 93 percent." 168/1
- Sociologist Dr. Phillips Cutright, Indiana University: "We find no evidence that the programs reduced . . . illegitimacy, because areas with weak programs or no programs at all experience smaller increases or larger declines (in pregnancy) than are found in areas with strong contraceptive programs." 169
- Dr. James W. Stout, Children's Hospital of Seattle: "Five studies conducted from 1980 to 1987 examined the effect of classroom sex education programs at the junior and senior high school level on teenagers from a variety of geographical areas and racial and socioeconomic groups. The researchers said: 'The programs had no discernible impact on pregnancy rates, a negligible effect on using birth control methods and insignificant influence on teenagers' decisions about when to engage the first time in sexual intercourse.' " 311
- Drs. James Stout and Frederick P. Rivara in the medical journal *Pediatrics*: "Our findings indicate that the expectations of altered adolescent sexual activity, contraceptive behavior and pregnancy are unlikely to be fulfilled by these [school-based sex education] programs, and we suggest that the effort to fight for sex education on these terms is not justified unless an effect is shown in further studies. To place the burden of counteracting the prevailing forces in our society toward premarital sex on our schools alone is both naive and inappropriate." 311/375-79
- Former Secretary of Education William Bennett: "There is no evidence that making contraceptive methods more available is the surest strategy for preventing pregnancy—to say nothing of preventing sexual activity. . . . Seventy percent of all high school seniors have taken sex education courses in 1985, up from 60 percent in 1976. Yet when we look at what is happening in the sexual lives of American students, we can only conclude that it is doubtful that much sex education is doing any good at all." 37
- Dr. Larry Cuban, professor of education, Stanford University: "Decade after decade . . . statistics have demonstrated the ineffectiveness of such courses in reducing sexual activity [and] teenage pregnancy. In the arsenal of weapons to combat teenage pregnancy, school-based programs are but a bent arrow. However, bent arrows do offer the illusion of action." 37

- Hansen, Myers and Ginsburg report in the *Journal of Marriage and Family* that their "findings suggest that knowledge as measured by birth control knowledge and sex education courses is not successful in reducing the chance of out-of-wedlock childbearing. . . . These findings have important implications for programs and policies addressing teenage pregnancy and childbearing. Although sex education is often promoted as a way to reduce the incidence of early pregnancy, our results suggest that simply requiring more students to take more sex education as it is currently provided is not the answer." 667/241-56

♦ Confessions of Planned Parenthood

Even Planned Parenthood admits that school-based sex education programs are not reducing pregnancies as had been hoped. In her article, "The Effects of Sex Education on Adolescent Intercourse, Contraception and Pregnancy in the United States" in *Family Planning Perspectives,* Dr. Deborah Ann Dawson says:

> *Nearly one-third of premaritally sexually active adolescents have had at least one premarital pregnancy.* The NSFG [National Survey of Family Growth] data reveal no significant relationship between exposure to sex education and the risk of premarital pregnancy among sexually active teenagers. . . . The final result to emerge from the analysis is that *neither pregnancy education nor contraceptive education exerts any significant effect on the risk of premarital pregnancy among sexually active teenagers*—a finding that calls into question the argument that formal sex education is an effective tool for reducing adolescent pregnancy [emphasis mine]. 141/168-9

Dr. Dawson was forced to admit that "the existing data do not yet constitute consistent, compelling evidence that sex education programs are effective in increasing teenage contraceptive use and reducing adolescent pregnancy." 141/162-63,168-69

In his commentary following a number of articles showing the failure of sex education to produce any significant effect on premarital pregnancy, L. D. Muroskin declared in Planned Parenthood's journal: "It is [increasingly usual] to hear that adolescent pregnancy is due to a lack of information or to faulty information about reproduction and contraception." 173/171

♦ Sex Education Abroad

Family planners would have us believe that "teenage pregnancy will be reduced if teenagers have easier access to contraceptives and better education on responsible sexual behavior and the proper use of birth control." 6/3 According to the Alan Guttmacher Institute, there is a basis for this assumption. In a study comparing the sexual behavior of teens in selected European countries with teens in America, the institute found that every year 86 of every 1,000 girls aged 15 to 19 in the United States become pregnant. This rate is nearly double that of Great Britain and France, and more than double that of Sweden.

The United States also leads in the rates of both teenage births and abortions. Six percent of American teens have had at least one abortion by the time they reach age 18. This is about twice the rate in Sweden and France. 159/90

The reasons for lower European teen pregnancy rates, according to this study, are intensive sex education and readily available contraceptives. The institute concludes that "it is likely that the United States has the lowest level of contraceptive practice among teenagers of all five countries." 159/90

However, the Guttmacher study omits certain contradictory data, including a report by the government of Denmark revealing that since compulsory sex education was adopted in Denmark in 1970, abortion rates doubled, illegitimate births nearly doubled and sexually transmitted disease rates more than doubled.

Another serious omission in the Guttmacher study is the sobering report on teenage sex in Sweden, a society in which sex education is universal and obsessively thorough, a country in which youngsters are literally bombarded with instruction in contraceptive use. Contraception is illustrated on television programs. Posters and street corner contraceptive vending machines abound. There is no question in any girl's mind as to where to go to be fitted with an IUD or to obtain the pill. And she has been taught that it is in very good taste to have condoms on hand to present to her sexual partners. 57/9

Roland Huntford, a Scandinavian correspondent for the *London Observer,* in his book *The New Totalitarians,* reports about how sexual liberation is affecting Swedish children:

> The new permissiveness has led to compulsive sexuality. There is among Swedish school children a pressure to have sexual intercourse, whether they want it or not. Even if a boy and a girl might prefer a platonic relationship, they will nevertheless usually force themselves into a sexual one. 408/332

A closer look at the data reveals that Sweden is anything but a sexual paradise. Huntford continues:

> License to copulate has led to a sexual obsession pervading the whole Swedish life. It has brought in its train a certain amount of mental illness. This is a subject on which the authorities are silent, and the organizers of sexual instruction prone to concealment. Nevertheless, it seems to have been established that much of expanding neuroses among school children and students is to be attributed to failure in the sexual rat race. Nervous breakdowns on this account are not uncommon. 408/339

Perhaps this problem is related to the suicide rate among Sweden's teenagers, which is the highest in the world–three times higher than the epidemic rate in our own country. 160/8 A common reason for teen suicide in the United States is pregnancy. As I examine the figures it seems clear that pregnancy prevention in most European countries has been costly in terms of abortion, sexually transmitted disease and suicide. Compulsory sex education and easy access to contraceptives has not been as beneficial to European teens as the Guttmacher study claims.

The foreign editor of *Look* magazine wrote an article on Sweden's battle over sex after ten years of compulsory sex education. He stated: "The rising incidence of venereal disease in Sweden over the past years, despite the virtual absence of prostitution, the presence of sex education and the easy availability of contraceptives that would prevent most cases of gonorrhea, baffles the experts." 161/3-8

Dr. Rhoda Lorand, psychotherapist and diplomate in clinical psychology of the American Board of Professional Psychology, provides greater detail:

> A comparison of the United States and Swedish graphs of the incidence of VD shows a steady upward climb in Sweden, beginning in 1954, the year sex education became compulsory there. . . . By 1964, after ten years of compulsory coed sex education and easy access to condoms (in accordance with the philosophy that children have the right to have intercourse), the increase in the incidence of VD and illegitimacy among youth had created alarm. A petition was signed by 200,000 people in support of an appeal to the Minister of Education, sent by 140 physicians, deploring the obsession with sex exhibited by the young people, declaring that the children misunderstood instruction in sexual matters for encouragement to practice. 57/7,8

Swedish authorities admitted to being baffled and discouraged:

> Despite all our efforts to educate the young people through lectures, brochures and other means, they just don't seem to care. They have a blind faith in penicillin and many of them even think it's "tough" to take a risk by deliberately refraining from using condoms or by carelessly selecting their sexual partners. 162

Comprehensive sex education isn't working in Sweden. We are in danger of replicating their mistakes if we don't abolish the myth about sex education and teen sexual activity.

♦ False Premises, False Results

Why have family planning, school-based clinics and comprehensive sex education curriculums failed in the United States as they have in Sweden? **We ended up with the wrong results because we started with the wrong premises.**

Wrong premise: Sex education reduces pregnancies.

Wrong results: Increased sexual activity, increased pregnancies, increased abortions.

Leon Dash, correspondent for the *Washington Post,* admits that he was misguided by the myth about teen sexuality:

> I had assumed that the problem of teenage pregnancy was one of youthful ignorance and male exploitation of vulnerable, emotionally needy girls. I was wrong on both counts. I found that teenage boys and girls as young as 11 knew as much about sex and birth control as I did. And, I found that the girls, far from being passive victims, were often equal—or greater—actors with their boyfriends in exploring their sexuality and desire to have a child. A child was a tangible achievement in otherwise dreary and empty lives. . . . Having a child is a rite of passage to adulthood for many boys and girls. In a world where few other goals can be obtained, it is a way of saying: I am a woman. I am a man. . . . I find it difficult to imagine—realistically—any government programs that will turn this situation around. 327/B1-B2

Dr. Stan Weed makes what I believe is an obvious but important conclusion:

> Awareness is growing that teen pregnancy is probably symptomatic of more fundamental factors in our society. There is also an increasing recognition that teenagers may be more impulsive, have a shorter time perspective and may be less likely to utilize adultlike decision-making processes. We can't expect teenagers to use birth control devices and seek counseling in the same manner as mature adults acting rationally about sexual intimacy. Even married adults are not always consistent and rational when it comes to something as volatile as sexuality. 146

♦ Right Assumptions, Right Results

What do we have to do to get the right kinds of results with our kids? We need to start with the right assumptions about sex education. Former Education Secretary Bennett says,

> Americans consistently say that they want our schools to provide reliable standards of right and wrong to guide students through life. In short, I think most Americans want to urge, not what might be the "comfortable" thing, but the right thing. Why are we so afraid to say what that is? 37

CHAPTER 11

Myth 5

"Comprehensive Sex Education Reduces Teen Abortions"

Many people believe that comprehensive sex education programs, school-based clinics and the ready availability of contraceptives help reduce the number of teenage abortions in our country. This idea is based on the assumption that the contraceptive practices promoted by family planning groups reduce pregnancies and thus decrease the need for abortions.

This is another sex education myth which is not supported by the facts. As we have already seen, the availability of contraceptives does not reduce teen pregnancies; it increases them. It is also true that the availability of contraceptives through sex education programs does not reduce teen abortions; it increases them. According to the Population Council Report, "Women who have practiced contraception are more likely to have abortions than those who have not, and those who have had abortions are more likely to be contraceptors than women without a history of abortion." 152

The Centers for Disease Control in Atlanta pointed out that close to 50 percent of the 15- to 19-year-old women who had abortions in 1976 were using contraception at the very time their pregnancy took place. Cited in 180 Dr. Dinah Richard, an educational consultant, reveals that, according to a study in the *Journal of Biosocial Science,*

> Repeat abortion seekers tend to have a better knowledge of contraception and tend to be more regular users of contraceptives than those seeking first abortions. The study notes further that the majority of repeat abortion

seekers perceive themselves as regular users of contraceptives and listed the pill and IUD as the predominant type of birth control used." 152

Pregnancies, births and abortions per 1,000 women, ages 15-19, United States, 1970–1980. 111

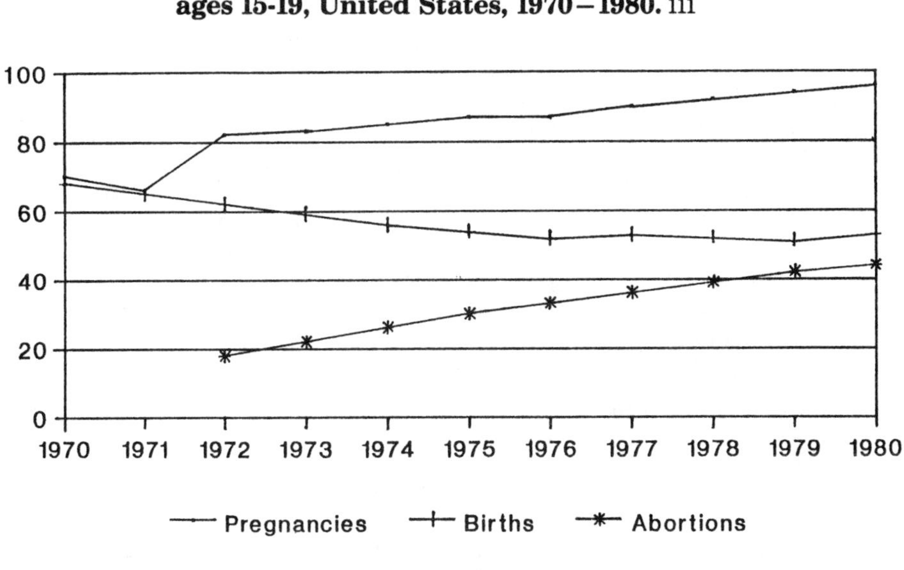

The above graph illustrates the dramatic increase in pregnancies (40 percent) and the alarming increase in abortions (123 percent) from 1970 to 1980. These increases are concurrent with the increase in numbers of comprehensive sex education programs and with the availability of contraceptives to teens. (See also the graph, "Impact of Teenage Family Planning Programs," and its explanation, in the previous chapter.)

During the 1970s, California instituted an eight-fold increase in family planning programs for teens. At that time the California abortion rate was equal to the national average. By 1984, with all the new programs operating and millions upon millions of dollars spent, the California abortion rate accelerated to 60 percent greater than the national average. 312

♦ Compounding the Problem

The Alan Guttmacher Institute, Planned Parenthood's researcher, projected a 180-percent reduction of teen abortions in response to comprehensive sex education programs and contraceptive availability. After five years, teen abortions had not decreased at all. Instead, they had increased 110 percent. 145 and 146 That's a 290-percent miscalculation–from minus 180 to plus 110! Yet, instead of admitting that its methods were not working to reduce pregnancies and abortions, the Planned Parenthood people insisted that the rising percentages simply meant more sex education was needed.

Planned Parenthood contends that the increase in abortions is not the result of the easy access to contraceptives. Faye Wattleton, president of PPFA, suggested in written testimony during the Title X hearings on March 31, 1981, that when contraceptive methods and practices are perfected, abortions will go down. She added, "It is well recognized by now that all contraceptive methods currently in use have serious drawbacks in their efficacy, safety and acceptability. . . . As a result, contraceptive use . . . is imperfect because of existing methods, and because human beings, too, are imperfect. Nevertheless, the inadequacy of contraceptive technology is reflected in distressingly high rates of recourse to abortion."

During those hearings Senator Dan Nickels asked Mrs. Wattleton if contraceptive failure was a key factor in the high rate of repeat abortions:

> *Nickels:* Do you have any statistics on the number of people who come in to have an abortion for the second time?
>
> *Wattleton:* I do not know what the statistics from our affiliates will be, but nationwide we are seeing a repeat rate of approximately 30 percent.
>
> *Nickels:* Does that say anything about your effectiveness as far as pregnancy prevention?
>
> *Wattleton:* It certainly says a great deal about our effectiveness in terms of pregnancy prevention technology that is available. . . . The (contraceptive) failures that we do see is (sic) a reflection of the shortcomings in technology. . . . Better technology would enable fewer to face an unwanted pregnancy. (P. 77 of hearings.)

The notion that better contraceptive training will reduce teenage abortion is false. The more comprehensive sex educators push contraception, the more teens will experiment with sex and terminate their unwanted pregnancies with abortions.

♦ Teen Pregnancy on the Decline

Comprehensive sex education is not the antidote to the teenage pregnancy and abortion issue. Dr. Jacqueline Kasun shows that "since 1970, pregnancy among American women 15 to 19 years of age has climbed by 32 percent (based on birth data from the National Center for Health Statistics and abortion estimates from the Alan Guttmacher Institute) although prior to that time it had been falling." 201/491

Dr. Kasun explains:

> The growing prevalence of abortion, more than doubling between 1972 and 1985, has prevented this rising rate of conceptions from resulting in a higher rate of births among women under 20. In 1986 there were 183,000 fewer births to women aged 15 to 19 than there had been in 1970 (National Center for Health Statistics). The rate of childbearing among United States teenagers fell from more than ninety per thousand in 1957 to about fifty in 1976; it has remained at this level, give or take a point or two, since then. Thus the growing prevalence of sex education has been accompanied by a marked rise in adolescent pregnancy, which had been falling, as well as by an explosive increase in abortions and a cessation of the previous decline in adolescent fertility. 201/491

♦ Seeing Abortion Clearly

Do we have a true picture of the enormity of the teenage abortion problem in our country? I don't think so. Our estimates are based on the numbers of abortions reported, but countless numbers of abortions go unreported! Even PPFA estimates that nearly two-thirds of teen abortions are never reported: "Respondents aged 15-19 are estimated to have *reported only 33 percent of the abortions they obtained in 1981* [emphasis mine]." 141/162-3,166

PPFA presented two studies (Marsiglio and Motts 140 and Deborah Anne Dawson 141) in *Family Planning Perspectives* concerning the effects of comprehensive sex education on the teenage pregnancy rate. Dr. Kasun points out that the authors of both studies admit their conclusions about contraceptives lowering the pregnancy rate are suspect because "they calculated pregnancies as the sum of live births plus abortions and the respondents to their surveys seriously understated the number of abortions they had had." Kasun explains, "The undercount amounted to 67 percent in one study, based on comparisons of the numbers reported by young people responding to the survey and national abortion data for their age group." 380 Kasun concluded, "Although young people who have had sex education clearly have an increased tendency to engage in premarital sex, the results of these studies do not indicate whether or not sex education affects the incidence of premarital pregnancy." 380

The obvious conclusion then, as PPFA admitted, is: "If failure to report pregnancies is associated with exposure to formal sex education—a question we cannot answer [or they don't want to answer!]—then our findings on the effects of sex education on pregnancy risk may be inaccurate." 141/166,168-69

I believe the sex education crisis in America is more serious than we admit because the abortion crisis is more staggering than we realize. It is estimated that there are 1.5 million abortions per year (4,000 a day), totaling more than 26 million unborn babies killed between 1973 and 1990. But where do these statistics come from? The activities of the abortion industry have gone largely unreported since 1973. Most states are not required to report abortions. All of our abortion statistics come from the Alan Guttmacher Institute, a source obviously biased in favor of Planned Parenthood.

According to Ken Freeman, the Alan Guttmacher Institute estimates abortion totals by extrapolating the reports of 800 clinics. Are these estimates correct, or is the problem much worse than we think? Remember, even PPFA admits that as many as two-thirds of teen abortions are never reported. I think the Guttmacher estimates fall far short of reality. Here's why.

An NBC special on the Roe versus Wade decision legalizing abortion reported that there are 4,000 abortion clinics in the United States. Are we to believe that each clinic averages only one abortion per day, totaling the current 4,000-per-day estimate?

Ken Freeman took an informal poll. He called several abortion clinics in Dallas to see how many women visit on an average day. The response? On a slow day, 10 to 20; on a busy day, 40 to 50. Not all these women come to have abortions, of course; some come for counseling.

Let's conservatively estimate that an average of 20 women visit each abortion clinic every day and that 10 of them receive abortions. That's not 4,000 abortions per day; that's *40,000* per day! Considering there are about 250 working days a year, that's 10 million unborn babies killed annually! One element which is not factored into the formula here is that some clinics may only be open two or three days a week. **We're not talking about 26 million lives snuffed out over seventeen years; we're talking about upwards of 170 million!** If these figures are anywhere close to being true, no wonder the abortionists don't want us to know exactly how many abortions are taking place.

Not only are family planning groups contributing to the skyrocketing abortion rate through comprehensive sex education, but they are also actively reaching out to counsel teenage girls to get abortions. Edward Brann, in an article for the Centers for Disease Control, explains how PPFA and health departments seek out pregnant girls for abortions:

> All involved a great deal of outreach. . . . The San Bernardino County Health Department employs four full-time social workers who conduct one-to-one, in-school follow-up counseling sessions with adolescent women who come to the health department for a pregnancy test. . . . Within one week . . . students are contacted at their school by what appears to classmates to be a routine call to the nurse or guidance personnel. Students are seen up to once a week in follow-up. The average is three to four visits

per student. . . . The rapid decline in fertility of teenagers in Hackensack and Bergen County is probably due . . . most of all, to readily accessible abortions. . . . Planned Parenthood . . . has an outreach department consisting of three full-time and three part-time employees." 215

The Alan Guttmacher Institute has had to confess, **"The decline in births is largely contingent on continued access to legal abortions." 367/5**

Using abortion as a birth control method is the height of decadence. I trust that you will carefully evaluate what type of sex education is introduced into our school system. If there is any chance that a program will encourage our kids to get abortions, I hope you will have the moral courage and convictions to say no to it.

CHAPTER 12

Myth 6

"Comprehensive Sex Education Will Succeed With Greater Funding"

Under the assumption that available contraceptives will reduce teenage pregnancy, the government has poured billions of dollars into family planning. Research shows that the total expenditure was in excess of $2 billion from 1971 to 1981.108/3 That amount does not include state or local expenditures.

All the experts and legislators sincerely believed the tremendous financial expenditures would decrease both teen pregnancies and teen abortions. However, the exact opposite is true. Although government spending increased by 306 percent during those years, teen pregnancy increased 48.3 percent, and teen abortions increased 133 percent. 176/6

♦ Spending and Failing

Dr. Jacqueline Kasun, author of *The War Against Population: The Economics and Ideology of Population Control* (Jameson Books) and "The State and Adolescent Sexual Behavior" in *The American Family and the State* (The Pacific Institute), has found that

> states that spend relatively large amounts on government birth control also tend to have high rates of teenage abortions-plus-unmarried births. For example, the rate of pregnancy in California is almost twice as high as the rates for North Dakota or Minnesota, and the level of per capita spending

on family planning in California is more than three times as high as in North Dakota and more than five times as high as in Utah. 176

According to her spring 1986 report, "Teenage Pregnancy: What Comparisons Among States and Countries Show," Dr. Kasun found that "four states led the rest in 1980 for (1) providing free access to publicly funded abortion, and (2) having spent higher than the national average amounts per person on publicly funded birth control. Those states are California, Hawaii, Georgia, and New York." 176 Table A below shows the teenage pregnancy and abortion-plus-unmarried birth rates for these four states. 176 and 409

Table A
Rates of Teenage Pregnancies and Abortion-Plus-Unmarried Births for States with FNCC

	Access to Birth Control		
State	Per Capita Public Expenditures on Birth Control as Percent of National Average, 1980	Teen Pregnancy Rate as Percent of National Average, 1981	Rate of Abortion-Plus-Unmarried Births to Teens as Percent of National Average, 1981
California	227%	133%	150%
Hawaii	170%	122%	134%
Georgia	142%	128%	131%
New York	111%	105%	135%

Dr. Kasun notes that all four states "provided free access to publicly funded abortion and also spent higher-than-national-average amounts per person on publicly funded birth control in 1980. *All four have higher-than-average pregnancy rates as well as higher-than-average rates of teenage abortions-plus-unmarried births* [emphasis mine]." 176

In contrast, Dr. Kasun says:

> Those states which spent the least on birth control and abortions tended to have the lowest rates of abortions-plus-unmarried births. Those states include Utah, South Dakota, Idaho, and North Dakota. . . . If history is any indication, **increasing public expenditures will not reduce the teenage pregnancy problem but rather increase it.** From 1971 to 1981 there has been a 306-percent increase in federal expenditure on family [planning] with a corresponding 48.3-percent increase in pregnancies and a 133-percent increase in abortions for women aged 15-19. 176

Table B tracks the ten-year history of rising federal expenditures for family planning and of concurrent increases in pregnancies and abortions: 407

Table B
Federal Expenditures on Family Planning:
Pregnancies, Births and Abortions Per 1,000 Women Aged 15-19
United States, 1970–1981

Year	Federal Expenditures on Family Planning ($ millions)	Births to Women 15-19	Pregnancies per 1,000 Women 15-19	Births per 1,000 Women 15-19	Abortions per 1,000 Women 15-19
1970	–	644,708	68.32	68.32	–
1971	80,000	628,000	64.66	64.66	–
1972	99,420	616,280	81.22	62.01	19.22
1973	137,280	604,096	82.61	59.69	22.91
1974	142,780	595,466	85.36	58.08	27.28
1975	148,220	582,238	87.77	56.28	31.49
1976	157,140	558,744	88.26	53.52	34.74
1977	184,620	559,154	91.87	53.69	38.19
1978	217,771	543,407	92.82	52.42	40.40
1979	233,031	549,472	94.7	52.3	42.4
1980	298,572	552,161	95.9	53.0	42.9
1981	324,977	527,392	N.A.	52.7	N.A.

The data clearly show that those states with higher per capita public expenditures on birth control have also experienced higher than average teenage pregnancy and abortion rates. One of the reasons for this correlation is that, as Dr. Kasun states, "Free birth control encourages sexual risk-taking and therefore a higher level of unintended pregnancy." 191

♦ A Foreign Comparison

Many family planning advocates such as PPFA point to the apparent success of sex education in selected other countries to validate their pleas for increased funding. But, as Dr. Kasun notes,

> In Europe, abortions are probably under-reported, because national health service physicians on government salary receive no extra income for extra procedures; there is a "shortage" of physicians in government practice, and government physicians remedy this "shortage" by providing medical services for a fee on a part-time basis; abortions, unreported to the government, which frowns on private practice, and available without bureaucratic formalities, appear to be one of these services. 176

Dr. Kasun has also compared various countries of northern Europe with those American states which "do not provide teenagers with free access to abortions and contraceptives, and spend lower-than-average amounts on government-funded birth control programs." As Table C illustrates, rates of abortions-plus-unmarried births in these American states are similar to the "low rates" reported for northern Europe. 176

Another factor which is seemingly overlooked by PPFA's Guttmacher study is the difference between birth control which is "readily available" in Europe and that which is free or government-supplied in the United States. Many American states provide free contraceptives and abortions to teens while many European countries—including Canada, England, France and Sweden—do not. As Dr. Kasun notes, *"There is a direct correlation between public expenditures for birth control and the rate of teen pregnancies* [emphasis mine]." 176

Table C
Rates of Teenage Abortion-Plus-Unmarried Births for Selected American States and Foreign Countries

(States selected do not provide teenagers with free access to abortions and contraceptives, and spend lower-than-average amounts on government-funded birth control programs.) 176 and 409

State or Country	Rate of Abortions-Plus-Unmarried Births per 10,000 Women Aged 15-19 1981	Per Capita Public Expenditures on Birth Control as Percent of National Average, 1980
Idaho	35	56%
Utah	27	31%
South Dakota	27	42%
Sweden	32	–
Canada	33	–
England and Wales	30	–
France	29	–

♦ Plying for Funds

School-based clinics are expensive. The Support Center for School-based Clinics reports that clinic operations run anywhere from $25,000 to $400,000 per clinic annually. 152 Mosbacher reveals that, for a proposed clinic program in Mecklenburg County, North Carolina, "an average of $79,000 would be spent annually for a single clinic to serve an average of six teens per day. That breaks down to $73.88 per student served each school day." 192 (Cf. 6 and 193/4.)

The agenda for family planning groups is to get sex education health clinics into the schools on private funds. Once clinic programs are up and running on private money, they appeal to the government for tax dollars to keep them running. These programs hope that once they are in place the government won't put them out. At an average of $100,000 a clinic, the transition from private to public funds is a staggering burden to lay on our school districts.

Joy Dryfus, in "School-Based Health Clinics: A New Approach to Preventing Adolescent Pregnancy?" (PPFA's *Family Planning Perspectives*), explains how to get a foot in the door with a school-based health clinic:

> Most school-based clinics began by offering comprehensive health care, then added family planning services later, at least partly to avoid local controversy. . . . Although private funds have played an important part in starting up these programs, almost all of the school programs look to public support for continuation. . . . Kathleen Arnold-Sheran, a former program administrator at the St. Paul clinic, estimates that $90,000 per year is needed to operate a full-time high school clinic once it has been equipped . . . roughly $100 per patient per year. 347/72-74

Dryfus warns, "Although it is not fashionable to suggest that long-term viability depends on federal funding, it is difficult to imagine that foundations will be willing to support these programs permanently." 347/75 In other words, "Don't let the school board or voters know that you will need public funds for continued operation. Keep that concealed until you are established. Once you're in, *then* "go for the taxpayers' dollars."

As a school board member who has responsibility to evaluate sex education programs, *please, be aware* of the subterfuge used by many sex education advocates. The PPFA's journal carries an article by Richard A. Weatherley (et al), associate professor in the University of Washington's school of social work, about how sex program advocates get into a school system through deception.

The first and most common strategy to avoid opposition is "to maintain a low profile . . . by giving names to programs that obscure their functions. Cyesis, Teen Awareness, Access, Service to Young

Parents, Healthworks, and Continuing Education to Young Families are some examples." 348/76 One might add to this list of deceptive names: Family Life Education, and Planned Parenthood.

The second strategy is to exaggerate the benefits: "Program advocates and service providers are more or less obliged to exaggerate the potential benefits of services in order to secure political and material support." 348/77

Weatherley cites a third strategy:

> One popular ploy was what we termed the "programming coattails" strategy. . . . [You should reveal] an incredible array of problems that allegedly would be solved by the provision of services for pregnant teenagers and adolescent parents. In claims reminiscent of those made for the patent medicine nostrums of the 19th century, it was argued that teenage pregnancy services would combat child abuse, crime, youth unemployment, sexual abuse, infant mortality, mental retardation, birth defects, drug abuse and welfare dependency. 348/77

Weatherley explains, however:

> Given the limited duration, scope and intensity of even the most comprehensive programs, it is not surprising that many of them fall short of meeting the more modest goals, let alone solving complex social problems. The empirical evidence suggests that many of the ill effects associated with adolescent pregnancy are rooted in poverty, a condition not explicitly addressed by any of the programs and services. . . . In reality, the programs are offered in the mode of crisis intervention. 348/77

My deep concern as the parent of four children is the realistic implications of the extent to which many comprehensive sex education proponents will go to implement their programs in a community. When Planned Parenthood's own *Family Planning Perspective* says that advocates often need to "exaggerate" and "conceal" their true intent, the problem, their content and the promised results, what does it mean to school board members, legislators and parents? Does it mean that everything they say and write is suspect because they

"exaggerate" the problem?
"exaggerate" the need?
"exaggerate" the results?
"exaggerate" teen sexual activity?
"exaggerate" the goals?
"conceal" their true motives?
"understate" the cost?
"exaggerate" their costs of clinics?
"exaggerate" community interest?
"understate" their grants from the government?
"exaggerate" statistics?
"understate" income from services?

Does it mean to our kids that in the classroom they

"understate" the dangers?
"understate" the failure rate?
"exaggerate" the protection factor?
"exaggerate" the benefits?
"exaggerate" teen sexual activity (i.e., "Everyone is doing it")?

Are sex educators actually trying to conceal their intentions to teach contraception in order to get funds for their programs? Yes. For example: Planned Parenthood's own journal says, "On the recommendation of its community advisory board, a midwestern program omitted the provision of contraceptives from the clinic's activities in the first year." 362/45 Douglas Kirby also warned sex educators: "Initially try to maintain a low profile." 369/18-21

Here are some additional questions to ponder:

- How do school board members realistically evaluate their programs (PPFA, etc.)?
- How do legislators realistically evaluate grant requests?
- How do concerned parents decide if their children should "opt out" of sex education or not?
- How do teens intelligently decide if what they are being taught is the truth or an exaggeration?

So often educators and parents are told that the sex education program promotes family values and premarital abstinence. However, marriage is hardly ever mentioned and abstinence is only presented as one of many types of contraception.

Be cautious in your evaluation of sex education programs because many of them redefine basic words and concepts. For example, there are various definitions for premarital abstinence, responsibility, core values, parental rights, etc. This is often done to conceal the true intent of a program. Keep these thoughts in mind when anyone appears before the Julian school board to present his program and intent for teaching about sex in our schools. Be sure to ask very pointed questions when these terms arise.

♦ Purposely Vague

Another deceptive strategy used by many sex education advocates to pitch their programs to legislators and parents could be called "double-speak." I've heard sex education double-speak with my own ears. For example, many sex education advocates refer to school sex classes as "required electives" in order to prevent kids and parents from opting out. Have you ever heard a more blatantly conflicting term than "required elective"? Yet the double-speak becomes a smoke screen to veil what's really going on.

Double-speak is also employed to give different messages to teens and their parents about values. For example, many sex educators assure parents that they will do nothing to change their children's values. But in the classroom they are openly out to get rid of the "junk" about morality kids are getting from their culture.

Furthermore, when sex education proponents tell school boards they are only interested in teaching anatomy and physiology, they really mean they want to teach the details and acceptability of all kinds of sexual response: erections, orgasms, etc. But they cover their intentions under the neutral terms "anatomy and physiology." That's more double-speak.

Sometimes double-speak means "forgetting" to inform kids and parents about such vital subjects as comprehensive sex education's contributing role in the rising epidemic of STDs. Instead, they cite the dangers of AIDS and other STDs in their desperate appeals for government funding as if sex education programs were helping to solve these problems.

When family planning advocates approach legislators for funds to initiate and maintain sex education programs and school-based clinics, they talk in the most alarming terms about teenage pregnancies. They tug at the heartstrings by urging that something must be done about "kids having kids." They pledge, promise and predict that by providing sex education programs and contraceptives, they will be effecting teenage pregnancy decline. They back up their claims with statistics showing the decline in the numbers of teenage births (while conveniently ignoring the figures showing the increase in pregnancies and abortions). Convinced that "somebody is finally doing something for our kids," legislators dole out millions to fund the very programs which are responsible for increases in teenage pregnancies and abortions.

The public, especially parents, are often misled to assume that "teenage mother" means "unwed mother." Various family planning groups are able to get funding for comprehensive sex education programs and school-based clinics by being purposefully misleading about the marital status of "teen moms."

The chart on the next page shows that of the 513,758 live births to females aged 15 to 19, more than half were to married mothers. Twenty-three percent were conceived out of wedlock and may have resulted in "forced" or "shotgun" marriages, but 28 percent were not. At the time the births took place, fewer than half of the teenage mothers were unwed.

OUTCOME	NUMBER	
Total live births (women aged 15-19)	513,758	100%
Conceived postmaritally	145,907	28
Born postmaritally	118,678	23
Born premaritally	249,173	48

Furthermore, the impression usually given is that all teenage pregnancies are unintended and unwanted. However, the research done by professors Zelnik and Kantner discovered that only 28 percent of pregnancies to teens were unintended. 110

Leon Dash, a *Washington Post* reporter, for his article "At Risk: Chronicles of Teenage Pregnancy," spent seventeen months researching and interviewing young adults and teenagers in Washington, D.C. He discovered that though many unwed teenage mothers first indicated their pregnancies "just happened," the truth was that nearly one-third of the mothers had gotten pregnant intentionally. Moreover, the family planning services in which they had participated offered no help in discouraging them from becoming pregnant intentionally. 109/2

♦ Pregnancy Ages

Another aspect that must be considered is the age of teens who become pregnant. Proponents of comprehensive sex education seldom mention that. They would like us to believe that the bulk of teen pregnancies occur to school-age girls, because it supports their plea for government funding of their programs. However, in charting the age rate of pregnant girls in the United States, researchers Venture, Saffel and Masher show that the greater number of pregnancies occur to older teens, those who are no longer school age. 107

Estimated Number of Pregnancies
Pregnancy Rates by Outcome, 1981

Age	All Pregnancies	Live Births	Induced Abortions
under 14	28,000	10,000	15,000
15-17 years	425,000	187,000	176,000
18-19 years	678,000	340,000	257,000

According to Dr. Jacqueline Kasun of Humboldt State University, much of the discussion of teenage pregnancy has reported in painful detail the alleged problems of teenage girls without stating that, of all girls under the age of 20 who give birth:

less than 2% are 11-15-year-olds
less than 4% are 15-17-year-olds. 108

This means that far fewer teenage pregnancies occur to school-age adolescents than those who are seeking funds for comprehensive sex education would like us to believe.

♦ Redoubling Futile Efforts

Planned Parenthood and other family planning advocates continue to plead for more money despite the fact that authorities like sociologist Dr. Philip Cutright reveal that **"areas with weak** [sex education] **programs or no programs at all experience smaller increases or larger declines (in pregnancy) than are found in areas with strong contraceptive programs."** [194]

The U.S. Congress's House Select Committee on Children, Youth and Family (December 1985) responded to these pleas by stating:

> By increasing rather than decreasing federal support for clinics that provide teenagers with effective and confidential services, we would make it possible for more teenagers to get responsible advice . . . [and] make it possible for adolescents to exercise responsibility and competence in their sexual behavior.

The committee also acknowledged that "there has been no change in the percent of sexually active teens who became pregnant, but there has been a huge increase in sexual activity which has led to a proportionate increase in pregnancies to unmarried teens."

By responding with more funds to support programs which are doing the opposite of what they promise to do, our legislators are behaving like the frustrated leader who was unsure of his goals so he redoubled his efforts.

They are responding like the sales manager who said in an address to his sales force, "Men and women, we are losing a dollar a box on our product. So I want you to pull out all stops, work twice as hard and sell twice as many boxes this next week."

Scott is a teacher in Illinois who, like so many other teachers, agonizes over the approach many in the education community are taking to teen pregnancy and abortion. He sees that the failure of sex education programs even to come close to projected goals means little to how our legislators spend our money. Scott observes:

> Whether [programs are] sufficient or not, advocates are asking for and receiving more money. It can be concluded that their main concern is not to find a way to really reduce the rate of teen pregnancy, but is simply to insist on indoctrinating students with a philosophy that has been shown to be in error. . . . It seems logical that programs that cannot prove their effectiveness should not be supported or funded. Any other program with a comparable failure rate would be quickly abandoned by policy-makers. For some reason, programs designed to deal with teen pregnancy seem to be exempt

> from the standards used to evaluate all other programs. Supporters of school-based clinics and other programs designed to meet the problem of teen pregnancy simply claim they need more and more money, more and more clinics, and increased access to young people. The time must come when policy-makers demand positive evidence. One would think the evidence is clear. These programs are part of the problem. New solutions should be explored. 139/5

Pouring more dollars into comprehensive sex education programs will not solve the teen pregnancy and abortion problem. In fact, the statistical evidence increasingly shows that these programs are doing more harm than good to our kids. It's time to move toward a viable solution.

Part Three

Seven Strategies for Resolving the Teen Sexuality Crisis

CHAPTER 13

Strategy 1

Include and Involve Parents

As previous chapters have shown, a value-free, morally neutral, facts-only approach to sex education is counterproductive to solving the problems of pregnancy, abortion and disease among our teenagers.

We must do more than teach reproduction and contraception if our kids are going to adopt a lifestyle of responsible moral behavior. The outside pressure is too great. Peers, television, movies, music and advertising constantly encourage kids to become sexually active. These negative influences often outweigh positive influences from other sources. Without consistent moral training from the school, church and home, our children will have a tough time incorporating positive values into their lives. Knowledge alone does not produce wisdom.

♦ Needed: A United Front

In the '50s and '60s the family, the church, the school and the media provided a clear, consistent, unified message to kids about morality. Parents teaching moral values at home were supported on the other fronts. But today parents often stand alone in the battle. The message promoted by the powerful entertainment and advertising media suggests that promiscuity is the rule and that the negative consequences from it are negligible. Surprisingly, even some of our churches are going soft on what I consider to be obvious positive moral values. Yet when the school system joins in the campaign by taking an alleged morally neutral position on sex education while failing to notify us or involve us in the process, we really feel like the rug is being yanked out from under us. When the school-based sex educators accuse us of not caring for our kids or not doing our job as parents, we're demoralized. We feel lambasted, criticized, undermined, ridiculed, ignored and excluded all at once. The school has abandoned the moral education of our children, but for some reason the parents come out looking like the bad guys.

Some educators insist that teens are going to be sexually active even if they feel guilty and that it would be better to get them to use contraceptives than it would be to allow them to become pregnant or to contract a sexually transmitted disease. For this reason, some professionals justify contraceptive information and services without parental consent. They contend that if teens were required to consult parents before receiving contraceptives, then the teens would not go to their parents and would proceed to suffer the consequences of unprotected sex. However, the opposite scenario is often true, for the fear of getting "caught" can serve as a constraint. For example, in the states and countries that require parental permission, the teen-pregnancy rate, abortion rate, and birth rate all have dropped.

As the parents of four school-aged children, Dottie and I have been very thankful that the teachers, administrators and school board members in our community of Julian have been our cohorts and not our adversaries in educating our children in all areas. We are better off as a family and our children are better equipped for facing life's struggles and challenges because of the years we've spent in the Julian school system. Our concern is that you stay as involved and interested in us as parents when it comes to our kids' sex education as you are in the other areas of their school life. As school board members, you make decisions about curriculum and programs that determine how our schools, teachers, counselors and administrators will relate to us and our children on the subject of sex. Don't shut us out at this critical point of our kids' lives. Include us and involve us in your planning. We need your help now more than ever.

♦ Parents Need to Be Included

Eunice Kennedy Shriver, vice-president of the Kennedy Foundation, says that the first step toward positive, healthy sex education is to "create a consistent, supportive network of parents, teachers, doctors, nurses, clergy, friends and counselors who work with adolescents over an extended period." Cited in 109 Notice that parents are first on the list. Parents need to be included in the decisions which affect the public sex education of their children. The U.S. Department of Education strongly emphasizes that

> if the use of condoms is to be discussed with young people, such a discussion must include the recognition of certain facts, *should take place with the approval of parents,* and should occur in an appropriate moral context. In particular, young people must know that the use of condoms can reduce, but by no means eliminate, the risk of contracting AIDS [emphasis mine]. 279

Including parents and seeking their consent in matters of morality are integral to effective sex education.

Parents also need to be included so the school program can help them deal with sex-related issues at home. The Educational Guidance Institute reports on the research of the Search Institute in Minneapolis on the parental role in sex education, saying that their studies show:

1. 80% of the parents surveyed believe it is their primary responsibility to give sex education to their children;
2. 80% of parents surveyed also said that they needed help;
3. Parents are concerned about what to teach, how to talk about sexual matters and sexual values (knowing less than their kids do about sex), and how to influence their behavior. 210

Parents need the resources and support the school can supply them for talking to their kids about sex.

Former Secretary of Education William Bennett recommended:

> [Educators] should welcome parents into sex education classrooms as observers. . . . They should inform parents of the content of these courses, and they should encourage parents and children to talk to each other about sex. Studies show that when parents are the main source of sex education, children are less likely to engage in sex. This should come as no surprise when one remembers that the home is the crucible of character, and that parents are the children's first and foremost teachers. . . . Sex education courses can help remind those parents of their responsibilities. 213

Often, lack of communication and cooperation between parents and school officials on the topic of sex education provokes unnecessary friction and alienation. Parents, antagonized by militant comprehensive sex education proponents, become suspicious of all sex educators and programs. Having not been included in school decisions about sex education, parents become outspokenly critical of teachers, administrators and school board members. Thus they live up to the label given them by former U.S. Commissioner of Education James E. Allen: "Damn parents." 211/11

Douglas Kirby, who is pro-comprehensive sex education, acknowledged that school sex education programs would be more successful if parents and their moral values were included in the planning: **"School programs are much more likely to be effective if the norms**

expressed in the school programs are supported and reinforced by the larger social environment." 204/602-3 In other words, if parents are involved and supportive of the program, and the curriculum complements the values of the parents, there is a real possibility of effecting positive sexual behavior.

♦ Parents Need to Be Involved

Strong family relationships tend to discourage teenage sexual activity. For example, studies show that a close mother-daughter relationship reduces the likelihood of premarital sexual activity by the daughter. 320/1 Girls growing up in households with both parents are less likely to be sexually active than those with a single parent. 321/16 When sex education programs take advantage of parental influence instead of ignoring it, they are likely to be more successful.

The journal *Pediatrics* reports on aspects of a sex education program that bring about positive effects on adolescent sexual activity. They found that projects that work "*help adults* improve their skills as parents and as role models in the community. It was found in the study that two and three years after the implementation of the program, the estimated adolescent pregnancy rate declined by 35 percent compared with the preintervention period, in contrast with a 5.5- to 13.9-percent increase in the rate in comparison communities." 313/378

Research shows that strained parent-child interaction and the lack of parental supervision are associated with greater chances of teenage pregnancy (shown by Chilman 1980*b*; Coffnel and Jacobson, 1971; Kantner and Zelnik, 1972; Klerman, 1980; Phipps-Yonas, 1980). When parents have good relationships and communication with their children, they are more likely to be "credible, significant, and influential" (Kar et al., 1979:151) in their children's lives. This influence may lead the children to delay sexual activity. 662/245

Studies 179/825-55 have found that "parental supervision of early dating was an extremely important predictor of teenage pregnancy. These researchers found that rates of teenage pregnancy were reduced when parents supervised:

(1) who the adolescent dated;
(2) where the adolescent went on dates; and
(3) the arrival time back home.

Thus, the influence of parents is an important component in the complex set of factors affecting teenagers' childbearing behavior." 662/251

The impact of parents' involvement is striking in light of research. Parents who show "more concern and have higher educational expectations for their children decrease the chances that their daughter will experience an early childbirth by 36 percent and 43 percent respectively. Teenagers' educational values and the values of their parents are also important for black teenagers' childbearing behavior. Results . . . show that having high educational expectations and concerned parents reduces the chances that a black teenager will experience an out-of-wedlock childbirth by 32 percent and 30 percent respectively." 662/248

A good example of parental involvement in a community-based sex education program is the Challenge Program, developed by the Educational Guidance Institute (EGI). When EGI planners designed their workshops, they did so intending to help parents assume their roles as authority figures in their children's lives. They held the conviction that Diana Baumrind writes about:

> For too long, parents have been led to believe that they must be permissive. Interestingly, studies show that when parents view themselves as simply a resource to be used as the child wishes and not as the ones responsible for shaping the child's future behavior, negative effects are likely to occur. *Children with overly permissive parents have difficulty believing their parents care about them; permissiveness is sometimes interpreted as rejection.* Studies show that children of overly permissive parents are less helpful to others and less willing to live by the moral standards of their parents. They are more likely to become involved in hedonistic behavior and more likely to seek out sexual materials for self-gratification [emphasis mine]. 322/256,261 and 323/87,91 . . . The same studies show that parents who are authoritative (not authoritarian) and exert moderately firm control and standards while affirming a child's own qualities and styles are more likely to produce children who are service-oriented, concerned about people, free from feelings of alienation and committed to a religious faith. Proper parental authority also enhances family closeness. The same study shows that if parents become overly strict, authoritarian and autocratic, children develop low self-esteem and heightened feelings of self-condemnation, and the family experiences greater disharmony. 323/87,91

The Challenge Program took these insights to heart, designing a sex education program which relies on parental authority and involvement. The program has been a resounding success. (The Challenge Program is described in greater detail in chapter 18–Strategy 6.)

I heartily encourage public schools to open the doors of their planning meetings and strategy sessions to parents. Their influence over their children's sexual behavior is greater than any other influence. Failing to include and involve parents in developing a sex education strategy is not only short-sighted but also foolish.

An excellent resource on how parents can be involved is Dr. Dinah Richard and Anne Newman's *Healthy Sex Education in Your Schools: A Parent's Handbook* (Pomona, CA: Focus on the Family Publishing, 1990).

CHAPTER 14

♦ A **key section** for busy parents.

Strategy 2

Teach the Consequences of Promiscuity

(with Dr. John Raney)

The teenage sexuality crisis will never be resolved until our kids understand the devastating consequences of sexual promiscuity. Casual sex may be safer with condoms, but it is definitely not *safe,* contrary to what many family planning groups and sex educators imply. We must teach our kids about the life-threatening risks they take whenever they forego virginity and abstinence.

In this chapter I want to describe several of the sexually transmitted diseases to which our kids are vulnerable when they become sexually active. I am indebted to Dr. John H. Raney, M.D., for helping me compile this information. Every teenager in America needs to be taught what's in this chapter.

♦ STDs Gone Wild

In recent times the interest and research in sexually transmitted diseases (STDs), formerly referred to as venereal diseases (VD), have mushroomed. First herpes and then AIDS were featured as the cover stories of major magazines. The public has become increasingly concerned about the hazards of these and some fifty other STDs to the point where public schools are now offering classes on how to avoid them. Doctors at the Centers for Disease Control in Atlanta currently recognize more than 13 million cases a year, up from 4 million in 1980. 387/234 The breakdown reveals that 35,616 Americans acquire an STD every day of the year. **At this rate one in every four Americans between the ages of 15 and 55 eventually will get a sexually transmitted disease.** 431/53

It is sobering to learn that our kids are contracting STDs at such an alarming rate. Pediatrician Mary-Ann Shafer of the University of California's medical school in San Francisco reports, **"Teenagers have more STDs than any other group in the United States."** 275/28 About 2.5 million people under 20 are infected with some form of an STD, including AIDS. 384/10A One panel of experts reported, "Americans under 25, and more specifically those in their teens, are the ones at greatest risk for STDs today." 275/28

Much has been written about AIDS and herpes, but there are many other diseases and conditions which are not as well known that can also wreak havoc in the lives of their victims. These other diseases are as serious a problem as AIDS and herpes. In the same eight years since AIDS appeared, "other STDs are thought to have caused 80,000 fatalities, not to mention fetal and infant deaths numbering in the millions." 275/28 In the pages to follow we will look first at AIDS and herpes, then explore several other STDs which our kids must know about.

♦ AIDS

Probably no other disease in recent times has caused as much fear or drawn as much of the public's attention as AIDS. This strange and deadly viral infection has rather obscure origins. Research indicates that AIDS may have begun in Central Africa. 538/2; 539/29; 540/150-51; 541/1357 It was in 1978 that the first known case of AIDS was reported to the Centers for Disease Control. 542/27 The first case among homosexual men was reported in 1979 and among intravenous drug abusers in early 1980. 542/27 It wasn't until 1981 that the first heterosexual transmission of AIDS was reported. 542/27

Experts say that although teenagers account for "less than 1 percent of all reported AIDS cases, their sexual behavior, including intercourse with multiple partners and infrequent use of condoms, may make them more vulnerable than many adults to HIV exposure." 273/1,12 According to the Centers for Disease Control, female adolescents are more likely than adult females to contract AIDS. The male-to-female ratio of adolescent AIDS cases is five to one; among adults, that ratio is twelve to one. 173 "The data show that the biggest single source of exposure to the virus reported by female adolescent patients was heterosexual contact, which was cited by nearly four out of ten such patients. Some 72 percent of the female teenagers with AIDS are black or Hispanic." 273/1,12

One-fifth of all people with AIDS are in their 20s. **Many of them were infected when they were in their teens.** 384/10A One study revealed that "three out of every 1,000 college students are infected with HIV." Former Surgeon General Koop said, "It's probable that most of those people contracted their HIV infection while still in high school." 85

Dr. Helene Gayle of the Centers for Disease Control revealed that, in 1988, 7 percent of the AIDS cases acquired HIV infection when they were adolescents. 434/757 It was also disclosed that "the proportion of females among adolescents with AIDS is greater than that among adults with AIDS (14 percent versus 7 percent)." 434/757

As might be expected, research has indicated that those who have a lifestyle involving multiple heterosexual partners are much more likely to develop HIV infection than those who have been involved in strictly monogamous heterosexual activity (such as in a marriage where neither partner is unfaithful). Of 400 heterosexual individuals involved in monogamous relationships only 0.25 percent were HIV positive while 5 percent of the men and 7 percent of the women in a group of 400 heterosexuals with at least six sexual partners annually for the five years prior to the study were HIV positive. 653/83

Infants born by mothers who have the AIDS infection have a 30- to 60-percent chance of testing positive for HIV. 665/16, 654/59

Some HIV-infected individuals may not test positive for the AIDS virus "for months or even years." 655/15

The HIV that causes AIDS attacks the body's defense mechanisms against disease by invading certain white blood cells, called T-helper lymphocytes, that ordinarily help the body fight infection. 543/131; 544/2; 545/66-67 After entering these T-helper lymphocytes, the virus multiplies extremely rapidly and in the process destroys the cells and damages the body's ability to fight off disease. 546/41-42; 547/82; 548/73-74; 544/2; 545/66 As a result, the individual is susceptible to all kinds of unusual infections that rarely infect human beings. 543/131-32; 549/13,17-18; 545/67

One such infection that is very common in AIDS patients involves pneumocystis carinii organisms which cause pneumonias. This infection can lead to shortness of breath, hypoxemia (low level of oxygen in the body) and death. Fortunately there are antibiotics which can effectively fight this infection. 550/9; 544/21; 551/6,10; 552/5,9

Another infection common in AIDS patients, but which rarely causes disease in healthy adults, is mycobacterium avium-intracellulare. In addition to causing a pneumonia, this kind of infection can cause open sores in the bowel, diarrhea, weight loss, persistent fever, and other problems. 543/135; 552/5,9-11; 553/20

AIDS patients may be victimized by a number of different kinds of fungus infections as well as by candida albicans (candidiasis) which can affect the mouth and throat, making eating very painful. 543/138; 550/9; 552/11,21 In some cases, old infections of TB (mycobacterium tuberculosis) have been reactivated or new infections have been incurred by AIDS victims. 554/86; 552/9-10 In addition, other bacterial pneumonias, and syphilis, are also seen in these patients. 555/1493

The severely damaged ability of AIDS patients to fight infections leads to very severe forms of common infections. For example, herpes infections may cause severe and extensive sores and ulcerations in the genital and rectal areas as well as in the mouth and esophagus of these patients. 543/139; 550/9; 552/21

Cancers have also been noted to be associated with AIDS infections. In particular, Kaposi's sarcoma causes a purplish lesion of the skin and lymphomas or tumors of the lymph glands, and has been found to be associated with the AIDS virus infection. 556/343; 543/136-38; 552/16,21

Severe brain damage and dementia have been found in these patients. 543/136-38; 557/77; 550/9; 552/14-16; 558/3003 They may suffer from disorientation, confusion, memory loss and seizures. 544/21; 559/87; 552/14-16 One psychiatrist observed that the dementia was "as severe as any Alzheimer's dementia I've ever seen." 558/87

It appears that an increasingly large percentage of individuals infected with the HIV virus will eventually develop AIDS. 560/7; 561/135; 563/54; 564/31; 565/13; 555/1493; 566/3012 Initially, many HIV-infected individuals will develop what is called AIDS Related Complex (ARC). 567/47; 559/87; 568/90; 569/13 They often experience such complications as unexplained fever, large lymph glands, diarrhea, weight loss, marked fatigue and a general sense of not feeling well. 567/47; 544/4; 549/18; 570/330 A few of these individuals may actually die from complications of ARC without actually going on to full-blown AIDS.

As of April 1988, the Centers for Disease Control estimated that 1 to 1.5 million Americans were infected with the AIDS virus. 571/1851 The CDC also has reported that, as of June 30, 1989, 99,936 individuals have been diagnosed as having AIDS. 572/784 The Public Health Service estimates that by 1992 there will have been a total of some 365,000 cases of AIDS diagnosed in the United States and that of these, some 263,000 individuals will have died from the disease. 571/1851 It has been estimated that in 1992 the medical costs of taking care of AIDS patients will be $5 billion to $13 billion. 571/1851 In the brief few years of its existence, AIDS has become the leading cause of death for single American men between the ages of 15 and 50. 567/44

A task force of insurance company medical directors concluded that AIDS may have catastrophic effects for health and life insurance companies which will have to pay out billions of dollars in benefits in the coming years. 573/52 Above and beyond these costs, it was estimated that the first 10,000 cases of AIDS resulted in the loss of $4.6 billion in future income. 574/210

Although AIDS has struck the homosexual community and the IV drug abusers the hardest, it has also crept into the heterosexual community. In 1986 there were 1,100 cases of AIDS that were thought to be due to heterosexual transmission. 578/31 More recently it has been estimated that some 3.6 percent of all cases of AIDS are due to heterosexual transmission. 571/1851

Tragically, in addition to being passed through sexual contact and among IV drug abusers, AIDS has also been found to be passed from infected mothers to their babies. In 1987 one out of every thirty-three babies born in New York City was infected with AIDS. 579/115

In recent years a tremendous amount of time, effort and money has been expended in an attempt to develop drugs to treat AIDS and a vaccine to prevent it. While no drug has been found that is able to cure the disease, a relatively new drug called azidothymidine (AZT) has been able to provide some temporary benefits by prolonging survival and decreasing the frequency and severity of infections that AIDS victims develop. Unfortunately AZT sometimes causes serious side effects, and recently there has been some evidence of viral resistance to the drug. 580/1281-82; 563/55; 581/558; 582/2409; 555/1493 Researchers have been experiencing great difficulty in developing an AIDS vaccine. 583/68-69; 545/73; 584/14; 585/13 Despite tremendous efforts in this direction, it appears that the availability of a safe and effective AIDS vaccine lies well in the future. 585/13; 558/3004-5

In view of the alarming statistics and frightening effects of AIDS infection, many secular leaders in our society have been calling for and promoting so-called safe sex practices. But as many have noted, such as Dr. Marcus Conant of the University of California at San Francisco, apart from a long-term, mutually monogamous relationship between two individuals who do not have the AIDS infection, there is no completely safe sex. 575/1340; 576/20; 577/2263 Theresa L. Crenshaw, M.D., president of the American Association of Sex Educators, Counselors and Therapists, told Congress in 1987, "For the sake of health, casual sex and multiple partners must be abandoned." 577/2263

A U.S. Public Health Service task force warned that "intercourse —even with a condom—with a person known to be infected with the AIDS virus is so dangerous to an uninfected partner that anyone in such a situation should consider alternative methods of expressing physical intimacy." 271 Our kids need to know the truth about AIDS.

♦ Herpes

Apart from AIDS, perhaps no other disease has jolted the casual sex movement in America as much as herpes. As recently as the 1950s the transmission of herpes during sexual intercourse was considered rare. 483/86 Between 1966 and 1979 the estimated number of consultations with physicians for herpes increased from under 30,000 to over 250,000. 484/169 By 1984 there were an estimated 20 million people in America with genital herpes. 485/41, 486/6, 487/59, 488/2417 The National Institute of Allergy and Infectious Diseases now estimates that about "30 million Americans are infected, and that 500,000 more catch the sexually transmitted virus each year." 432 (See also 658/3509.)

In addition to this huge number of symptomatic cases there are many cases of genital herpes infection in which the individual has no symptoms. 658/3509

So-called free sex no longer seems attractive as huge numbers of Americans find themselves to be victims of this modern-day plague. Victims feel shock, panic, shame, hopelessness, bitterness and rage upon learning they have contracted herpes. 489/24, 490/1 Searches for the guilty sex partner are made, and in some cases lawsuits are initiated. 491/39; 490/11

Studies show that 25 to 65 percent of all women carry the virus unknowingly, (433) **averaging almost 50 percent of all women over 18**. *USA Today* reported a study indicating that up to one-third of all adults carry the genital herpes virus in their blood system.

One study of pregnant women in several large American cities indicates that up to 65 percent have silent (symptomless) herpes infections. 658/3509

The herpes-causing organism is a virus that is closely related to the one which causes chicken pox and shingles. Like other viruses, it cannot be successfully treated with antibiotics, although a new antiviral agent called Acyclovir can be quite helpful in suppressing the infection and helping to prevent recurrences.

Herpes can be divided into two types: I and II. In the past, type I was associated with infections above the waist, such as the common cold sore on the lip. Type II was associated with infections of the genital area. However, with the increased practice of oral sex, this distinction has changed. 487/59; 492/63; 488/2417; 493/1044 According to one group of studies, from 26 to 40 percent of genital herpes involve type I. 492/63

It has been estimated that one-third to one-half of the initial herpes infections are either without symptoms or so mild they go unnoticed. 494/76; 484/182 Those victims suffering symptoms typically experience painful blisters beginning two to twelve days after sex with an infected person. The blisters then break down to form ulcers and generally heal within about two weeks. 484/170,175; 493/1044 Primary or initial infections can be much more severe, causing swelling, lymph node enlargement, fever, headaches, muscle aches and discharge or drainage from the genitals. 494/26; 495/88; 493/1044 Once the acute infection is over, the herpes virus migrates up the sensory nerve endings to the nerve ganglion and there goes into a latent state.

Later, after some stress, emotional upset, sexual intercourse, menstrual period or for no apparent reason, the virus will migrate down the sensory nerve endings to the surface or skin and form new blisters, thus creating a recurrence of the initial herpes infection. 501/48; 496/39; 497/144,148; 498/148; 499/359,364-65; 500/8; 493/1049 The frequency and severity of these recurrent attacks of herpes vary considerably. 484/193 During the acute attack, it has been recommended by doctors that patients remain sexually abstinent to avoid the spread of the infection. 502/56; 503/89; 497/150 It should be noted, however, that the infection can be passed even when an infected individual has no symptoms, as individuals have been found to shed viruses up to 20 percent of the time, even during symptom-free periods. 493/1049; 504/8; 505/142; 506/24W; 507/153 In fact, according to one medical source, it may be that most herpes infections are passed during these periods. 507/153

While condoms offer partial protection against the spread of herpes infection, this protection is not complete. Herpes can be spread even when condoms are used. 493/116,1049; 505/142; 506/24W; 508/117; 509/56 Also, while Acyclovir may help modify or suppress an infection, it will not completely prevent the transmission of the infection from one person to another. 510/146; 511/20

In addition to the pain and discomfort from the infection itself, herpes can cause other problems. It has been estimated that a baby delivered by a mother with an active infection will have a 40- to 60-percent chance of contracting the disease. 512/50; 488/2417 Because of their poorly developed immunologic systems, some 40 percent or more of the infants who contract herpes will die, and many of the others will suffer brain damage. 513/1; 514/7; 488/2427 To avoid these tragic problems, doctors deliver babies by C-section if the mother has an active infection or is shedding herpes viruses.

Although it is a rare problem, herpes sometimes infects the brain, causing a localized encephalitis, which can lead to severe brain damage or death. 493/1045; 515/444; 516/182 Also, there is the possibility that herpes may help to cause genital cancers, serving as a co-factor in this regard. 517/41-42 In cervical cancer, definite association between herpes viruses and the cancer cells has been noted. 514/7; 518/110; 519/6 Also, more recently an association between herpes viruses and vulvar (external portions of the female genitalia) cancer were noted. 493/1046; 520/13-14

The pain and problems associated with herpes infections point to the importance of avoiding casual sexual encounters, as even one sexual experience with an infected but symptom-free person may lead to years of intermittent suffering and trouble with this infection. Our kids must be taught the truth about herpes.

♦ Pelvic Inflammatory Disease (PID)

PID is an infectious inflammation of the female organs which strikes approximately one million women in America each year. 445/50; 446/1735; 447/47 A number of different kinds of organisms or bacteria can cause this infection, such as gonorrhea or chlamydia trachomatis. In some cases a severe infection forms within the womb and fallopian tubes. If this infection is not treated adequately or in time, a pocket of pus may form that eventually will burst, spreading the infection throughout the abdominal cavity. When this occurs, the victim may first notice a sudden increase in pain and very quickly begin to go into shock. 448/24; 449/32 If she does not have surgery quickly to deal with the infection, she may die within a matter of hours. 450/909 Such surgeries can involve the removal of all of the internal female organs, thus leaving her unable to bear children. In addition, because of the removal of the ovaries, she will need to be on estrogen, a hormone medication, for many years. 451/104; 452/139

In some cases, PID may involve a very mild infection, particularly if chlamydia trachomatis is involved. This organism is too small to be seen by a light microscope and is difficult to culture. Consequently it has been a difficult organism to detect until recent times. These infections can be so mild that the woman may not even be aware that she has any infection. 453/1-2; 454/86 Nevertheless, over a period of time this infection may lead to a complete blockage of the fallopian tubes and infertility due to the scarring of the infection. 453/1-2; 455/157; 456/5 Many women in this situation will not know anything is wrong until they try to get pregnant and find that they are unable to. 455/157

Chlamydia trachomatis is not only a major cause of PID, but frequently also causes miscarriages and premature labor. 457/149; 458/46; 459/34 Women with this infection also tend to have more stillbirths and postpartum infections. 458/46; 459/46; 460/20 In the newborn child, chlamydia can cause eye infections and pneumonia. 461/2; 462/3369; 457/149

In men, chlamydia can cause chronic prostate infections and other infections of the male genitals, such as epididymitis, which can seriously affect a man's fertility. 455/164; 463/2; 464/88; 465/66; 466/88 (The epididymis lies next to the testicles and serves as a storage vessel for sperm cells.)

It has been estimated that a quarter of a million cases of acute epididymitis each year are caused by this organism. 463/2 While most women do not have symptoms with chlamydia, most men develop a milky discharge and pain on urination. It has been estimated that one in twenty adult males is a silent carrier of the infection. 455/164 There are an estimated several million new cases of chlamydia trachomatis each year in this country. It is more common than gonorrhea and syphilis combined. 467/38; 468/18; 469/15; 470/32; 471/67

Of those women who developed PID as a result of chlamydia, gonorrhea or some other bacterial infection, it has been estimated that 10 to 15 percent who have a first-time infection will become permanently infertile. Those who develop PID a second time have an estimated 30- to 35-percent chance of becoming infertile. And those who have a third episode of PID have an estimated 60- to 75-percent chance of becoming infertile by this infection. 472/2; 449/28; 473/109; 474/112

Infertility, however, is not the only problem that these women face. One research study found that women with PID were five times more likely to have abdominal operations and three times more likely to have abdominal pain or pain during intercourse than would normally be expected. 475/10 Unfortunately, many women do not realize that a single casual sexual involvement can lead to chronic pain and sterility. 474/112 Women with multiple sexual partners are have a much higher incidence of PID. 445/50 For teenagers who have multiple sexual partners, their risk of getting PID increases fivefold. 281/50

PID can lead to other tragic problems such as ectopic pregnancy. An ectopic pregnancy involves the development of the fertilized ovum or fetus in some other place in the mother's body besides the womb, such as the fallopian tubes. However, the fallopian tubes are unable to expand as the womb is to contain the ever-growing fetus. Usually at around six to eight weeks the developing baby is so large that the fallopian tube suddenly ruptures, leading to rapid bleeding and shock. 478/94,101; 479/951 Typically the victim experiences severe pain and may even pass out. Without treatment, this condition can lead to death. 478/103; 480/3,96 While ectopic pregnancy can be caused by a variety of medical problems such as pelvic adhesions from previous surgery or endometriosis, some 50 percent of women with this condition appear to have had PID previously. 474/112; 476/1729; 477/48

Due to the tremendous increase in the number of ectopic pregnancies in this country, ruptured tubal pregnancy has now become a major cause of maternal death. 481/3 According to one source, the number of ectopic pregnancies has increased from approximately 18,000 in 1970 to 68,000 in 1980. 477/48 The increase in the number of ectopic pregnancies in this country has been so great that it has been referred to as an epidemic. 477/48; 480/3 Half of the women who have ectopic pregnancies will be infertile afterward. 478/92

It appears that PID can cause ectopic pregnancies by partially blocking the fallopian tubes. In such a case it is possible for the tiny sperm cells to make their way up through the narrowed and scarred fallopian tube to the female egg and fertilize it. But it is then impossible for the much larger fertilized egg to traverse the constricted fallopian tube to the womb where the fetus would normally develop.

It should be noted that surgeons have had only limited success at repairing damaged tubes. 455/174; 482/92 It should also be noted that in vitro fertilization (fertilizing the woman's ovum with her husband's sperm outside of her body and then placing it back into the womb) has also met with rather limited success. 482/92

Although use of condoms has been encouraged as a means of protecting against the spread of STDs, a recent Rutgers University study of students with genital complaints who were seen at the student health center cast doubt on their efficacy in protecting against chlamydial infections. Of those who used condoms, 35.7 percent had chlamy compared with 37 percent who used oral contraceptives and 44 percent who used no contraceptives. 656/19,23

♦ Cytomegalovirus (CMV)

The risk of infection with cytomegalovirus is an additional reason to avoid casual sexual encounters. While CMV is found in the saliva and apparently can be transmitted in a variety of ways, it is also found in male semen and in female cervical secretions and can be transmitted through sexual intercourse. 511/22,26,28; 521/74-75; 522/23 Frequently CMV infections produce no symptoms, but they may cause illnesses similar to the flu or mononucleosis. 523/29; 521/75

A much more serious situation arises when a pregnant woman becomes infected and then transmits the infection to her unborn child. An estimated 40,000 to 80,000 babies were born in 1982 with congenital CMV infections. 523/29 Of these infected children, 10 to 20 percent will have significant and permanent handicaps such as microcephaly (small headedness) or hydrocephalus, seizures, hearing problems, psychomotor retardation and learning problems. 523/2,29; 524/9

Other babies infected during pregnancy will die before birth, be born prematurely or have fatal problems with liver and spleen disease. 521/75; 524/9; 525/1,74; 526; 527/2 **In the United States, congenital CMV infections are now one of the leading causes of hearing problems in children.** 527/2 Infected mothers can also transmit their infection to their babies during delivery. 527/29 CMV may also cause pneumonia and respiratory problems in babies. 521/75

♦ Hepatitis B

Hepatitis B is another viral infection that can be transmitted sexually. 511/23; 528/99; 529/94 The incidence of hepatitis B goes up dramatically with an increase in the number of sexual partners. One study found that those with only one or two sexual partners had a less than 1-percent incidence of hepatitis B, while those with ten or more sexual partners had a 7-percent incidence. 530/50 **Some 60 percent of homosexual men have had hepatitis, while some 85 percent of homosexual males have become infected by age 40.** 531/49; 530/50 Fortunately a vaccine protecting individuals against hepatitis B became available in 1982, and the U.S. Public Health Services recommended that the high-risk groups, such as prostitutes, homosexually active males and heterosexually active persons with multiple sexual contact, should receive the vaccine. 530/44; 532/27

Some victims have such mild cases of hepatitis that they are unaware of it, suffering only flu-like symptoms if any. 511/23; 530/41; 533/27 Others experience severe, sometimes fatal liver damage. Hepatitis-B virus infection also has been found to lead to primary liver cancer in a significant percentage of cases. 530/41,44; 534/46

Hepatitis can also be transmitted from a mother to her unborn child, resulting at times in the death of the fetus, a stillbirth, premature delivery or hepatitis in her newborn child and an ongoing infection through childhood. 535/PC52,35 Other research indicates that 90 percent of the babies whose mothers are chronic hepatitis-B virus carriers will be infected at the time of their birth. Of these babies, some 90 percent will go on to become chronic hepatitis-B virus carriers. 534/46 Left untreated, a significant percentage of carriers will eventually develop cancer of the liver. 534/46 Fortunately, immunization of these exposed babies shortly following their birth can prevent this in a high percentage of cases. 536/36, 537/240, 534/46

♦ Venereal Warts

In comparison to AIDS and herpes, venereal warts (caused by the human papillomavirus) have received little publicity. Yet in recent years there has been a tremendous increase in the incidence of this disease. **Data indicate that during the time visits to doctors for herpes increased 300 percent, visits for venereal warts increased 1,100 percent.** 593/84

There are an estimated one million or more cases of venereal warts a year in the United States. 586/31 It is estimated that some 10 percent of adult men and 5 percent of adult women will have venereal warts at some time in their lives. 587/64

In one study 48 percent of the women in an STD clinic (with normal pap smears) had evidence of this infection, and in another study 17 percent of an otherwise normal group of individuals also had evidence of this infection. 659/23

Sixty percent or more of the sexual partners of patients with the human papillomavirus infection have the infection themselves. 659/23

While VD warts are very common, it is felt that perhaps infections with the human papillomavirus that do not cause warts, or are asymptomatic, are more common than those that do. 588/47; 589/160 Evidence also suggests that homosexual males have a higher than average incidence of venereal warts. 587/64

Venereal warts are readily passed during sexual intercourse. 590/31; 591/2 They typically occur about two to three months after exposure. However, they have been known to occur as soon as a few weeks after sexual contact and as long as two years after exposure. 592/94; 593/65

The warts can occur on different parts of the male or female genitals, even inside a woman's vagina or cervix or inside a man's penis. 594/3,84; 595/21 VD warts grow quickly during pregnancy and may interfere with the delivery of the child. 588/55; 595/54; 596/54 Though it is quite unusual, babies born to mothers with warts may develop warts around their anus or in their vocal chord area, which can cause hoarseness or difficulty with breathing. 588/47; 595/54; 597/3

In addition to being unsightly, warts can be troublesome to treat successfully. 598/48 Even when they are burned off, frozen off or surgically removed, warts frequently seem to recur. 598/48 Other sexually transmitted diseases such as syphilis, gonorrhea and trichomoniasis are often found along with the VD warts. 595/21; 593/65

In addition to the human papillomavirus, a poxvirus can also cause a different type of wart called molluscom contagiosum. 599/103; 600/11 This smaller wart usually occurs in clusters, and while often no bigger than a fifth of an inch in diameter, it may grow to be as large as an inch in size. 601/103,107 This wart can also be found in other parts of the body and be spread by contact. Between 1966 and 1983 the incidence of molluscom contagiosum increased ten-fold. 600/11

♦ Pelvic Cancer

While doctors used to believe that VD warts were harmless, more recent research indicates that this is not the case. Dr. Ralph Reichert of Columbia University College of Physicians and Surgeons notes that women who have VD warts secondary to the human papillomavirus infection are 1,000 to 2,000 times more likely to get cervical cancer than women without the warts. 602/150, 603/3 Dr. Orth, at the Second World

Congress on Sexually Transmitted Diseases in 1986, noted that certain types of the human papillomavirus were found in over 90 percent of the cervical cancers studied. 604/6 At a state medical meeting of family physicians, Dr. Austin predicted that **"an epidemic of cervical cancer among women is likely to occur if liberal sexual lifestyles continue."** 605/3

Medical research has indicated that there are a number of risk factors which increase a woman's chance of developing cervical cancer. These include multiple sexual partners, having sex with someone who's had multiple sexual partners and beginning sexual intercourse at an early age (18-20). 606/144,148; 607/3012; 603/3

The associate chief of staff of the Boston Hospital for women, Dr. Robert Kistner, noted in 1972 that "early and frequent coitus, especially with multiple partners, seems to increase the incidence of this cancer precursor." Dr. Kistner added, "Carcinoma in situ in women under 25 made up only 30 percent of the total cervical cancer cases in 1950-51. However, by 1967-68 this figure had increased to 92.2 percent of the total." 435

Surprisingly, beginning sexual activity at an early age is considered an even greater risk factor for the development of cervical cancer than having multiple partners. 657/135 This rather surprising finding seems to be related to the immaturity of the cells that line the cervix in younger women. 608/10, 606/148

Another study found cases of cellular abnormalities in the cervixes to be five times greater in a group of promiscuous teenagers than in a group of virgin teenage girls. 435 Medical researcher I. D. Rathin of the Kaiser Foundation Research Institute reported, "There is enough material in recent literature to caution young women against sexual intercourse at early ages. These several studies are concerned with causation of cancer of the uterine cervix, and results are all in the same direction. . . . All studies agree that cervical cancer risk is increased by . . . first coitus at early ages. . . . **By observing abstinence the adolescent female is on reasonably valid biological ground, which requires no moral or religious support."** 436/486

Rodkin also reported, "Twice as many patients (i.e., the subjects with cervical cancer) as controls began coitus at ages 15-17. . . . Patients also differed strongly from controls with respect to . . . number of husbands and total number of coital mates. . . . Many more patients than controls had multiple sexual mates." 437/603

In regard to women having sex with an individual who has had multiple sexual contacts as a risk factor, women with cancer of the cervix were more likely to have had husbands who had visited prostitutes or who had extramarital affairs. 609/39 Dr. Irving I. Kessler of Johns Hopkins found that "extramarital sexual practice by either the woman or her spouse is also associated with cervical cancer risk." 438/1912-19

Prostitutes have been found to have very high rates of infection with the human papillomavirus and have a 12-percent rate of cervical cancer, making this a real "occupational" risk. 594/84 Research indicates that there are also high-risk males, referred to as "carcinogenic (cancer-causing) Charlies," who have given large numbers of women positive pap smears in regard to cancerous or precancerous conditions of the cervix. 603/9

In addition to apparently helping to cause cervical cancer, it appears that the human papillomavirus is also associated with increased incidences of vulvar cancer, cancer of the external genitals in women. To a lesser extent it is associated with penile cancers in men. 610/163; 604/6; 611/42; 594/3,84 Furthermore, it appears that cancers of the anal area may be associated with warts, and those who develop warts as a result of oral sex may be at increased risk to get cancers of the esophagus and larynx, or vocal cord area. 604/6; 611/42

Gynecologist Dr. Joe McIlhaney declares, **"I have begun telling those patients of mine who seem interested in knowing the cause of their cervical dysplasia, cervical cancer or venereal warts, that they are sexually transmitted diseases almost entirely."** 297/28-30

Dr. S. L. Barron, in his study of the consequences of sexual activity in teens under 16 years of age, shows that "the risk of carcinoma of the cervix doubled in women who became involved sexually before 17. He strongly concluded that there is both a medical and a moral basis to promote abstinence." 439/787

♦ Syphilis

Although the exact origins of syphilis are unclear, evidence suggests that the sailors who accompanied Christopher Columbus brought it back from the New World. 612/235-37; 613/3-4; 614/27 Whether it was a new disease or a more severe form of syphilis than was already present in Europe is not known, but this disease spread quickly to various parts of the world through armies and prostitution. By 1496 it had spread to France, Germany, Holland and Greece, by 1497 to Scotland, by 1498 to India, by 1499 to Russia and by 1505 to China. Each country tended to blame another. The Italians referred to it as the "French Disease," the French referred to it as the "Italian Disease" and the Indians and Japanese referred to it as the "Portuguese Disease," etc. 612/239-40 In the American colonies, however, where there were strict moral standards regarding sexual activity, the first case of syphilis did not occur until 1646, some twenty-six years after the landing at Plymouth Rock. 612/240-41

The *New York Times* reported that in 1987 syphilis cases were up 35 percent over 1986. 440 *Education Week* reported that syphilis cases **"for teenagers between the ages of 15 and 19 rose from 15 per 100,000 in 1984 to 21.9 per 100,000 last year."** 273/1,12

While the exact number of syphilis cases is difficult to obtain because of underreporting, it appears that, with the discovery and use of penicillin, the number dropped dramatically until about 1957. 613/6 However, **between 1957 and 1981 there was an apparent fourfold increase in the number of reported cases.** 613/6 This increase appears to have coincided with the so-called "sexual revolution."

In addition to increased rates of syphilis among adults, the rate of congenital syphilis (infections in newborns that developed prior to birth) increased fourfold over a three-year period of time, 1985 through 1987, and continued to rise after that. 658/3509

While capable of causing severe disease and complications, syphilitic infections typically begin with rather mild signs and symptoms. In the first of three stages, not including the latent stage which occurs between the second and third, a small bump may appear from nine to ninety days after the transmission of the infection by sexual contact. This bump slowly breaks down, forming a painless ulcer. 613/7-8; 615/1756 During the second stage, which often occurs three weeks after the development of the first, the individual may experience a flu-like illness with fever, headache, runny nose, aches and pains, sore throat and, at times, a generalized skin rash. 613/10-11; 615/1756-57 After awhile these symptoms disappear and the individual goes into what is called the latent stage, feeling completely free of illness or disease. 615/1757; 616/86

Some of these individuals who have a latent infection will go on in time to develop tertiary syphilis. For some this third stage may take the form of destructive lesions, called gummas, which involve the breakdown of tissues, such as skin and bone. 616/86; 617/25-29 As much as ten years after the onset of the latent stage, other infected individuals may develop severe problems with the heart and major blood vessels. Heart valves may be damaged and the aorta, the major artery through which blood flows from the heart, may begin to balloon because of damage, forming an aneurysm. In other cases obstruction of circulation may occur, leading to angina. 617/29-32; 618/89,93

In still other patients, severe damage to the brain and spinal cord may occur. Some of these patients may experience marked memory loss and confusion or dementia, while others may become psychotic. It appears that syphilis of the brain can mimic almost any psychiatric disorder. 617/32-36; 615/1757-58; 619/14 Severe damage to the spinal cord may lead to loss of position sense in the legs and a very unsteady gait. Spinal cord damage can also lead to incontinence and impotence. 617/33-35; 615/1758

Also disturbing is the data that links syphilic infection with increased rates of HIV (AIDS) infection. 660/51,977

Syphilis in a pregnant woman can lead to disastrous consequences for her unborn child. Studies indicate that approximately one-fourth of these children will die before birth, another one-fourth will die shortly after birth and still others will develop various complications and medical problems from the syphilis. 620/37 Fortunately, congenital syphilis, the infection of the baby in the mother's womb, is a rather unusual occurrence. While accurate estimates of the true number of children born with congenital syphilis are difficult to obtain, it appears that the number has been climbing in recent years from a reported 115 in 1978 to 158 cases in 1983. 621/1750 These cases tended to involve mostly unmarried young women who received little or no prenatal care. 622/1721

♦ Gonorrhea

Medical researcher Dr. Gordon Muir reports that **gonorrhea has become "the most common reportable disease in school-age children, surpassing chicken pox, measles, mumps and rubella combined."** 441 "In 1987," explains *Education Week,* "gonorrhea was reported in more than 1 percent of young people aged 15 to 19. Although people between the ages of 20 and 24 had an infection rate of more than 1.5 percent, the CDC found that 'when adjusting for sexual-activity rates, **adolescents 15-19 actually have the highest rates of gonorrhea of any age group.' "** 273/1,12

H. Hunter Handsfield, director of the sexually transmitted disease control program for the Seattle-King County Department of Health, called the gonorrhea rates "truly phenomenal," especially for black, inner-city teenage girls. 273/1,12 Handsfield warned, "If a black girl (in King County) becomes sexually active at the age of 13 or 14, her risk of getting gonorrhea is 25 percent every year. If the same girl delays her sexual activity until the age of 15, she has a 50-percent chance of getting the disease by the age of 18." 273/1,12

Unlike syphilis, which causes some of its most severe problems many years after the initial infection, gonorrhea tends to cause problems early on. It commonly causes discharge or drainage from the penis or vagina as well as frequent and painful urination. In females gonorrhea can spread into the uterus and fallopian tubes, causing pelvic inflammatory disease. These infections can lead to infertility, abdominal pain, pain during intercourse and ectopic pregnancies. 623/68; 624/185-86 Serious and uncontrolled infections may lead to a need for surgery.

According to Dr. Grimes of the University of Missouri at Kansas City School of Medicine, gonorrhea is the primary cause of arthritis in young adults. 625/71 It is also the most common cause of infectious arthritis in the general population. 626/45 Although it occurs rarely, gonorrhea may also cause infections of the heart or of the lining of the brain and spinal cord. 625/71-74; 627/10-11

In addition to gonorrhea of the genital organs, individuals can develop gonorrhea of the rectum and pharynx (throat) if they're involved in oral or anal sexual practices. 626/44-47

About 60 percent of the women and 20 percent of the men who have a gonorrhea infection will not have any symptoms. 626/44-45; 615/1750 This makes it difficult to control the spread of infections, as an infected individual without symptoms may pass it on to somebody else without even knowing he or she had it in the first place.

In the past, gonorrhea was readily treated by a shot of penicillin, but many strains of gonorrhea have become resistant to this medication. In recent years a number of different kinds of resistant strains of gonorrhea have developed, making treatment increasingly difficult. 628/3,16; 629/48

It is difficult to know the exact number of cases of gonorrhea in this country because of underreporting, but between 1960 and 1980 the number of reported cases of gonorrhea rose from about 259,000 to slightly over a million. 630/43 It is thought that there were actually twice that number of cases–two million–in view of the tendency of this disease to be underreported. 630/43

It is apparent that, although some have had a tendency to think of gonorrheal infections as rather trivial and unimportant, in view of the above facts and data, this is not at all the case. A great many of the more than "70 percent of people who are sexually active by the age of 19 may have an initial exposure to an STD, become infected, and pass the infection on without ever feeling ill or knowing they've been infected." 343/3509

♦ Miscellaneous STDs

While a complete description of all sexually transmitted diseases is beyond the intent and scope of this chapter, there are several others that should be mentioned: trichomoniasis, T-mycoplasma, scabies and pediculosis pubis.

Trichomoniasis. Trichomoniasis is a tiny, one-celled protozoan that affects about one-fifth of all women who are sexually active with multiple partners during their reproductive years. 631/33; 632/18; 633/138 There are an estimated 3 million or more new cases of this infection in the United States each year. 633/138; 631/33 One study in the *Medical Aspects of Human Sexuality* reports that "an estimated 8 million Americans each year develop trichomoniasis." 661/73

Trichomoniasis seems to be easily passed through sexual activity as it is found in 85 percent of the women who are sexual partners of infected males and in 70 percent of the men who are involved sexually with infected females. 661/73 While men frequently do not have any symptoms, they may develop a discharge from the penis. Research has shown that mobility of the sperm may be decreased by the infection, tending to decrease the ability to father children. 631/33; 633/138-39

In women this infection is rare in virgins, although it can be transmitted non-sexually. 633/138 About one-quarter of women do not have any symptoms while others may have a heavy yellowish or greenish malodorous vaginal discharge and also experience severe itching. 633/139 The infection can cause pain on urination and intercourse as well as menstrual problems. 631/33; 632/20; 633/139 **It appears that trichomoniasis can increase infertility in women.** 633/139; 634/7; 635/13-14 Trichomoniasis typically can be successfully treated with Metronidazole. Recently, however, some strains of trichomoniasis have developed resistance to low doses of this drug. 633/139

T-mycoplasma. In spite of the fact that T-mycoplasma infections have received very little publicity, they are very common. This infection is not found in young adults who are virgins, but it has been found in over 40 percent of men, and over 70 percent of women, with three to five sexual partners. 636/164; 637/55 Recent research indicates that it is at least a temporary cause of infertility in women. 636/165,169 T-mycoplasma infections may also play a role in miscarriages. 636/165; 638/2

In men, T-mycoplasma infection is thought to cause some infertility problems as well as penile discharge, pain during urination, and itching. 636/169; 639/17; 637/57 Also in males it appears that this infection may lead to Reiter's Syndrome, which involves inflammation of the eye, or conjunctivitis, urethritis and arthritis. 637/57-58,63; 640/73 The arthritis in this syndrome can sometimes recur for years. 640/78

Scabies. Scabies is caused by a tiny, eight-legged mite. 641/111 While this infection is often contracted during sexual intercourse, it can be passed through non-sexual means. 641/112 Typically the female mite burrows into the skin of the infected individual to lay her eggs in areas of the body such as the male genitals, breasts, buttocks, armpits, wrists, elbows and near the naval. 641/112; 642/1248 Itchiness, which is thought to be due to the body's reaction to either the eggs or the mite's feces which are deposited in the skin, is often very marked at nighttime. 642/124B Fortunately, prescription lotions are effective in curing this particular infection.

Pediculosis pubis. Pediculosis pubis is an infection similar to scabies, but one that is caused by a tiny, wingless insect called a crab louse which is barely visible to the naked eye. 641/116-17 This louse has claws on the second and third pair of legs which allow it to hold onto pubic hairs while moving about. 641/118 Frequently there is a one-week to one-month delay between the infestation and the onset of symptoms, which involve itching that at times can be severe. 643/55; 641/118 This pubic louse feeds frequently on the blood of the infected individual by sticking its mouth down into tiny blood vessels. 641/118 Prescription lotions are frequently effective in the treatment of this infection. 641/120

* * *

From this brief review of some of the more significant sexually transmitted diseases, it is apparent that promiscuous or casual sexuality can lead to numerous problems. These problems not only involve the immediate symptoms of the disease, but also can create such long-term problems as infertility and cancer. No wonder Paul, inspired by the Holy Spirit, warned, "Flee from sexual immorality. All other sins a man commits are outside his body, but he who sins sexually sins against his own body." 644

Dr. McIlhaney explains the need for monogamous relationships in light of STDs:

> **If sex is avoided until marriage and then engaged in only in marriage, all these sexually transmitted diseases would be of no importance at all because they could not enter into a closed circle relationship between husband and wife.** Such an approach is not only not naive, it is also not moralizing, but it is now necessary. 297/28-30

More research is not the answer. "No matter how much money we pour into studies, we'll never completely control STDs medically because there'll always be a new one. The bottom line is changing behavior." 344/3510

Former Surgeon General Koop explained, "Sexual abstinence is a *very good idea* for youngsters of school age. Today–in the presence of the deadly AIDS epidemic–I think we, as adults, must step forward and help our children address the phenomenon of their own sexuality in a caring, developmental way." 442 Koop explained to the conference of school administrators, "For the rest of us . . . abstinence may not be the behavior of choice. What then? Then the next best thing is monogamy . . . one person, one mate; find someone to whom you can give your love and respect and trust . . . someone who will give the same in return . . . and stay with that person forever." 442

If we faithfully teach our teenagers about the devastating consequences of promiscuity, they will more clearly understand the value of virginity and abstinence in promoting a healthy life now and a healthy, happy, rewarding sex life in marriage.

CHAPTER 15

Strategy 3

Teach Moral Values

Hopefully by now you agree with me that sex education is neither value-free nor morally neutral. Even those programs which claim to be such are promoting certain moral values (e.g., "You're going to do it anyway, so wear a condom and protect yourself"; or, "You're the only one who can decide what's best for you sexually"). Values are being communicated; the question is, what values or whose should be communicated? **Should school-based sex education programs continue to ignore traditional moral values of sexual behavior while our kids stumble blindly through their relationships without a clue as to what's right and wrong?**

There is a growing number of educators and administrators who are answering that question with a resounding *no*. Educational consultant Dr. Dinah Richard says, "By the 1980s, many educators realized morality is not as subjective as people are sometimes led to believe and that sex education can reinforce parental values and societal norms." 206/570 Many agree that it's time to reinstate the teaching of moral values in conjunction with our sex education programs.

♦ Kids Need to Know Right From Wrong

Children have a psychological need to be taught positive values. Psychiatrist Melvin Anschell points out that "today's children and adolescents need an educational system that upholds the family . . . a morality that supports the struggle for existence and sustains civilized life, rather than undermining it." 26

The U.S. Department of Education issued a statement declaring that "the surest way to prevent the spread of AIDS in the teenage and young adult population is for schools and parents to *convey the reasons adolescents should be taught restraint in sexual activity. . . . The most important determinant of children's actions is their understanding of right and wrong* [emphasis mine]." 269

Dr. Dinah Richard observes that the educational movement which was designed to help our kids clarify their moral values has backfired:

> In the 1970s, values clarification became the main approach to sex education, and its traces can still be found in many courses, not simply in sex education. However, the values clarification approach usually did not result in students gaining a better awareness of their values. Instead it produced confusion over what are right and wrong behaviors and left students with the impression that ethics were situational. This form of education likewise has little meaning to it. 206/570

Dr. Frances Davis, M.D., sees the lack of values in the teens he works with:

> The teenagers I see in clinic are not ignorant of contraceptive use, but *they are ignorant of the value of sex beyond a biological event that brings self-gratification*. . . . Let's not sell our children short by spending millions of dollars on contraceptive awareness, but *let's take the time to plant principles, morals, and a vision for their future.* It is a higher price to pay but what we teach our children now will not only affect them but will influence generations to come [emphasis mine]. 295/IV-20

Steve Potter, a sex educator who has become curriculum coordinator for an abstinence-based program called Teen-Aid (see chapter 18–page 208), saw the need for teaching values after his experience of teaching a sex education program. Potter said the program "concentrated on the mechanics of birth control and . . . characterized sexual intercourse more as a biological act rather than as a profoundly meaningful human experience." 319

The U.S. Department of Education also saw the need to maintain a moral context when teaching young people about sex. Their directive about condoms stated:

> Any discussion of condoms must not undermine the importance of restraint and responsibility in the minds of young people. It is important to remember that condoms have long been widely available and that most teenagers know about them, yet the teen pregnancy rate has still risen. This is not only because condoms do fail, but also because teenagers who know about condoms often fail to use them. *Teenagers' beliefs and convictions about proper sexual behavior are more effective in shaping their behavior than mere knowledge about devices such as condoms.* Indeed,

promoting the use of condoms can suggest to teenagers that adults expect them to engage in sexual intercourse. This danger must be borne in mind in any discussion [emphasis mine]. 279

♦ A Surprising Turnaround

The cry for value-based, morally positive sex education is finding increasing support among nationally recognized authorities. The *Washington Post* recently reported a surprising and unusual consensus that the nation's schools abandon the value-free teaching approach which has been widely used for two decades:

> The consensus is that schools should . . . take clear positions on right and wrong behavior and personal morality—teaching, for example, that students should not engage in sex.
>
> This reconciliation of normally opposing camps was evident . . . when support for "values education" was voiced by such diverse leaders as California School Superintendent Bill Honig, District of Columbia Superintendent Floretta D. McKenzie, liberal television producer Norman Lear, former education secretary Terrel H. Bell and White House domestic policy adviser Gary L. Bauer.
>
> "After thirty or forty years of seeing the dangerous results," Honig said, "we are coming back together in consensus."
>
> "We have not done a good job in the last fifteen years in teaching values," Honig said. . . . "There has been a belief that pluralism means you can't take a stand. That is death to young people." . . .
>
> School superintendent Floretta McKenzie said she began her career believing schools neither could nor should teach values. "I have taken a 180-degree turn on that matter," she said. "I don't think we can separate out the teaching of values from public education." . . .
>
> The consensus of the educators was that **"schools cannot teach values adequately by simply adding a course on the subject, but must weave lessons of virtue and morality throughout the curriculum."**
>
> "Teaching values does not mean asking children to write 'I shall not lie' 1,000 times," said Bauer, former chairman of the Working Group on the Family and a former undersecretary of education. "Morality should be implicit in whatever subject a teacher is teaching." 319

In his book, *Sexuality Education: An Evaluation of Programs and Their Effects,* Dr. Douglas Kirby summarizes the reason for this consensus shift: **"When specific values were not clear goals of the course, there is much less evidence that sex education had any impact upon the students."** 318 (See also 204/595.) We must return to teaching values because value-free sex education isn't working.

♦ Values to Be Taught

According to Eunice Kennedy Shriver, moral values are critical to effective sex education. She claims that, second only to creating a network of supportive adults, the most important step toward positive healthy sex education is to "emphasize the affirmation of moral values, building self-esteem, strengthening family relationships, providing education, preparing for jobs, and the assumption of personal responsibility for the results of one's actions." Cited in 109

Margaret Whitehead, co-founder of the Educational Guidance Institute, believes that sex education should not be limited to the physical dimension of a teen's life. Rather, teaching about sex should relate to the whole person and his or her values. Whitehead states:

> There are five aspects of a whole person: the intellectual, the physical, the spiritual, the emotional and the social. A successful sex education program should deal with the spiritual aspect *which includes questions of right and wrong and whether there is a greater meaning to life,* the emotional aspect which includes the need for mature people to control their emotions and feelings, and the social aspect which includes how friendships are developed and how the person interacts with the community [emphasis mine]. 292

Dr. James Dobson, psychologist, author and former associate clinical professor of pediatrics at the University of Southern California, comments on the dangerous separation of sexual physiology and sexual morality:

> I have been strongly opposed to sex education courses as they are usually taught in public schools. The typical program attempts to teach the technology of sex without discussing the morality of sex. In my opinion, these components should never be separated. When you teach physiology and facts without ethical consideration, it's like showing a kid how to shoot a pistol without telling him where to aim it. I think a well-designed sex education program in a school could make a valuable contribution, but it would have to incorporate more than "how to." 282/3

♦ The Impact of Church Attendance

When considering the importance of teaching values and morality in sex education, the impact of church attendance cannot be ignored. Advocates of value-based sex education are not saying that public school programs should *promote* church attendance. However, **considering the positive influence church attendance has had on curbing teen sexual activity, in no way should any teacher, school, curriculum or program** *discourage* a teen's involvement in church. Consider the following evidence.

A study by Marsiglio and Mott discovered that the strongest determinants of first intercourse at the age of 15 are:

(1) church attendance no more than several times a year;
(2) parental education of fewer than twelve years;
(3) black race.

They discovered that at age 16, any combination of these variables plus several others (e.g., having a fundamentalist Protestant upbringing, or being an economically disadvantaged white) all have stronger effects than does prior exposure to a sex education course. 140/151,158-60

According to a 1986 Lou Harris/Planned Parenthood poll, 79 percent of young people who frequently attend religious services have never had sexual intercourse. 27 The National Research Council reports that young people who hold strong religious views are less likely to become sexually active. 236/17 And in his famous 1948 report, Dr. Alfred Kinsey found a direct correlation between being "actively connected with church activities" and abstaining from non-marital intercourse. 237

After scrutinizing all the studies, Dr. Jacqueline Kasun observed that regular church attendance is the strongest positive influence on the sexual behavior of girls over the age of 17. 380 Her conclusions are confirmed by the 1986 Lou Harris Poll for Planned Parenthood. PPFA's own research, performed by Dr. Deborah Anne Dawson, agrees that "church attendance one or more times a week reduces the odds of first coitus at all ages." 141/162-63

The Why Wait? Teen Sex Survey in the Evangelical Church showed that 21 percent of those who attended church regularly had had intercourse, compared to 37 percent who considered themselves "religious" but did not attend church regularly. Students who identified themselves as "born again" had an even lower rate of intercourse: 19 percent—as compared to 49 percent on the low side and 65 percent on the high side for the teenage population as a whole. 410

The results of a study by Garris, Steckler and McIntire should cause serious concern about the reverse effect of school-based health clinics on the religious interests of teens. They discovered in a California test clinic that there was a disturbing shift away from religion among the teens they served. When asked at the beginning of the family planning program to respond to the statement, "I enjoy participating in religious studies," only 39.6 percent disagreed. But after six to eight months involvement in the clinic's program, 56.2 percent disagreed. These clinics may claim to be value-free and morally neutral, but they are producing negative attitudes about religion which are counterproductive to positive influences on teen sexual behavior.

♦ Morality Is Not Fanaticism

William Raspberry, syndicated columnist for the *Washington Post,* seriously questions the critic of value-based sex education who accuses chastity advocates of being fanatics. I want to close this chapter with his response to this narrow view:

> There is a tendency among liberals to cast opponents of public school sex education into the same bag as book-burners, creationists and religion-in-school advocates.
>
> Obviously, some people subscribe to all these things. But it occurs to me that one can have reservations regarding sex education, as it is frequently handled, without being automatically eligible for membership in the Flat Earth Society.
>
> Like my liberal friends, I have trouble understanding people who seem to suppose that sexual ignorance promotes chastity. Like my conservative friends, *I have trouble with the notion that sex education can be properly taught without also teaching at least the rudiments of morality.* I'm not talking about the biology of human reproduction, which can be taught in a morally neutral context. School children ought to be taught "where babies come from," how they develop and so on. But **I have grave doubts about the wisdom of teaching teenagers about their own sexuality without teaching them something as well of the morality of sexual activity.** 294

Mr. Raspberry also takes issue with those who propagate the concept that abstinence is a religious subject:

> There seem to be one-and-one-half arguments against the teaching of morality in the public schools. The one is that morality is indistinguishable from religion and, as such, has no place in the public schools. I suppose I would buy the argument if I knew religions that advocate promiscuity or theft or murder or the other things that the society generally considers immoral. But it seems to me that *there are moral precepts that are held by adherents of all faiths—even by agnostics and atheists—and that these include strictures against adolescent sex.* I find it hard to imagine a religious group that would be offended by a public school teacher who told her students it was better to postpone sex until marriage.
>
> The half argument is that a classroom may include children whose own parents were never married and that it is, therefore, not possible to describe premarital or extramarital sex as immoral without condemning the parents of these children. But we are talking moral advice, not condemnation, and my guess is that even *unwed parents would prefer their children postpone sexual activity at least until they are mature enough to handle it.* In short, I don't see moral instruction as offensive to anyone [emphasis mine]. 294

As a health teacher and educator, Coleen Mast correctly observes, "Contraceptives are a poor substitute for the difficult and costly work of teaching adolescents to be responsible adults who can make moral distinctions. . . . How are adolescents to learn self-control, fidelity, responsibility and moral courage when so many adults fail to teach and model such qualities themselves?" 202/550-51

Mast is very realistic when she observes, "[Adolescents] deserve moral support and encouragement because remaining chaste is not easy in the face of so many biological and cultural forces pressuring them to have sex. They need a sex education program that will bring out the best in them." 202/547

Based on all evidence presented, if we are sincerely concerned about reducing teen promiscuity and pregnancy we should immediately and unashamedly return moral values to sex education curriculum and not discourage our young people from church attendance.

Don't be swayed by the statistics and warnings by PPFA and many sexologists that teens are irrevocably involved sexually and it doesn't matter what you teach, kids are going to do it anyway. Many studies show that about half of the 18-year-olds have not had sexual intercourse. (B. C. Miller, "Teenage Pregnancy: A Comparison of Certain Characteristics Among Utah Youth," Utah State Office of Education, 1981; Melvin Zelnik and John F. Kanter, unpublished tabulations from the National Longitudinal survey of youth, 1983, as cited in Barrett Mosbacker, "Teen Pregnanacy and School-Based Health Clinics," Washington, D.C.: Family Research Council, Aug. 1986 8; U.S. House Select Committee on Children, Youth, and Families, "Teen Pregnancy: What Can Be Done? A State-by-State Look," Washington, D.C.: GPO, 1986 395; C. D. Hayes, "Risking the Future: Adolescent Sexuality, Pregnancy, and Childbearing," National Research Council, 1987, pp. 54-55 186; and the Why Wait? Teen Sex Survey in the Evangelical Church by Barna Research Group, 1987.)

It is also important to note that many who have had sex have had only one partner, or just one experience. Among black adolescents sexual activity is actually decreasing.

Not only do teenagers *need* moral values, but most of them also *want* a value-based sex education. In the 1987 Survey of High Achievers by *Who's Who Among American High School Students,* 59 percent of the girls and 49 percent of the boys stated that the discussion of values and morals in sex education would be valuable help to students in deciding about having sex. 27

CHAPTER 16

➧ A **key section** for busy parents.

Strategy 4

Teach Abstinence

Dr. Dinah Richard, who consults with schools on abstinence programs, defines abstinence-based sex education:

> It teaches that human behavior, including the sex drive, is controllable and that the sex act itself is a beautiful expression of love properly occurring between a husband and wife. Besides the unitive role of sex, the procreative aspect within a marriage is presented as an exciting event that brings forth new life. Abstinence education helps teens realize that sex in the wrong context will result in unfortunate consequences. By stressing avoidance, teens can enjoy greater freedoms in their present and future lives. 206/574

For abstinence education to be accomplished effectively, the commitment to teach it must be long-term, and the abstinence education program must be designed to achieve long-term goals.

- Is teaching abstinence merely preaching to kids that sex is bad?

Dr. Richard very pointedly resists that notion:

> Many teachers believe that abstinence education is simply preaching to kids and not teaching them about issues related to sexuality. Actually, however, **abstinence education is factual sexuality instruction placed within a moral context.** It covers information about human anatomy and development, pressures to be sexually active, consequences of sexual activity, resisting the pressures to become involved in sex, freedoms that accompany abstinence, building positive friendships, appropriate dating behaviors, resolving conflict, communication with parents, future

plans, marriage, parenting and family life. It covers many of the same topics found in other sex education courses, but differs in the direction the teacher leads the students and the perspective it offers on the issues. 206/573

♦ Teens and Parents Want Abstinence Education

- Is abstinence education unpopular with teens and parents because of its stringency or narrow moral focus?

Not according to Dr. Richard. **"Because abstinence is the only 100-percent effective means of preventing pregnancy and the spread of sexually transmitted disease, abstinence education is quite attractive from a health perspective."** 206/573

- Is it unrealistic to believe that abstinence will have an impact on the teenage pregnancy rate?

Again, Dr. Richard responds, "Studies indicate that abstinence education has changed the attitudes and behaviors of teens and has helped reduce the pregnancy rate." 206/573

- Will teaching abstinence offend parents who are themselves promiscuous? Should schools exempt from abstinence education students whose parents do not reflect that lifestyle?

As an educator who strongly believes in parental involvement, Richard says:

> Even parents whose own lifestyle is not consistent with the theme of abstinence education tend to agree that their own children should be taught self-restraint. But even if some parents disagree, the school's role is to teach young people about the healthiest choices in life. Though some parents might drive recklessly, abuse alcohol or perhaps use drugs, schools nevertheless are obligated to promote the safest behaviors, regardless of whether or not some adults serve as poor role models. 206/573

One study shows **parents want three major values instilled in their children: self-restraint, compassion and commitment.** 411 These three values form the basis of abstinence education. Former Secretary of Education William Bennett points out that another study shows "70 percent of adults want their children taught sex education from the morally based abstinence perspective." 316/162

Bennett adds, "Not only do parents want this perspective, teachers likewise want abstinence to be the focus of instruction. . . . And in spite of what people might think about today's teens, nine out of ten of them indicated that they want help in resisting pressures to be sexually active." 316/164

That sex educators lack an understanding of the value of abstinence is obvious in the Mathtech study funded by the U.S. Centers for

Disease Control and authored by Douglas Kirby, et al. The executive summary of the study, *An Analysis of U.S. Sex Education Programs and Evalution Methods,* lists their goals (notice, **not one mention of abstinence, or of its being, in any way, a desired goal of sex education**):

> The goals of sex education are both numerous and varied. A sampling of them follows:
>
> - To provide accurate information about sexuality.
> - To facilitate insights into personal sexual behavior.
> - To reduce fears and anxieties about personal sexual developments and feelings.
> - To encourage more informed, responsible, and successful decision making.
> - To encourage students to question, explore, and assess their sexual attitudes.
> - To develop more tolerant attitudes toward the sexual behavior of others.
> - To facilitate communication about sexuality with parents and others.
> - To develop skills for the management of sexual problems.
> - To facilitate rewarding sexual expression.
> - To integrate sex into a balanced and purposeful pattern of living.
> - To create satisfying interpersonal relationships.
> - To reduce sex-related problems such as venereal disease and unwanted pregnancies. **669/3**

The "executive summary" acknowledges that the various sex education programs "do not appear to affect the students' personal values which guide their own behavior." **669/7**

However, they admit that the programs "tend to increase the students' tolerance of the sexual practices of others." **669/7**

The research showed that with near unanimity the professionals believe the discouragement of all premarital sexual activity is not important. Some [professionals] even volunteered that such discouragement was counterproductive." **669/9**

♦ Learning Self-control

The U.S. House Select Committee on Children, Youth and Families honed in on the real problem of teenage pregnancy. They expressed several key insights about society dealing with–and not dealing with–the adolescent crisis:

> Why does the problem seem so much more difficult in this generation? Are babies born today different from babies born 50 years ago? Or is the difference in the adults who are raising them? Or is it truer to say that we have abandoned them? Teaching our children to be adults is perhaps the

most difficult job we have. *Teaching them self-control, respect for themselves and others, fidelity, courage and patience requires constant and tireless efforts* [emphasis mine]. 283

I believe the only long-term program that will turn young people around is one that provides a sound basis for abstinence. To some people that may sound hopelessly naive, but sex and the family will never be restored to their rightful place in our society until we help young people control sexual activity and stop merely trying to prevent pregnancies or live births. Ellie Tottie comments:

> The thrust of teaching the young about sex should be to instruct them that there is strength in restraint and that freedom is not doing what you want but what you ought. Parents must teach their children the need to say no, because the unwillingness or inability to say that little word makes us slaves to others and, still worse, slaves to our passions and fears. 45/A8

Learning to say no is a mark of maturity. The subject came up one day when my two oldest children, Sean and Kelly, who are in their early teens as I write this, teamed up on me. Their question was, "How old do we have to be before we can date?"

As part of my reply I said, "You are not ready to date until I believe you have developed the character and moral maturity to go out on a date with someone you really like, and when that person pressures you sexually, you can look him or her straight in the eyes and say no, and then act upon it. If I don't think you can do that, I wouldn't be a truly loving, caring father if I let you date." Amazingly, they agreed with me.

A large part of maturity is the ability to postpone immediate satisfaction. We must help our young people learn to do that when it comes to their sexuality.

Those who promote comprehensive sex education don't have the same agenda. Their goal is not to help kids say no, but to prevent unwanted pregnancies. Faye Wattleton, president of Planned Parenthood, states, **"We are not going to be an organization promoting celibacy or chastity. Our concern is not to convey 'shoulds' and 'should nots,'** but to help young people make responsible decisions about their sexual relationships. . . . *We've got to be more concerned about preventing teen pregnancies than we are about stopping sexual relationships* [emphasis mine]. 296 Ironically, there is a direct correlation between stopping teenage sexual relationships and stopping teenage pregnancies.

One of the finest summations on the need for implementing abstinence programs is from Coleen Mast, the developer of the effective abstinence-based program called Sex Respect (see chapter 18, page 202):

> Sex education should defend the institution of family by helping students understand that maturity and responsibility must be prerequisites to parenthood. It should point out that if they are not ready for commitment and fidelity in marriage, they are not ready for parenthood. If they are not ready for parenthood, they are not ready for sex. 202/546

Teaching kids to say no to promiscuity is also the only proven way to keep them from contracting sexually transmitted diseases. Former Surgeon General Koop and former Secretary of Education Bennett issued a joint statement outlining the importance of abstinence in combatting AIDS:

> An AIDS education that accepts children's sexual activity as inevitable and focuses only on "safe sex" will be at best ineffectual, at worst itself a cause of serious harm. Young people should be taught that the best precaution is abstinence until it is possible to establish a mutually faithful monogamous relationship. 270

There are numerous benefits to be enjoyed by the teenager who learns to abstain from premarital sex. In Part Four you will find a chapter listing 28 positive reasons teens should practice abstinence and parents, schools, sex education programs and churches should teach abstinence.

♦ Abstinence Works

Dr. Douglas Kirby, a comprehensive sex education researcher, of the research group ETR and the Center for Population Options, concluded that

> programs clearly emphasizing specific values, and especially those designed for younger youth that emphasize abstinence, may be effective. The research in several fields including smoking and drug abuse also suggests that "value-free" approaches may be less effective, and that programs emphasizing important, widely held values may be more effective. 204/601-602

The journal of the American Medical Society published the results of a study from an area of South Carolina reporting both high rates of sexual activity and pregnancy. The study, concentrating on an educational goal of teaching premarital abstinence, showed a significant and sustained decrease in pregnancies in a population depicted as high-risk for teenage pregnancy. 285/3382

Many in the medical profession are beginning to see the medical and emotional benefits of advocating and teaching abstinence to teens. The American Medical Association's House of Delegates has developed "policy positions that favor chastity as a prophylactic measure. . . . The delegates endorsed 'abstinence' for single people and 'fidelity and continence' [Note: *continence* means self-restraint or the ability to refrain from some bodily activity] for married couples." 284

In 1984 the California Medical Association (CMA) passed a resolution titled "RX: Adolescent Abstinence." The resolution recognized that unwanted teen pregnancy is a serious problem and that the California Medical Association ought to support teens who want to say no to premarital sex by providing health education activities for them. The resolution concluded:

> **Be it resolved** that CMA recognizes that premarital abstinence is an effective means of precluding unwanted pregnancy; and be it further resolved that CMA suggests that the media, appropriate public agencies and all concerned professional groups, in their educational campaigns to the public, emphasize the effectiveness of premarital abstinence as a means of reducing the incidence of unwanted pregnancy. 286

A similar resolution was adopted by the Texas Pediatric Society on May 17, 1987, to be forwarded to the American Academy of Pediatrics (AAP) as of September 1987:

> **Whereas**, over one million teenage girls become pregnant each year, and
> **Whereas**, the incidence of sexually transmitted disease in the adolescent population remains a major health concern – herpes and AIDS currently have no cure and venereal warts are recognized as carcinogenic viruses – and
> **Whereas**, teen use of contraceptives has been shown to be unreliable, and
> **Whereas**, abortion with its immediate and long-range health consequences is a poor method of birth control, and
> **Whereas**, the AAP should set an example for media, public agencies and concerned professional groups,
> **Be It Resolved**, that the AAP recommends that adolescents postpone, until marriage, sexual activities that may lead to pregnancy or sexually transmitted diseases. 109/11-12

Increasing numbers of national and state legislators and policy-makers are recognizing the need to present an abstinence-based message in sex education. When Congress passed the Adolescent Family Life Act in 1981, "it did so with the clear intention of promoting abstinence to teenagers." 206/570

Many states are beginning to realize not only the medical and emotional value of abstinence, but also the educational value. California's Superintendent of Public Instruction and Board of Education have issued guidelines for family life/sex education which affirm sexual abstinence outside the context of marriage: "Sex education programs which do not emphasize sexual abstinence are inconsistent with society's concern for reducing unwanted teenage pregnancy, AIDS and other sexually transmitted diseases."

Then California Senate Bill 2394 added Section 51551 to the Education Code. It reads:

> All public elementary, junior high and senior high school classes that teach sex education and discuss sexual intercourse shall emphasize

100-percent effective against unwanted teenage pregnancy, sexually transmitted diseases and acquired immune deficiency syndrome (AIDS). . . . All material and instruction in classes that teach sex education and discuss sexual intercourse shall be age appropriate.

Course material and instruction shall stress that abstinence is the only contraceptive method which is 100-percent effective, and that all other methods of contraception carry a risk of failure in preventing unwanted teenage pregnancy. Statistics based on the latest medical information shall be provided to pupils, citing the failure and success rates of condoms and other contraceptives in preventing pregnancy.

Course material and instruction shall stress that pupils should abstain from sexual intercourse until they are ready for marriage.

Course material and instruction shall teach honor and respect for monogamous heterosexual marriage. 288

The Illinois General Assembly passed a strong abstinence law on October 31, 1989. The principle features of the new Illinois Sex Education and Family Life Education law are:

All public elementary, junior high and senior high school classes that teach sex education and discuss sexual intercourse shall emphasize that abstinence is the expected norm in that abstinence from sexual intercourse is the only protection that is 100-percent effective against unwanted teenage pregnancy, sexually transmitted diseases and acquired immune deficiency syndrome (AIDS) when transmitted sexually.

Course material and instruction shall teach honor and respect for monogamous heterosexual marriage. . . .

Course material and instruction shall stress that pupils should abstain from sexual intercourse until they are ready for marriage. . . .

Course material and instruction shall include a discussion of the possible emotional and psychological consequences of preadolescent and adolescent sexual intercourse outside of marriage and the consequences of unwanted adolescent pregnancy. . . .

Course material and instruction shall stress that sexually transmitted diseases are serious possible hazards of sexual intercourse.

Course material and instruction shall advise pupils of the laws pertaining to their financial responsibility to children born in and out of wedlock.

Course material and instruction shall advise pupils of the circumstances under which it is unlawful for males to have sexual relations with females under the age of 18 to whom they are not married. 289

Parents in Illinois schools have the right to examine the instructional materials "and to remove their children from all comprehensive sex or family life courses or AIDS instruction without action against the student by the school." 289

♦ Teach for Behavioral Change

The value-free, morally neutral approach to sex education advocated by so many today starkly contrasts the way our nation responds to other problems which threaten individuals with pain and death. The staff of the Department of Education, in response to questions on safe sex, observed,

> With lung cancer, for example, we seek to motivate people to stop smoking, not merely to protect themselves with filters. Moreover, we focus the messages primarily on behavioral change (in that case, stopping smoking), only secondarily on making smokers more knowledgeable about lung cancer. 225

The same message of behavioral change—namely forsaking promiscuity and contraception for abstinence—needs to implemented with our teens.

> Similarly with drugs we teach our young people to "just say no," rather than accepting their habit and encouraging them to practice 'safe drugs.' (In some cases, even this is changing, toward the teaching of 'safe' drug use, as in a large city where the health department advises drug users about how they can clean their needles). 225

Principal Joe DeDiminicantonio of the San Marcos (California) Junior High School said, "A knee-jerk reaction to the problem of teenage pregnancies would be to haul all the girls into one gym and all the boys into another gym, show them some movies and to tell them where to buy prophylactics. But what we really want to do is change behaviors and influence attitudes, and that will take some time." San Marcos Junior High saw a phenomenal drop in teenage pregnancies after implementing an abstinence-based, self-worth enhancing sex education program. (The San Marcos program is more fully explained in chapter 18—Strategy 6—p. 211.)

"Premarital abstinence," writes S. DuBose Ravenal, M.D.,

> must be taught as the norm, as the only safe, effective way to prevent teen pregnancies, and as in the case of drug education, not compromised just because some will persist in the behavior despite the best efforts to dissuade them. . . . For the sexually active, resumption of abstinence is not only possible, but often welcomed and successfully adopted when teens are presented a clear, uncompromising message. 287

Our "clear, uncompromising message" to teens must include that they make a behavioral change in the face of all the pressure to conform to society's declining moral standards.

A couple approached me with a pointed question I have heard from countless numbers of starry-eyed college students: "We love each other; we're engaged and we're going to get married next year. The pressure to have sex is so great. Should we wait?" Their expressions mirrored the sincerity of their inquiry.

I responded to them as I have to so many others, "I definitely encourage you to wait. Of all those I've counseled to wait, so many of those who didn't ended up deeply regretting getting sexually involved. They've confessed to me that they wish they had waited. However, of all those who did wait, I cannot recall one person who later said, 'I wish I hadn't.' "

States are beginning to uphold the standard of abstinence in sexuality programs and AIDS instruction: Illinois, Indiana, Washington, California, Rhode Island, Florida, etc. 371

Illinois requires that "public school sex courses teach sexual abstinence until marriage as 'the expected norm' and honor and respect for monogamous heterosexual marriage." H.B. 2634 was passed over Governor James Thompson's veto by large majorities in both houses (94-12 in the House and 38-14 in the Senate) and took effect immediately.

The most controversial portion of the new statute is the requirement for "evaluating and measuring effectiveness" of all sex and family life courses used in Illinois. 289/1

What is amazing (and is true in almost every situation nationwide) is that "despite the tens of millions of dollars that Illinois taxpayers have poured into such programs through both the schools and the public health and welfare agencies to combat the high rate of teenage pregnancy, no evaluation of results has ever been made.

"The state-funded agencies fought bitterly against H.B. 2634, saying that 'the stress on abstinence was unnecessary.' They were strongly against any evaluation requirement."

CHAPTER 17

Strategy 5

Eliminate Mixed Messages About Abstinence

A pregnancy prevention strategy must send a clear, consistent message about the acceptability or unacceptability of adolescent sexual behavior. No pregnancy prevention program can be expected to work if it sends a mixed message or if the surrounding culture undermines its message. Indeed, the effectiveness of any program is largely dependent on the consistency of its message.

What is a mixed message? Margaret Whitehead, founder of the Educational Guidance Institute, says, "Sex education programs that say 'Don't have sex; but if you do, use a contraceptive' are conveying a double message that undercuts the desired message about sexual abstinence." 292 Whitehead cites an example of her concern:

> "What can people do to make sure they don't get it [AIDS]?" asks an AIDS curriculum that many high schools use. The curriculum supplies "two simple rules" as answers. Its first is, "Don't take any body fluids directly into your body during any kind of sexual intercourse. Use condoms (rubbers)—they are able to stop the AIDS virus when used correctly." The other is, "Don't share needles for IV drugs or tattoos ever." Neither says, "Abstain from sex." 292

Whitehead stresses, **"In order to influence children's behavior, parents and teachers need to provide a clear and consistent message in support of premarital abstinence**. . . . Kids say they need help and support for saying 'no'; instead, adults are making contraceptives available [emphasis mine]." 292

♦ Emotional Starvation

The mixed message, which is really a recommendation for contraception, harms teens both physically and emotionally. First, due to the statistical failure rate of all contraceptives except abstinence, the mixed message can result in physical complications that teens didn't bargain for: pregnancy, cervical cancer, abortion, unwanted birth or sexually transmitted disease.

Second, the mixed message almost always results in emotional starvation. Kids need to escape their loneliness and find acceptance and security through love, but too often these needs are confused with what the surrounding culture presents as the "need" for sex. Even when kids are successful at the game of sexual roulette (they have sex and beat the odds against pregnancy and STDs), they still come away from the encounter with their needs unmet. Coleen Mast compares this experience to people who eat junk food:

> There are enough calories in a can of pop and a bag of potato chips to satisfy one's hunger. But these foods do not meet the individual's nutritional needs. Usually, the result is that one eats more and more junk food to satisfy these needs. While a person may certainly feel full after eating junk food, such a diet will, in fact, leave him undernourished. In the same way, the deep human need for love cannot be met by sex alone—even by "protected" sex. Too often people seek to fill their need for love with "junk food," more partners and a greater variety of sexual experience, only to find frustration, emptiness, and self-destruction. **Contraception contributes to the confusion between a perceived need for sex and the true need for love and acceptance.** 315

Other psychological and emotional consequences of premarital sex can be equally serious. These include feelings of guilt, fear, self-hatred, doubt, disappointment, the pain of exploiting or being exploited by another person, and the stunting of growth in personal identity and social relationships. Teens may be successful at preventing pregnancy during promiscuity, but **there's no such thing as a condom for the mind and the heart which are always vulnerable to great injury when the message about premarital sex is unclear.**

♦ Vulnerable to Bonding

Many teens are surprised and sobered to learn that contraceptives also offer no protection against the powerful emotional bonding that takes place during sexual intercourse. The sensations and emotions that intercourse stimulates leave a deep impression on the memory. A person retains memories of the sex partner, the circumstances and the emotions long after intercourse has taken place and the relationship has dissolved. In marriage, the experience and memories of intercourse create a desire in the partners to know each other more completely, to maintain and deepen their relationship. Outside the commitment of marriage, the emotional bonding from sex can have devastating effects.

The student workbook for Sex Respect, an abstinence-based sex education program, points out:

> Premarital sex can prolong an infatuation by giving a couple the illusion of knowing and caring about each other more than they actually do. Unmarried couples are also apt to become so engrossed in their physical relationship that other aspects of the relationship cannot develop. Indeed, sexual activity can even become a way to avoid any other kind of intimacy. Teens who are involved in a sexual relationship can easily be fooled into marrying the wrong person for this very reason; the pleasure and emotional bonds that result from intercourse blind them to the emptiness and lack of meaningful communication in the relationship. 315

Teens involved in premarital sex get caught in a "double bind." Either they marry for the wrong reasons, or they break up instead of marrying, in which case they face the overwhelming pain of tearing their sexual/emotional bond. "Some teens will try to ease the pain by quickly entering another relationship," writes Coleen Mast,

> only to discover that the new relationship is plagued by memories of the previous one. If the new relationship ends, there is another rending of the sexual bond. Each time the bond is torn, the ability to bond becomes weaker. That ability cannot be fully restored even after the person wants to establish a lasting relationship in marriage. 315

Others will feel fearful of becoming vulnerable in another relationship and will hold back part of themselves. The inability to trust another contributes to making sex nothing more than a momentary pleasure. When two people cannot share themselves completely, intercourse loses its deepest meaning, and it may not be restored even within marriage, when the partners want sex to be something special again.

♦ Fighting the Wrong Enemy

Coleen Mast writes:

> By offering teens a mixed message, adults enjoy the illusion that they are taking effective action against the rising number of illegitimate births among teens. Like the bull in a bullfight, who spends all his energy attacking the matador's cape until the bull, weakened by repeated spear wounds from his actual enemy, receives the final, fatal blow, the concerned adults in our society have been distracted from the root of the problem by the babies being born to unmarried teens. Adults are spending a great deal of time, talent, energy and money trying to eliminate the unwanted babies. But the real enemy – the uncontrolled sexual desire in teens which is causing the babies – is not being addressed. Meanwhile our society is being wounded by the "spears" of death, disease, guilt, mental illness, sexual

boredom in marriage, immaturity, lack of commitment, abortion and social breakdown. Contraception is not the answer for sex education because illegitimate births are not the only problem.

Further, contraceptives reinforce the idea that adolescents are no better than animals, compelled to mate whenever they feel the sexual urge. By giving contraceptives to teens, adults are telling them that, although chastity is by far the best choice, teens probably won't be able to control themselves and therefore need contraceptives. Ironically, teens have responded to that implied message with an increase in both pregnancies and abortions since contraceptives have become widely available.

The sad lesson many teens have learned is that **sexual gratification, even when it is experienced repeatedly, is not the same as sexual fulfillment.** Contraception, technology's despairing answer to adolescent sexual activity, has intensified the loneliness, frustration and emptiness of our young people. Their anguish can be seen in the alarming statistics on drug and alcohol abuse, pregnancy, sexually transmitted disease, abortion and suicide among teens. Contraceptives are no substitute for the difficult and costly work of teaching adolescents to be responsible adults capable of making moral choices. 315

♦ Broken Homes Equal Double Trouble

In an interview with Dr. Onalee McGraw, vice-president of Educational Guidance Institute, reporter Susan Olesak asked about the impact of the mixed message on teens from broken homes. She writes:

> When asked about teens without a stable, two-parent home, [McGraw] says that "they need clear guidance twice as much." The double message, recommending abstinence while teaching about birth control, "is infinitely worse for kids without family support. It is twice as important to present a clear, coherent message that it is better if you don't give in to urges, to kids without family support." 290

Ms. Olesak had good reason for asking the question. Research shows that girls from one-parent or divorced homes have a 60-percent greater chance of becoming sexually involved. 291/60 What Dr. McGraw was emphasizing is that teens from broken homes need an even greater emphasis on the why's and how's of abstinence.

In 1988 I visited several educational organizations in Washington, D.C. One group was preparing a national sex educational curriculum and brought together about fifty educators as consultants. When they began talking about the rising number of kids coming from broken homes, the curriculum developers said they didn't want to bring any undue pressure or hurt on these kids by promoting in their materials the traditional two-parent home. They were surprised when the educators urged them to hold up the traditional home as a healthy model. According to the consultants, kids from broken homes especially need the message that a monogamous marriage relationship is normal.

♦ Unnecessary Pressure

Dr. Dinah Richard warns about the undue pressure teens feel when they receive the mixed message that contraceptives are okay:

> Unfortunately, teens have the false notion that "everyone is doing it," and when educators promote contraceptives, they fuel this misconception. A Lou Harris poll showed that **the main reason teens have sex is perceived pressure. And when teachers begin to talk about contraceptives, they add to that pressure.** In the same poll, 87 percent of teens said that they did not want family-planning services on their campuses, and 72 percent did not even want the services near the school. 27/21-24; 71

They're asking for a clear message, but they aren't getting it.

The pressure continues on teens who have lost their virginity and who don't want to get sexually involved again. Dr. Richard says:

> Many teens who have had sex return to abstinence, usually because they fear pregnancy or want to avoid guilt or emotional hurt. This return is often called "secondary virginity," but it is a choice rarely mentioned in comprehensive sex education. When teachers promote contraceptives, they are passing up a prime opportunity to reach teens who are struggling with decisions. Instead of using the student's sense of guilt, hurt or fear as a pivotal point for changing behavior, the teacher is unknowingly trying to dismiss those feelings. 206/571-72

A number of educators, along with family planning groups such as Planned Parenthood, intentionally try to eradicate feelings of guilt and fear in young people by encouraging them to use contraceptives instead of practicing abstinence. Educational consultant Dr. Richard takes issue with those who promote this kind of "compliance-training":

> At compliance-training workshops, some educators, counselors and nurses receive instruction on how to get teens to comply with contraceptive usage. The intention of compliance-training is to learn how to get adolescents to recognize denial, overcome guilt about being sexually active and acknowledge their sexuality by acting responsibly. There are some major limitations to this type of approach, and professionals should take seriously its ethical implication when using it. Because the source of guilt for teens could be that their sexual activity conflicts with their parents' values, their religious upbringing and other factors that influence their morality, educators need to realize that they would be undermining the forces that could otherwise work to move students forward to abstinence. 380; 387

♦ It's Okay to Tell Them No

In an article covering a presentation by Margaret Whitehead, reporter Ed Bauer relates that Whitehead told of a 16-year-old girl

> who went to school personnel for help because she was pregnant. The girl was repeatedly told about contraceptives, *but was never told that she should*

stop having sexual relations because it could ruin her life. Whitehead said that some girls say they have premarital sexual relations because "no one ever told me not to." She believes that such girls are crying out for clear and consistent direction from responsible adults [emphasis mine]. 292

... [Whitehead] said that the most common objections to an abstinence-based program are that (1) the children won't respond to it, and (2) the parents won't get involved. She responded by referring to studies that show the failure of programs that use the "option" approach, which gives children the option of abstinence or using contraceptives.

She also described studies of drug education methods which show that mixed-message drug education programs didn't work. Significant success was achieved when a clear and consistent drug-abstinence message was taught. She said that these results would be as applicable to sex education as to drug education.

A result of presenting moral issues to children as being "options" is that children develop their own personal moral codes. Whitehead quoted Dr. Lillian Rubin, a sociologist and psychologist at the Institute for the Study of Social Change at the University of California at Berkeley as saying that teenagers today have "a sense that they alone call the shots on their sexual behavior." 292

Please keep in mind when teaching values and positive sexual behavior that students, especially leaders, carry a tremendous influence over their peers. Include students in the program presentation. The role of peers is critical. Douglas Kirby writes:

Adolescents can not only give classroom presentations, they also can help shape the program, design the materials, write letters to the school newspaper, conduct surveys of risk-taking behaviors, and serve as role models for responsible behavior. When many student leaders openly and consistently express norms against risk-taking behavior, schoolwide norms may change. 204/601

Though Kirby's reason for advocating student involvement is to promote contraception use, etc., student involvement can be even more powerful in promoting abstinence.

An essential characteristic of an effective sex education program must be to provide adolescents with clear and specific directions. Adolescents need a set of guidelines that will help them discover who they are and help them form healthy relationships. "Be careful" is not enough, nor is it enough to tell teens that premarital sex is acceptable if they are "ready" or "responsible," or if they "think through" their decision before taking action. We must not assume that an adolescent understands these concepts in the same way an adult would. We must instead provide information and directions that can be understood on the concrete level of reasoning.

CHAPTER 18

➧ A **key section** for busy parents.

Strategy 6

Implement Abstinence-Based Programs

The parents, educators and school board members who are unhappy with the philosophy and results of so-called value-free, morally neutral sex education in public schools have two possible alternatives. The first is to eliminate sex education from the public school system. Many argue that, since sex is such a personal and intimate subject, children should learn about it in a setting that embodies these same characteristics: the home. Why take the chance of infringing on the modesty, privacy and innocence of children by giving them information about sex in the secular public school setting?

This objection certainly applies to children up through age 12. When preteens learn about sex in a positive, healthy way from their parents, they also get the message that sex is a part of love and family. At this age level, children are better served by schools which provide training for their parents in how to teach their children at home about sex and sexuality.

However, adolescents benefit from receiving at least some of their sex education in the public school. Teens characteristically test and evaluate in the outside world what they have learned inside the home. They need to verify what their parents have taught them about truth and morality by checking it against what they hear from other authority figures, particularly teachers. Therefore the second alternative is to keep sex education in the schools, but change the content from value-free to value-based.

If sex education in the classroom presents positive moral values which promote physical, emotional and spiritual well-being, the school becomes an important ally to parents by reinforcing what many teens have already learned at home. Teens will be doubly equipped to make the decisions that will help them build moral character now and establish sound families of their own in the future. Those students whose home situation is morally negative in teaching and/or example will benefit even more from a value-based public school sex education curriculum.

♦ Evaluating Sex Education Curriculum

So where does a concerned, involved parent, educator or school board member begin? What kinds of questions must you ask in order to determine the appropriateness of an abstinence-based sex education course for public school use? Dr. Dinah Richard, who consults with schools and parent organizations on abstinence-based programs, provides a 30-question checklist for evaluating sex education programs and materials:

1. Are parents included in the school's process of setting policies and guidelines and of selecting materials?
2. Does the program have tangible means of direct parental involvement other than the superficial means of simply opting to have their children taken out of the class?
3. Are parents presented respectfully, as a valuable resource, as persons to turn to for help and as persons with whom to discuss sensitive issues?
4. Does the program have a moral perspective that teaches what is right and wrong, directing students toward the right choices?
5. Does the program use correct, not slang, terminology?
6. Does it teach that the sex drive is controllable and that abstinence is realistic?
7. Does it define abstinence as restraint from all sexual activity, not simply one form of intercourse?
8. Does the program use the phrase "premarital abstinence" rather than terms such as "postponing" or "delaying" sex (or premarital sex)?
9. Is abstinence presented as positive behavior and premarital sex as destructive behavior?
10. Does the program refute the myth that "everybody is doing it"?

11. Does the program promote secondary virginity?
12. Does the program teach the techniques of saying no?
13. Does the program present the tragic physical as well as emotional consequences of premarital sex?
14. Is the program free of double messages? Does the program omit a discussion or demonstration of contraceptive devices?
15. Does the program refute the notion of "safe sex," telling students about contraceptive failure?
16. When questions about alternative lifestyles or deviant behaviors are brought up, does the instructor refrain from discussion, referring students to their parents for information instead?
17. Is the latency period (elementary school age) protected?
18. Do materials avoid sexually explicit content?
19. Is the word "marriage" used rather than "monogamous relationship"?
20. Is marriage presented as a legal, moral and spiritual commitment?
21. Is sex presented as a favorable and enjoyable act occurring within marriage for unitive and procreative purposes?
22. Are love, fidelity, and commitment presented as standards within marriage?
23. Is the family defined as a blood or legal relationship?
24. Is pregnancy presented as an exciting event within a marriage?
25. Is the family presented as a source of love, nurturing and stability?
26. Does the program respect the student's privacy and the family's privacy?
27. Do materials and films use positive role models instead of pop stars?
28. Is the teacher an appropriate role model?
29. Are students asked to portray or write about only wholesome topics?
30. Are all materials age-appropriate? **206/574,5**

Dr. Richard also suggests asking some fairly pointed questions of the school board and school administration:

1. Has the school stepped back and taken an objective look at the various approaches to teaching sex education?
2. Has it determined the basis on which it will choose a particular approach?

3. Does the approach have a sound rationale?
4. Has the school devised a strategy for allowing the greatest amount of community input?
5. Has it developed a procedure for carefully evaluating all materials before implementing them?
6. Has it devised a system for assessing the extent to which the program is working?
7. Is it willing to make changes? 206/577-78

By answering these important questions up front, schools will find that they will be forced to develop a strategy. That strategy will help them attract parents as allies and establish an effective abstinence-based sex education program.

There are two general approaches to affecting teen sexual behavior with abstinence-based programs. The **first** is a school-based approach and the **second** is a community-based approach. In the pages that follow, I want to acquaint you with two school-based programs–Sex Respect and Teen-Aid–and two community-based programs–The Challenge Program and Why Wait?

♦ Sex Respect

Sex Respect is a program for chastity education written from a public health perspective. This program provides logical arguments for the healthy practice of sexual abstinence and is being used by more than 1,000 public school districts throughout the country. Sex Respect is a positive, down-to-earth program that gives teens a clear message: Say no to premarital sex and yes to love. This course, by health educator Coleen Mast, was created in 1983 as a curriculum project under the auspices of the Committee on the Status of Women (directed by Kathleen Sullivan). The project was part of the program for Mast's master's degree in Health Education. In the fall of 1985, the Sex Respect curriculum was selected by the Department of Health and Human Services, Office of Adolescent Pregnancy Programs, to receive a $300,000 grant for studying the effects of teaching chastity in junior high and high school students.

The effectiveness of the Sex Respect program testifies to the fact that adolescents do respond when the truth about sex is presented clearly and positively. While not much data is yet available about behavioral changes in students who have taken the Sex Respect course, attitudinal changes have been demonstrated. Out of 1,841 students from six Midwestern states who completed the course, only 20 percent indicated at the outset that they could "always" control their sexual feeling. At the end of the course, this figure rose to 39 percent. The percentage of students who indicated sex is "all right as long as there's no resulting pregnancy" fell from 36 percent to 18 percent. There was also a 48-percent increase in the number of students who felt sex should be saved for marriage and an 80-percent decrease in those who "probably wouldn't say anything and just let sex happen."

Since attitudes form the basis for actions, attitude changes such as these can be expected to bring about similar changes in behavior.

For example, Ron Musgrave, principal of Bradley Bourbonnais Community High School, noted in an interview with syndicated columnist Mike McManus that **the teen pregnancy rate for his school declined 50 percent in the first three years Sex Respect had been taught in freshman health classes.** 315

Parental Involvement

The goal of Sex Respect is not to replace parents in sex education but to assist them in teaching their teens about sexuality. Parents are provided with their own workbooks which include the complete student text. The workbook includes helpful information about communicating with teens and contains assignments to be completed by parents and teens at home. These assignments open the way for deeper discussions between parent and child about specific moral values. The confidence-building materials encourage parents to talk to their teens about more controversial topics.

Sex Respect's emphasis on parental involvement has produced some extraordinary results. In one case a single mother and her older teenage daughter (who was sexually active) became interested in the Sex Respect course being taken by the eighth-grade daughter. By the end of the course all three had decided to support one another in keeping a pact to abstain from sex until marriage.

In another instance the father and mother of a teenage boy attended a parents' meeting introducing the Sex Respect course their son was about to take in school. The father was so impressed with the meeting that he went home and read the entire course text that same night. His verdict was, **"I only wish they'd had this kind of course when I was young."** He told his wife that the material covered by the text was so important that he couldn't afford not to be involved in working through the material with his son. Working together on Sex Respect assignments, the father and son developed a warmth and intimacy which had previously been lacking in their relationship. Their improved relationship also had a positive impact on the marriage and ultimately enabled the whole family to experience better communication and greater intimacy.

Sex Respect Topics

The Sex Respect course provides ample material to fill ten hours of classroom time covering the following topics.

Aspects of human sexuality. The program stresses that human sexuality is much more than biological. The subject of sexuality is treated respectfully and with dignity. Students are shown how to respect others, themselves and their own sexuality.

Parents who are concerned that their children's privacy and innocence will be offended in a sex education course are assured that the Sex Respect program seeks to protect the modesty of teens. For example, biological information is presented as a quick review of material already learned in science classes rather than being emphasized as the most important aspect of sex. Students are directed back to their parents for discussion about topics that are more controversial or sensitive such as masturbation, homosexuality and abortion. The program recognizes that parents are the experts in determining the level of understanding, sensitivity and maturity of their own child and guiding the discussion accordingly.

Mature love and sex. Instead of telling teens that premarital sex is okay as long as the couple love each other, Sex Respect tells teens that they must be mature in every respect–not just the physical–before they can handle a sexual relationship. The program emphasizes that it is only in the life-long commitment of marriage that sexual intercourse can bring fulfillment. Outside of marriage, sex has many negative emotional, psychological, physical, social and spiritual effects which can cause serious and often irreversible harm. Teens are also told that unless they are ready for fidelity and commitment in marriage, they aren't ready for parenthood. And if they aren't ready for parenthood, they aren't ready for sex.

How to say no to sex. Clear directions are given to help teens "just say no" to premarital sex. For example, the Sex Respect text lists ways to build self-confidence and assertiveness and provides an exercise that challenges students to think up effective responses to "lines" they might hear from members of the opposite sex. They are also shown how their speech, actions and personal appearance can say no to sex, and how a host of little decisions made during the course of a date can either lead toward or away from sexual activity. For example, a choice to drink on a date may weaken a teen's resolve and lead to later sexual activity. A decision not to watch a sexually explicit movie on a date may keep a couple from getting aroused and involved.

Students are taught that sex doesn't "just happen." It is the result of a number of little decisions made along the way. Throughout the Sex Respect course teens are challenged to think about the choices they will confront and plan their dates carefully instead of drifting aimlessly into sexual situations. Sex Respect emphasizes specific information about how to avoid the many pressures to engage in premarital sex that young people face.

Secondary virginity. For teens who are already sexually active, the course introduces the concept of "secondary virginity": the decision to stop premarital sexual activity. Sex Respect challenges students by reminding them that they are human, not animal, and humans have the ability to reason and to choose. A teen is capable of deciding not to engage in premarital sex at all. Even those teens who have made some poor decisions about their sexual behavior in the past can decide to practice abstinence in the future. Teens are advised that practicing secondary virginity is not easy, but that it is possible and tremendously rewarding.

A sexually active sophomore girl, whose unmarried mother was also promiscuous, confided in her health education teacher after the chapter on secondary virginity, "I never knew I could say no." Sex Respect helps teens realize they have the power to say no whether or not their virginity is intact, or whether or not they have positive sexual role models.

Other topics covered in the Sex Respect course are sexual freedom versus sexual impulsiveness, consequences of teenage sexual activity, and dating guidelines.

Challenged to Think

Throughout the text, students are challenged to think seriously about the issues of human sexuality and to respond in ways which help them make the concepts and language their own. One popular exercise, for example, challenges teens to make a critical evaluation of the music they listen to. Students are asked to evaluate the message of the music as it relates to such topics as love, lust, self-control and selfishness.

One freshman boy complained that his Sex Respect homework was hard. "I even had to think to do the exercises," he confessed. "In all my other classes, the answer to the first question is usually in the first paragraph, the second question is answered in a following paragraph, and so on. But for this course, I actually had to think about what I read and how it applied to me." Students soon discover that thinking isn't so difficult and that it can be a rewarding and confidence-building exercise.

Tapping Youthful Idealism

Another strong quality of the Sex Respect program is that it taps into the idealism of youth. Many teens are aware of sex-related mistakes made by their parents, older siblings and peers, and they want something better for themselves. A number of these young people recognize that they should wait until marriage to become sexually active. **They are looking for adults who will tell them that abstinence is the best choice and that it is possible to save sex for marriage.**

For example, one exercise appeals to teens' idealism by asking, "What are some of your goals for the next 10 years?" and "How might involvement in premarital sex prevent you from realizing these goals?" The chapter on parenthood explains that a healthy marriage is the ideal environment for raising children and points out the negative impact on children when they lack loving, caring parents—a situation which many teens have experienced themselves and wish to avoid when they have children of their own. Sex Respect is designed to bring out the best in teens and to give them higher moral standards to reach for.

Teens respond positively to Sex Respect's message that sex is good, not bad, when experienced in the right context. Early chapters explain that sexual intercourse is meant to express a union on the mental, social, emotional and spiritual levels as well as the physical. When the sexual union involves all these dimensions, both partners experience the fulfillment of their human need to love and to be loved. Idealistic teens are hungry to hear that their sexuality takes on its deepest meaning and offers its greatest fulfillment within marriage and that married sex is well worth waiting for.

A Sex Respect instructor tells the story of a 13-year-old girl in Texas whose big goal in life was to have a baby by the time she was 15 because the cousin she admired had done so. Her mother had been completely unable to dissuade her. When the girl took the Sex Respect course as a freshman, she was rather quiet and participated very little. When the course was completed, however, the girl's mother came to the teacher in tears to tell her that her daughter no longer wanted to have a baby and intended to wait for marriage before experiencing motherhood.

Sex Respect offers true sexual freedom to adolescents by providing clear information about human sexuality, clear motivation to remain a virgin or to change their behavior if they are not, and clear directions about how to achieve these goals.

Signs of Success

The Sex Respect course is changing lives, giving hope and helping people learn about and practice chastity, not through fear, but through understanding. In testimony before the Virginia General Assembly in February 1988, Dr. Joseph Zanga, pediatrician at the Medical College of Virginia and professor of pediatrics at Virginia Commonwealth University, stated:

> The Sex Respect program adopted at a number of our nation's schools . . . has had notable and noticeable success in reducing not just births to teenagers (often accomplished in other programs by increasing the number of abortions among teenagers), not just pregnancies among teenagers (often accomplished in other programs by increasing their use of birth control, thereby exposing them to other often deadly risks), but by decreasing their sexual experimentation—the only way we can ever hope to achieve success. 372

Participants in the program also had positive words to say about Sex Respect:

> This program doesn't just teach the students how not to get pregnant. It teaches that virginity is okay; it's okay to say no to sex [school principal in Illinois].
>
> I've already had a sexual relationship, but I'll choose secondary virginity after taking this course. Thank you! I feel better about myself now [high school girl in Missouri].
>
> I'm much more confident with a program that includes parental involvement [mother in California].
>
> My friends and I want you to know this program is great. We kind of thought it was okay to be a virgin, but we liked hearing why it's good to save sex for marriage [high school boy in Hawaii].
>
> I'm delighted at how easy it is to teach [physical education teacher in Maine].

The *Washington Times* magazine, *The World and I,* reported on the success of the Sex Respect program in Lamar, Missouri, a quiet little town of about 4,000 residents:

> Although Lamar does not have the troubles of a growing metropolis, it nevertheless experienced a teen pregnancy problem, having two or three unwed pregnancies per year. For such a small town, even one teen pregnancy is considered one too many.
>
> The change for the better began in Lamar when a group of concerned parents came across Sex Respect. . . . Unlike the type of information about contraceptives that health teachers and nurses receive in college, this curriculum talks about abstinence, changing former behaviors, true love and other topics that will help teens build healthier lives now and in the future.
>
> Based on this foundation of common concern, a committee was formed. . . . The committee invited a person trained in the Sex Respect curriculum to come to Lamar and demonstrate it to parents. The demonstration convinced the community that Sex Respect was the approach they wanted. After the board approved the curriculum, the school nurse and director of instruction attended a teacher-training workshop and then began using the program in the school.

> During the two years that the program has been used in Lamar . . . some [teen] pregnancies have occurred in Lamar, but not among [the 500] students who took the course.
>
> Students in Lamar are asked to complete anonymous evaluation forms after the program. . . . Student responses are almost always favorable and indicate that students realize they are important people, that what they do and feel matters, and imply that they intend to say no to premarital sex. These comments show that the self-esteem of students can be heightened by participation in the program. 206/580-81

Teaching Sex Respect

The Sex Respect teacher's manual, parent's guide and student's workbook, written by Coleen Kelly Mast, **revised, expanded and updated** for Fall 1990 are available from the publisher: Respect, Inc., P. O. Box 349, Bradley, IL 60915, (815) 932-8389; or Project Respect, P. O. Box 97, Golf, IL 60028, (312) 729-3298.

♦ Teen-Aid, Inc.

The purpose of Teen-Aid is to reduce the many adverse physical, emotional and social consequences of premarital sex among teens by encouraging abstinence as a premarital lifestyle, by increasing the understanding of fertility and respect for the power to create life, and by promoting effective parent-teen communication. Teen-Aid advocates:

- Premarital abstinence gives the teen time to mature.
- Respect for authority is essential to maturity of teens.
- Teens need to be involved in character-building activities.
- Love is a decision, not a feeling. Marriage is built on that kind of love.
- Postponing sexual relations until marriage helps establish strong families.

Born Out of Concern

In 1981 two teachers, taking time off from teaching to be mothers, became concerned about the quality of the sex education their children were receiving in the public schools. LeAnna Benn and Nancy Roach wanted their children to know that sex is not dirty or bad but a celebration of love and new life to be enjoyed within marriage.

Their misgivings about the sex education courses being presented in public schools nationwide moved them to conduct a conference in eastern Washington to evaluate the problem. They learned that existing sex education programs, which were almost exclusively of the contraceptive variety, seemed to aggravate the very problems they were supposed to solve! The conference generated interest in the desire to seek alternatives. Professionals were contacted and the board of directors of Teen-Aid was formed. The board members included an obstetrician/gynecologist, a psychiatrist, a coach, a high school sex education teacher, a natural-family-planning instructor, and a few college-educated mothers.

The unifying theme of Teen-Aid was to research the subject of sexual behavior and determine if abstinence is a viable, preferred alternative for unmarried teens. Specifically, the following subjects were given high priority: family unity, parent-teen communication, consequences of sexual activity, pregnancy and teen parenthood, abortion, sexually transmitted diseases, peer and media pressure, refusal skills and the much forgotten emotional and social consequences of sexual activity.

A Plan of Attack

The Teen-Aid vision is comprised of four main elements. The first is the development of an affiliate program to facilitate replication of Teen-Aid activities so that many local communities can have resources for quality sexuality education, information and services. Teen-Aid hopes eventually to have affiliates in every state.

The second element is the provision of locally-tailored services to meet community needs. Spokane opened the first office in 1983 to fill a need for pregnancy testing and support services. Volunteer counselors were trained to help teens evaluate their sexual activity and its consequences. Providing services is one way to reach young people who are making decisions about becoming sexually active. As the service program has grown, family counseling, parenting classes for teen moms and for adults with problem teens have been provided.

The third element, public presentations, is the backbone of the local education program. Parent seminars and teen presentations are provided to public schools, service clubs and churches. Parents who know that premarital abstinence is a viable lifestyle need skills to help them train and support their own children.

The fourth element is quality sex education materials with family values at the core. Teen-Aid researches and develops family life educational materials suitable for public schools. **Teen-Aid is one of the few organizations taking an academic approach to teaching the value of and the skills to achieve abstinence.** Teacher training seminars are also available.

Providing a Value-Based Curriculum

At the outset the founders of Teen-Aid were astonished to find that virtually no value-based family life materials were in print, and they soon realized that great opposition to this philosophy existed. Value-free comprehensive sex education was firmly entrenched, and any other approach was foreign to many educators. Teen-Aid was convinced that abstinence-based materials had to be offered in the marketplace to address the many shortfalls of the prevailing ideologies. Teen-Aid met the challenge by developing a sex education curriculum based on a personal responsibility/abstinence model.

The junior high curriculum is called *Me, My World, My Future,* and its companion parent program is called *Teaching Responsible Sexual Behavior.* The student materials cover such topics as friendship and dating, adolescent physical changes, reproductive anatomy, fetal development, pregnancy, abortion, sexually transmitted diseases, AIDS, tobacco, drugs and alcohol, decision making, communication skills, caring, advantages of premarital abstinence, nutrition, exercise, peer pressure and refusal skills. Parents are informed of what is being taught in class through "Parent-Grams" which provide a format for discussing personal family values at home.

Teen-Aid's senior high curriculum, *Sexuality, Commitment & Family,* was first published in 1982. This fifteen-day program has been used in all fifty states, in all ten Canadian provinces and in seventeen other countries. This course of study includes the topics of love, friendship and dating, reproductive anatomy, fetal development, abortion, sexually transmitted diseases, marriage, parenting, setting family goals, career choices as they relate to future family plans, listening and communication skills, assertiveness skills, consequences of adolescent sexual activity, advantages of premarital abstinence, the media and its effect on shaping attitudes, peer pressure and leadership. Parents are encouraged to discuss these topics and share their values with their children at home through "Parent/Teen Communicators."

The parent course, *Teaching Responsible Sexual Behavior,* helps parents understand premarital abstinence as a lifestyle and how they can help their teenage children achieve that lifestyle. Some of the topics covered are the ineffectiveness of contraceptive education, helping kids who are already sexually active, helping kids remain virgins when their parents were promiscuous as teens and helping kids deal with peer pressure. The course can be presented in such places as PTA meetings and church groups. In 1989 the National Parent Teacher Association (PTA) presented the Bingham PTA in Sandy, Utah, with an award for parental involvement in AIDS curricula while using the Teen-Aid parent workshop and school programs.

Positive Results

In 1987 Teen-Aid was awarded a grant by the Office of Adolescent Pregnancy Programs of the U.S. Department of Health and Human

Services. The grant was provided so Teen-Aid could study the effectiveness of its junior high curriculum and the parent workshop in reducing teen sexual activity and its harmful consequences. The study measured student values and attitudes regarding premarital sexual activity before and after the course of study. Students moved 10-15 percent in the direction of abstinence on all the critical issues dealing with the onset of sexual activity. In fetal development knowledge the shift was as high as 75 percent. Researchers note that a shift of as little as 5 percent is highly significant after only fifteen hours of instruction.

Issues found to be most important were the teen's focus on the future (taught in lessons on setting goals and health issues), decision-making, consequences of sexual activity, and refusal skills. The program was found to have a significant impact on both females and males, on sexually active students and virgins, and on students from minority groups or from broken families. It is apparent that truth is attractive for young people no matter what their situation may be.

Objective data shows that Teen-Aid programs give positive results. *Sexuality, Commitment & Family* was shown to be highly effective in the San Marcos, California, school district. During the 1983-1984 term, one out of five teenage girls in the district became pregnant, one of the highest rates in California. School officials decided to do something about it. Dr. Dinah Richard analyzed the Teen-Aid approach:

> The concerned school officials in San Marcos acted responsibly and wisely. Administrators called together parents, school staff and clergy in order to decide what needed to be accomplished. The group realized that the seventh-grade science unit on human reproduction was simply inadequate to address the entire problem. The junior high principal acknowledged that simply lecturing students on contraceptives would have been an ineffective response; instead, the educators wanted to shape attitudes and change behaviors.
>
> The community was in almost complete agreement that abstinence education was the perspective to teach. . . . After setting up a committee, the school then proceeded to examine resources consistent with the goals they were trying to accomplish. They selected the abstinence curriculum *Sexuality, Commitment & Family,* developed by Teen-Aid of Spokane, Washington. . . . Unlike most sex education curricula, *Sexuality, Commitment & Family* places information within a moral framework. It is based upon traditional ethical views, strongly supports the family and teaches that the deepest meaning of the sexual act derives from the marriage commitment. . . .
>
> Besides the abstinence curriculum, San Marcos Junior High adopted "How to [Study] Notes," "How to Be Successful" and "How to Be You," all of which are designed to help students improve their study skills, self-image and decision-making ability. The educators decided to include these items too because they wanted students to learn how to set goals and discover effective means to achieve them. Though these units were not part of the sex

> education program per se, the school believed that the combination of these materials would enhance all areas of learning and help alleviate a wide array of problems, including drug and alcohol abuse, suicide and sexual activity. 206/578-80

The following remarkable results have been achieved in the San Marcos program (Teen-Aid has applied for a grant from the U. S. Department of Education to replicate this study and to verify these results):

	1984	1986	1988
Total female student population	600	800	1,000
Teen pregnancies	147	20	15
Pregnancy percentage	20%	2.5%	1.5%

Furthermore, in 1988 the San Marcos program won the California award for the lowest student dropout rate. The percentage of *A* students increased from 2.2 percent to 4.5 percent and the number of scores in the lowest percentile decreased from 16.4 percent to 11.7 percent.

In 1989 the National School Boards Association published a journal which named the San Marcos (California) School District's curriculum, *Decision Making: Keys to Success,* one of the nation's 100 best curricula—the only family life course listed out of 1,000 North American entries. The Teen-Aid curriculum, *Sexuality, Commitment & Family,* was part of that curriculum.

The Institute for Research and Evaluation was commissioned by the Office of Adolescent Pregnancy Programs (OAPP) to study the effects of Teen-Aid's abstinence-based program. This second-year evaluation showed that the shift toward abstinence in attitudes and values was statistically significant.

Upon completion of the abstinence-based Teen-Aid curriculum, the students "were more likely to affirm that abstinence was the best way to avoid pregnancy and STDs, that premarital sex was against their values and standards, and that it was important to them not to have premarital sex." 56/35

The study showed they also were "more likely to reject the permissive notions of sex being OK if their partner wants it, if they are in love, or if they just use birth control. While this pattern was similar to what was found for girls last year, the pattern for the boys this year was equally strong."

Information about the San Marcos program can be obtained from Teen-Aid. The two three-week Teen-Aid courses, one for junior high and one for senior high, can be ordered from Teen-Aid, North 1330 Calispel, Spokane, WA 99201, (509) 328-2080.

♦ Implementing a School-Based Program

A school-based program like Sex Respect or Teen-Aid can be implemented in several ways. Concerned parents can initiate the process by contacting school administrators and school board members. Teachers can talk to other teachers who work in departments where sexuality or family life skills are taught. Persistence is important when working through the chain of command of a school district.

Another method of placing value-based materials into schools is by holding parents' meetings within the community. Present the materials to community leaders and parents to familiarize them with the value of abstinence-based programs. Some parents are unaware that it *is* possible to provide value-based sex education in their schools. They often comment that programs like Sex Respect and Teen-Aid are like a breath of fresh air.

♦ Challenge Program

The second approach to affecting teen sexual behavior is community-based programs such as the Challenge Program initiated by Margaret Whitehead and Dr. Onalee McGraw. Seeing that families were rapidly losing their influence over their children's sex education, Whitehead and McGraw founded the Educational Guidance Institute (EGI). EGI is a non-profit organization established to promote abstinence-based educational programs in human sexuality for teens. The programs offered by the Institute emphasize family involvement and parent-teen communication and the positive value of human sexuality within the context of marriage. EGI states that their programs are abstinence-based, community-centered and family-oriented.

Under a grant from the Office of Adolescent Pregnancy Programs, Department of Health and Human Services, EGI has developed the Challenge Program for young teens and their parents. The four sessions help parents and teens face and discuss the following issues:

1. *The Challenge for Parents:* Importance of parent-teen communication; need for parent guidance; understanding abstinence-based education.
2. *The Challenge of Sexual Freedom:* The value and dignity of the human person; sexuality issues; decision-making; premarital abstinence; maturity; love, marriage and family.
3. *The Challenge of the Teen Years for Parents and Teens:* Positive aspects of premarital abstinence; negative aspects of promiscuity; dealing with today's pressures on teens; threat of AIDS; friendship, dating and maturity; communication issues.

4. *The Challenge of Living Sexual Freedom:* Teen panel discusses their experiences; how to handle pressures (media and peer); dating, friendship and living the challenge of freedom.

A Partnership Between Parents and Professionals

EGI is involved in developing K-12 curriculum guidelines for family life education that are based on a positive rationale for sexual abstinence until marriage and for the central importance of the family and parental involvement. The process utilizes current research in child development and adolescent psychology. The EGI guidelines spring from the philosophical view of the person as a social being who can think and make decisions.

EGI challenges parents and professionals to work in partnership to appeal to the best qualities in young people and to help them make decisions that are beneficial to them and society. EGI is available to implement community-based family life education programs. Related professional services to communities include curriculum development and teacher training.

Changing Attitudes Through Communication

According to project coordinator Margaret Whitehead, the four-session parent-teen Challenge Program brought about "a dramatic increase in the communication between parents and teens concerning sex, dating and social pressures with both groups showing increased confidence in their respective abilities to understand the value of premarital sexual abstinence and to deal with negative social pressures." Tables A and B illustrate the success of the first phase of a multi-year EGI project. The data is based on the responses of 54 parents and youth who were tested at two points in time: the first prior to a two-week program on sexual values and the second at the conclusion of the program.

Table A
EGI Program Impacts:
Attitudes of Parents About Teen Sex and Sexuality

Question	Percentage	
Right now are you prepared enough to teach your child about human sexuality? (Yes)	51%	Before
	91%	After
Have you discussed the way to behave on a date? (Yes)	60%	Before
	95%	After

Question	Percentage	
Have you discussed sexual intercourse? (Yes)	56%	Before
	76%	After
Have you discussed sexually transmitted diseases or AIDS? (Yes)	69%	Before
	88%	After
Young people can control their sexual feelings. (Strongly agree)	34%	Before
	53%	After
I feel confident in my role as a moral teacher of my children. (Strongly agree)	48%	Before
	71%	After
My attitudes about human sexuality influence my teen's attitudes about human sexuality. (Strongly agree)	44%	Before
	71%	After
Have you talked with your child about human sexuality within the context of marriage? (Yes)	53%	Before
	75%	After
Have you talked with your child about the difference between love and infatuation? (Yes)	40%	Before
	71%	After
Have you talked with your child about the sexual pressures that are on kids today? (Yes)	65%	Before
	80%	After

Table B
EGI Program Impacts:
Attitudes of Young People About Sex and Sexuality

Statement	Percentage	
Young people who date in supervised groups will not get involved with sex. (I agree)	54%	Before
	80%	After
Television and movies influence what teens do on dates. (I agree)	64%	Before
	80%	After
Getting involved with sex interferes with long-term goals. (I agree)	61%	Before
	86%	After

Statement	Percentage	
I feel comfortable talking with my parents about sex. (I agree)	30%	Before
	44%	After
Sexual intercourse among unmarried teens is wrong. (I agree)	66%	Before
	86%	After
Young people who have already had sex outside marriage should stop and wait until they are married. (I agree)	76%	Before
	89%	After
Has your parent talked with you about the difference between love and sex? (Yes)	51%	Before
	77%	After
Has your parent talked with you about sex within marriage? (Yes)	67%	Before
	80%	After
Has your parent talked with you about the long-range results of decisions you make daily? (Yes)	73%	Before
	86%	After

To obtain the four-part Challenge Program, write:
Educational Guidance Institute, 927 S. Walter Reed Drive, Suite 4, Arlington, VA 22204, (703) 486-8313.

♦ Why Wait?

Another successful community approach to abstinence-based sex education is called Why Wait?, a national campaign I helped launch which is designed to penetrate communities, families and churches.

As I spoke on high school and college campuses in the early '80s, I became acutely aware that premarital sex had become rampant, even among church-going adolescents. Kids talked to me about their deep hurts. **They needed love, acceptance and intimacy, and they believed that sex would satisfy that need.** But sex only brought them deep emotional grief, unwanted pregnancies and sexually transmitted diseases. I realized that the sexual revolution was actually a quest for intimacy.

A Three-Step Plan

In 1984 I developed the core vision for the Why Wait? campaign and Dave Bellis was appointed national Why Wait? coordinator. By November 1985 we had developed a three-step plan.

The first step was implemented in 1986. A symposium was held in which leaders from twenty-three major church denominations came together in an effort to mobilize for action.

The second step was a media blitz. It began in October 1987 and was designed to raise the level of church awareness of the problem. Since then I have spoken more than 1,000 times on radio and television, in churches, at universities and at conventions as part of this effort to make people aware of the need for a positive, abstinence-based approach to teenage sexuality. We offer the Why Wait? "action packet" for additional information on how to mobilize a community for a city-wide Why Wait? rally. By spring 1989, more than fifteen United States cities had hosted city-wide rallies. Another dozen were scheduled for fall 1989 in conjunction with the Petra tour.

The topics I cover in a Why Wait? talk are summarized in titles like "Why Should I Wait?" "How to Say No" and "A Clean Heart for a New Start." The message is very positive and usually lasts less than two hours. A follow-up conference includes intensive all-day workshops for teens, parents and clergy. I recommend Sex Respect author Coleen Mast for conducting teacher training workshops.

The third step is equipping people with tools to effect positive change: audiovisuals, books and other resources. These tools are designed to help parents and youth workers train young people in the area of human sexuality and to instill in them a solid foundation upon which healthy, successful lives can be built. One resource, a video titled **"No, the Positive Answer," has been shown in more than 60,000 churches and seen by more than two million teens.** The adult training series, "How to Help Your Child Say No to Sexual Pressure," has been viewed by more than a million parents. Resources like these are available for small-scale uses or to follow up a city-wide rally or conference.

The educational resources produced by our Why Wait? team are designed for ongoing education. Why Wait? rallies and conferences may be one-time events, but working with young people is a continual task. The adolescent sexuality crisis is too complex and far-reaching to be solved easily and quickly. The problem did not arrive overnight, so we must approach a solution with a long-term commitment.

Focusing on the Church

Studies confirm that, although a multitude of variables are influencing today's youth to become sexually active, there are ways to overcome these pressures. Young people are more likely to abstain if the following conditions occur:

(1) The adolescent lives with both parents;
(2) Parents teach the value of premarital abstinence;

(3) The teen personally believes that premarital sex is wrong;
(4) Parental discipline is moderately high;
(5) Parents have moderately strict rules about dating;
(6) Parents are interested in the teen's grades and personal achievements;
(7) The teen has attained high academic grades;
(8) Teens have made future plans for higher education;
(9) Parents have good communication and a close relationship with their children; and
(10) The teen has strong religious convictions about premarital abstinence. See 324 and 323/72

While classroom education and community-based workshops are successful approaches to addressing these issues of teenage sexuality, our Why Wait? campaign has taken a comprehensive approach which enlists the help of churches. I believe the church is still a viable instrument for instilling spiritual foundations about sexuality. When we first launched our Why Wait? campaign, we were able to gain the support of youth pastors because most of them realized that many church teens were having sex, but by and large senior pastors refused to recognize this.

Our Why Wait? study, "Sexuality and the Evangelical Church," has changed that. The study showed that 43 percent of churched youth have experienced sexual intercourse by age 18. Considering that the national average for all teens is roughly 50 percent, it's obvious that many churches have neglected their responsibility for shaping the morality of the youth in their congregations. The results of the survey made leaders look more closely at the problem.

The Why Wait? campaign has been so effective in the United States that leaders abroad have taken notice of it. Church leaders throughout the United Kingdom have already met with our team and developed their own initiatives for Why Wait? campaigns in their churches.

* * * * *

As you can see, there are many avenues available to concerned parents, educators, school board members and church congregations for implementing abstinence-based programs with today's teens. Our kids don't need to remain the victims of the pregnancies, abortions and diseases which accompany so-called value-free, morally neutral sex education. The tide can be turned if we will act.

CHAPTER 19

➧ A **key section** for busy parents.

Strategy 7

Use Commercially Available Resources for Abstinence Education

There are a number of excellent resources available for teaching abstinence-based sex education.

A must resource for anyone evaluating a sex education curriculum is Dr. Dinah Richard's study, *Has Sex Education Failed Our Teenagers? A Research Report* (pages 45-46). The study is available from Focus on the Family Publications, 801 Corporate Center Drive, Pomona, CA 91799, (714) 620-8500.

Richard's analysis is so excellent, I asked for and obtained permission to reproduce her description of five programs. 206

1. **AANCHOR** is an acronym for **An Alternative National Curriculum for Responsibility**, and it was designed for junior and senior high students in public schools under a grant from the OAPP [Office of Adolescent Pregnancy Programs]. The curriculum is concerned with primary prevention in teaching youths to abstain from premarital intercourse. It is designed to help them learn to live responsible and wise lives by learning criteria by which to assess the quality of one's behavior, thoughts and feelings.

AANCHOR consists of six modules: responsibility, ethical thinking, the family, communication, the law and human reproduction.

Unlike most sex education courses, AANCHOR begins with a discussion of meaning, not merely the learning of facts. It uses case studies and role playing to help students develop moral decision-making abilities. It is not a values clarification approach; rather, it helps students realize why some choices are better than others. Parents are involved through parent-child discussions and homework assignments. For more information, contact Dr. Terrance Olson, Department of Family Sciences, Brigham Young University, Provo, UT 84602, (801) 378-2069.

2. **Family Values and Sex Education (FVSE): A Curriculum on Family and Citizenship for Middle School Students.** Designed for public junior high school health, family or social studies classes, FVSE invites students to live in ways that promote their futures, strengthen their family relationships and foster personal health and well-being. The curriculum lays a foundation of understanding quality family relationships; explores communication and decision-making; acknowledges the relationship of the family, society and law; and discusses human reproduction, AIDS and how to foster future families of high quality.

   The curriculum has three modules: Family and Individual, Family Communication Skills, and Family and the Next Generation (human reproduction). Parental involvement is central. Parent-teen worksheets are included to help guide family discussion of important topics and values.

   The curriculum is not problem-centered. Instead, it focuses on how to live a wise and happy life, which helps young people avoid crises. It offers positive ways to say no. The curriculum gives clear endorsement of premarital abstinence. Contraceptive usage by unmarried teens is not promoted.

   The curriculum was written by Terrance Olson, Ph.D., and Christopher Wallace, and was under the supervision of more than 100 academic and health experts. It can be obtained from Focus on the Family Publishing, 801 Corporate Center Drive, Pomona, CA 91799, (714) 620-8500.

3. **Me, My World, My Future** is one of the newest programs receiving a grant from the OAPP. The curriculum contains fifteen lessons appropriate for public middle schools. This value-based program encourages the postponement of immediate gratification in exchange for healthier future goals in the areas of sexual activity, drugs, alcohol and tobacco. Concrete learning

activities are used to introduce the complex concepts of decision-making and communication.

To facilitate parental involvement, parent-teen communication worksheets accompany each lesson. The daily take-home sheets are designed to deepen the transmission of values from parents to teens by giving the opportunity to discuss important subjects together. For more information, contact Teen-Aid, Inc., North 1330 Calispel, Spokane, WA 99201, (509) 466-8679 or (509) 328-2080.

4. **Sex Respect: The Option of True Sexual Freedom** is a curriculum [pilot-tested] through a grant under the Adolescent Family Life Act (AFLA), which is administered by the Office of Adolescent Pregnancy Programs (OAPP) of the U.S. Department of Health and Human Services.

The curriculum teaches that the best way to enjoy true sexual freedom in the long run is to say no to premarital sex. The units define human sexuality; recognize influences on sexual decision-making; identify emotional, psychological and physical consequences of teenage sexual activity; discuss dating guidelines; teach how to say no; show how to change former sexual behavior; and explore the responsibilities of parenthood. Approximately ten hours of classroom time are needed to cover the material.

The curriculum includes three separate workbooks—one for students, one for teachers and one for parents—that cover the same content and are used simultaneously. Originally intended for eighth- and ninth-graders, Sex Respect is now being used successfully in grades seven through eleven.

Sex Respect was written by Coleen Mast of Respect, Inc. The Committee on the Status of Women, directed by Kathleen Sullivan, is the grant recipient and field tester of the curriculum; the grant project is called Project Respect. Both Respect, Inc. and Project Respect have developed separate high school curricula. Project Respect's new high school curriculum is **Facing Reality**.

For more information about the curricula, contact Respect, Inc., P. O. Box 349, Bradley, IL 60915-0349, (815) 932-8389, or Project Respect, Committee on the Status of Women, P. O. Box 97, Golf, IL 60029-0097, (708) 729-3298.

[An excellent resource on how to teach abstinence is "Everyone Is Not Doing It," a set of four video tapes (available for $125 plus shipping) narrated by Mike Long and produced and distributed by Project Respect. Mike Long is available as a consultant on how to teach abstinence through Project Respect.

Colleen Mast, through Respect, Inc., is a vital resource in this area of premarital abstinence education to work with both educators and parents. Both Long and Mast have conducted workshops to train teachers, parents and community leaders on how to incorporate successful abstinence education in the schools.]

5. **Sexuality, Commitment and Family** is a public high school curriculum that emphasizes the deep meaning of sexuality in the context of the family, of self-respect, of respect for others and of respect and love for one's future spouse and children.

   The curriculum is designed for a three-week program, which includes one day of introduction, one day of testing and thirteen days of instruction. Areas of emphasis include: basic anatomy and maturational changes of adolescence; types of love; advantages of premarital abstinence; peer pressure; consequences of premarital sex; communication skills; and the fundamental purpose of marriage. Contraceptive risks are discussed, and students are steered away from usage.

   Each lesson includes a worksheet to be taken home to keep parents informed about classroom lessons and to foster parent-teen communication. For more information, contact Teen-Aid, Inc., North 1330 Calispel, Spokane, WA 99201, (509) 466-8679 or (509) 328-2080.

A sixth resource, **WOMANITY**, is a grass-roots educational organization promoting traditional family values, especially sex-appreciation (chastity for teens). They publish creative, candid, appealing brochures and booklets on abstinence, chastity, dating, virginity, etc. *Abstinence Works, a Notebook on Premarital Chastity* is one of their approximately twenty-two resources, and I highly recommend it.

WOMANITY conducts community seminars and produces several excellent resources in video format (e.g., "Just Wait"; "Saving Sex for Marriage"; "A Real Man Talks About Sexuality"; etc.).

One of WOMANITY's strengths is the desire to network with groups and individuals who also promote respect for sex as belonging in heterosexual, monogamous marriage. Much of their material can be used alone or as a supplement to other chastity/abstinence-affirming curriculum.

You can obtain a free catalog and also order a sample packet of this organization's publications ($9.00 prepaid) from **WOMANITY**, 1700 Oak Park Blvd., Annex, Pleasant Hill, CA 94523, (415) 943-6424. Patricia Driscoll is the director.

The following organizations promote abstinence-based sex education for schools, and they provide numerous excellent resources. I encourage you to look through this list of audiovisuals and other resources listed by Dr. Richard that can be used in the public school classroom.

Respect, Inc.
Sex Respect, publisher
P.O. Box 349
Bradley, IL 60915
(815) 932-8389

Citizens for Excellence in Education
P.O. Box 3200
Costa Mesa, CA 92628
(714) 546-5931

The Department of Family Sciences
Brigham Young University
Provo, UT 84602
(801) 378-2069

Educational Guidance, Inc.
907 S. Walter Reed Drive, Suite #4
Arlington, VA 22204
(703) 486-8313

Focus on the Family Publishing
801 Corporate Center Drive
Pomona, CA 91799
(714) 620-8500

Project Respect
Box 97
Golf, IL 60029-0097
(312) 729-3298

Couple to Couple League
Box 11084
Cincinnati, OH 45211
(513) 661-7612

Teen-Aid, Inc.
North 1330 Calispel
Spokane, WA 99201
(509) 466-8679

Part Four

Resources for Evaluating Abstinence Education

CHAPTER 20

Resource 1

A Case Study of Comprehensive Sex Education: "The Virginia Family Life Education Program"

In this chapter you will be introduced to the Family Life Education (FLE) curriculum guidelines for sex education in Virginia, which was in the first tier of fifteen states targeted by Planned Parenthood to have K-12 sexuality mandates by 1990. 668 In 1987-1988, Virginia established its FLE mandate for kindergarten through the tenth grade (K-10) and required implementation in all public schools in the 1989-1990 school year.

The Virginia FLE program is regarded as a model of the kind of sex education that family planning and other networking groups are striving to institute in every public school in the country.

In light of the overwhelming evidence that "comprehensive," non-directive sex education does *not* reduce teen promiscuity, pregnancies or abortions, or reduce sexually transmitted diseases (STDs), decision-makers and citizens must ask, *"Is the Virginia FLE model promoted by Planned Parenthood a viable sex education program for our schools?"* 668

The failure rate—that is, the rise in teen pregnancy rates in the FLE "model localities"—provides convincing evidence of the inefficiency of the "safer sex" approach of sex education.

♦ Curriculum Objectives and Content

The FLE course objectives for students in kindergarten through grade ten reveal the wide range of sex-related topics to which the children of Virginia are exposed:

- Fourteen separate objectives beginning as early as grade 6 deal with contraception.
- Three separate objectives beginning as early as grade 7 deal with homosexuality.
- Nine references beginning as early as grade 5 encourage abstinence from "premarital" sex. The original term was "premature" sex, but it was changed to "premarital" sex by the Board of Education only after a tremendous outcry from citizens and legislators during the 1988 legislative session.
- Two objectives beginning as early as grade 8 deal with the use of condoms to prevent AIDS.

Abstinence is cited only as a method of contraception. Abstinence also was redefined as including such behavior as "sexual outercourse."

Graded curriculum topics are equally revealing:

- In grade 1 children learn explicit genital terminology in mixed groups.
- In grade 3 children receive a detailed explanation of human reproduction including fertilization of the egg by the sperm. Mr. Brook on the Campbell County School Board wisely pointed out that third-grade teachers will also be talking about intercourse because the inquisitive third-graders will ask, "How does the sperm get there?"
- In grade 4 the menstrual cycle is discussed and students make presentations about the male and female sex organs.
- In grade 5 sexual intercourse and sexually transmitted diseases will be discussed.
- In grades 5 and 6 children will learn about masturbation, erections and nocturnal emissions (wet dreams).
- In grade 7 birth control, AIDS and homosexuality and lesbianism will be taught.
- In grade 8 children will be taught how to use condoms to prevent AIDS.

A number of local curricula under the Virginia FLE mandate include worksheets or questionnaires on values clarification techniques (most schools have redefined or renamed the techniques previously called "values clarification." They are now referred to as "peer counseling," "decision-making skills," "role playing," etc.) with questions like the following, which were used in a girls' eighth-grade class in Roanoke, Virginia: (1) Do you wish birth control methods were available without your parents knowing about it? (2) Do you frequently wonder what the sex act is like? (3) Are your parents still in love?

At Cave Spring Junior High in Roanoke, girls were asked to write reports on lesbianism, incest and rape. Sanitary napkins, tampons, lubricants and contraceptive devices—including IUDs and unwrapped condoms—were passed around the room for girls to touch. Question boxes were made available in classes so that anonymously submitted topics could be discussed openly, topics such as oral and anal sex, douching and the frequency of adult intercourse.

The Roanoke sex education program began in the early '70s. The city now has a teen pregnancy rate which is twice the national average.

♦ Program Results

What does the Virginia FLE program hope to accomplish? Is pregnancy prevention among its goals? Jeanne Bentley, the Director for Health and PE, is a key member of the Virginia Department of Education FLE program development team and one of the leading advocates of the program. Yet, in a public discourse, Bentley admitted that "there is no goal stated that K-12 FLE will reduce teen pregnancy, because we're not sure it will." 412

"We're not sure that FLE alone is going to reduce teenage pregnancy significantly," remarked Jim Bailey, FLE educator for the Department of Health, to a joint subcommittee on teen pregnancy. "There are several other ingredients that need to be put into this formula . . . school-based clinics, for example." 413 Bailey's comment reveals more of the program's true objectives: comprehensive sex education *plus* school-based clinics. Maryland State Representative Robert O'Donnell, who also testified, agreed that "such programs (FLE) alone will not reduce teen pregnancy." 414

Bailey and O'Donnell have seriously understated the facts. Anne Marie Morgan, a Virginia capitol correspondent, reports: "Teens who have had 'comprehensive' sex education (birth control included) are much more likely to engage in premarital sexual intercourse than those who do not have 'comprehensive' sex education or those who have no sex education at all." 198

♦ Medical Consequences of FLE

Several medical doctors, psychologists and psychiatrists have commented on the negative effects of comprehensive sex education on children. Their testimony clearly warns that the Virginia FLE program, and others like it, are doing more harm than good to our kids.

William McGrath, M.D., a psychiatrist in Phoenix, Arizona, writes:

> There is a phase of personality development called the latency period, during which the healthy child is not interested in sex. This interval from about the age of five until adolescence serves a very important biological purpose. It affords a child an opportunity to develop his own resources, his beginning physical and mental strength.
>
> Premature interest in sex is unnatural and will arrest or distort the development of the personality. Sex education should not be foisted on children; [it] should not begin in grade schools.
>
> Anyone who would deliberately arouse the child's curiosity or stimulate his unready mind to troubled sexual preoccupations ought to have a millstone tied around his neck and be cast into the sea. 415

Just think of all the child molesters and pedophiles already running loose in our country. Can you imagine how childish innocence coupled with a premature, unnatural interest in sex can turn some of our kids into willing targets for these sexual deviants?

New York psychologist Rhoda L. Lorand, Ph.D., states:

> Twenty-five years ago, I and many other child analysts might have enthusiastically endorsed school sex education. . . . We have since learned that it is harmful to force sexual preoccupation on children of the elementary school grades. . . . Forcing of sexual preoccupation on the elementary school child is very likely to result in sexual difficulties in adulthood, and it can lead to disturbed behavior in childhood. 415

"Trying to teach children about sex without arousing sensuous feelings," comments Melvin Anchell, M.D., of Los Angeles, "is about as hypocritical or naive as trying to describe the nature of fire without acknowledging the heat produced. . . . Shattering the fantasies and doubts of children without proper aging can act as a premature seduction causing irreparable psychological harm including perversion." 415

Max Levin, psychiatrist with the New York Medical College, commented on the issue of statewide mandating of value-free, morally neutral sex education in Virginia:

> Many of our sex educators . . . are leading our youngsters astray. I disagree with the SIECUS (Sex Information and Education Council of the United States) position that sex education "must not be moral indoctrination." . . . I speak not as a clergyman but as a psychiatrist. There cannot be emotional health in the absence of high moral standards and a sense of human and social responsibility. I know that today morality is a "dirty

word" but we must help our youth to see that moral codes have meaning beyond theology; they have psychological and sociological meaning. 415

The American Academy of Pediatrics (AAP) is concerned about the negative impact of comprehensive sex education on children. Recently the president and vice-president of every chapter in the United States signed the following resolution:

RESOLVED, that the Academy (of Pediatrics) recommend that adolescents postpone, until marriage, sexual activities that lead to pregnancy or sexually transmitted diseases. 416

In a letter objecting to the mandate for comprehensive sex education, Dr. Joseph E. Zanga, M.D., chairman of the division of general pediatrics and emergency care at the Medical College of Virginia, Virginia Commonwealth University, writes:

What we need for the State of Virginia is to teach the original program supported by the majority of citizens of the Commonwealth, which was proposed by the State Board of Education. That program told the children *to say "no"* and advised them that if they had further questions in that regard, they should speak to the teacher, the school nurse, their physician or their parents *privately* after class. That approach gives us the opportunity to encourage that majority of teenagers who are not sexually active to continue in their resolve and to influence those who are to take a more reasonable approach, or at least protect themselves as much as that may be possible [emphasis theirs]. 417

Dr. Mark L. Johnson, a urologist, wrote a personal letter to Virginia parents expressing his agony over the devastating consequences of teen sexual promiscuity:

To the parents of Virginia:

As a physician who treats sexually transmitted diseases, I would like to comment on the Virginia Family Life Education program. I am in favor of sexuality education that will spare our teens the bad consequences of sexual activity, but I do not believe that Virginia Family Life Education will accomplish that goal.

The educational strategy that will be used in Virginia has been used in various forms around the country for the last fifteen years. **This strategy has never been shown to lower teen pregnancy rates or venereal disease rates, but it has been associated with increased rates of sexual activity.** My greatest concern about this program is the false impression it conveys about the risk of premarital sexual activity.

The majority of parents in our state would encourage sexual abstinence until marriage as the ideal choice for their child. The state, through the FLE program, is going to offer two ideals for behavior. Abstinence is mentioned as an acceptable choice, but the impression is also strongly conveyed that it is acceptable to choose to have sexual intercourse as long as a reliable contraceptive is used. Allow me to comment on what the state considers "responsible sexual activity."

A sexually active teen faithfully using birth control pills has an 11-percent chance of becoming pregnant each year she is sexually active. **Teens who faithfully use condoms have an 18-percent chance of pregnancy per year**. Those using foam, diaphragms, etc., have higher chances of becoming pregnant. The odds of becoming pregnant even while faithfully using a "reliable" birth control method are the same odds one has playing Russian roulette with one shell in the chamber each year. If no contraceptive method is used, you play the game with two shells in the chamber.

Perhaps a greater concern is sexually transmitted disease. Gonorrhea and syphilis can be cured easily, but herpes is a lifelong infection which may necessitate a C-section birth in women. Chlamydia causes pelvic inflammatory disease, which leads to sterility and ectopic pregnancies, both of which are now very common among young women. Condyloma has recently been shown to be the causative factor in cervical cancer in young women. In our city in the last two years, a number of women in their teens and 20s have been treated for cervical cancer, most by local therapy, but some by hysterectomy. Each of the above sexually transmitted diseases is common among sexually active teens, with chlamydia and condyloma, the most dangerous ones, being most common.

Birth control pills, considered a "responsible" choice by sex educators, offer no protection against disease. In addition, recent scientific studies show a possible fourfold increase in breast cancer among early users of birth control pills. What about condoms? Recent studies show up to 30 percent of condoms leaking enough to transmit bacteria and viruses. A recent scientific study of condom use for disease prevention was discontinued because of the high failure rate of condoms. They offer some protection, but not as much as sex educators would have your child to believe when they term condom use "responsible."

According to a recent poll, 71 percent of Virginia parents think that the Family Life Education program will decrease teen pregnancies. This course gives parents a false sense of security. Students who support this course are counting on it to help them avoid the consequences of premarital sexual activity. This course gives them a false sense of security. How "responsible" is it for the state to offer this program to the people of this state as the best solution to the consequence of teen sexual activity?

There are sexuality education programs based on a different educational strategy which have a proven ability to reduce rates of teen sexual activity, and the attendant consequences. I hope that the parents of Virginia will take the responsibility for demanding of their state government an educational program that works.

Mark L. Johnson, M.D. 415

Many physicians strongly endorse abstinence as the best sex education advice they can give. Notice the critical issue of values which is reflected in key phrases from these testimonies: "encourage that majority of teenagers who are not sexually active to continue their resolve" (Dr. Zanga); "trying to teach children sex without arousing sensuous feelings" (Dr. Anchell); "there cannot be emotional health in the absence of high moral standards" (Dr. Levin). The medical profession is issuing fair warning:

1. Sex education will inevitably arouse sexual and sensual feelings in children and teens.
2. Arousing sexual feelings will in no way aid in reducing teen pregnancy or STDs.
3. Rather, sex education will lead to a conflict of values within the teen about what is right, especially if it is taught as morally neutral, meaning anything is okay.
4. Morally neutral, "do what is best for you," sex education will serve to weaken any resolve the teen might have about trying to stay away from premarital sexual involvement.
5. Whatever values the teen may have held will then seem unfair, unpopular, undoable or wrong.

This regression is inevitable.

♦ Media Opinion of FLE

How has the media responded to Virginia's attempt at comprehensive sex education? Consider the following reports and testimonies submitted after Virginia's FLE program was implemented.

In an editorial urging Virginia to look closely at states that have no mandatory sex education and have decreasing pregnancy rates among teens, the *Richmond Times-Dispatch* stated:

> Rosemary Evans, a health teacher from Ettrick, eloquently refuted the idea that ignorance (i.e., lack of sex education) is mainly to blame [for teen pregnancies]. She said that many teens who are knowledgeable about contraception choose to discontinue use and become pregnant. With scant prospects to raise their esteem (from those in poor communities especially), they conclude that having a baby would be a tangible achievement. Pregnancy-prevention information is a "quick fix," she argued, that does not ease such underlying causes as poor self-image, youth unemployment, lack of training in sound values, discipline and "instruction for parents on how to be good parents." 312.

On October 10, 1989, the headlines of the *Fairfax Journal* proclaimed, "Pregnancies Rising Among Northern Virginia Teens." Catherine Toups reported:

> Alexandria's teen pregnancy rate jumped 26.4 percent in 1988 over the previous year, the most dramatic increase in Northern Virginia, according to the Virginia Department of Health Statistics.
>
> Comparatively, teen pregnancy increased by 5.9 percent in Arlington, 6.3 percent in Fairfax County and 9.4 percent in Falls Church in those years.

The statistics are for pregnancies of girls between the ages of 10 and 19. There were 57,850 girls and young women in that age group in Northern Virginia in 1988. That number had declined from 1987, when 59,083 lived in the Northern Virginia suburbs.

But while population declined, more teen pregnancies occurred. One of every 24.4 Northern Virginia girls–4.1 percent–got pregnant in 1988. That compares to one in every 27.2–3.7 percent–who became pregnant in 1987.

The majority of those pregnancies–62.3 percent–were ended by abortions. That compares to the 1987 abortion rate of 60.6 percent, a 2.8-percent increase.

Alexandria's abortion rate among teens increased between 1987 and 1988 from 50.3 percent to 58.7 percent.

The number of pregnancies continued to rise, despite an increased emphasis on sex education in all public schools. 199/A1

It is important to note that Alexandria implemented a "comprehensive" FLE/Sex Education program some years before the recent Virginia FLE mandate. The Alexandria program was used as a "model" for the state program. However, in 1986 Alexandria had the third-highest increase in the rate of teenage pregnancy in Virginia at the same time the city had a school-based health clinic–two years next to the school and one year in the school.

The Virginia Department of Health Statistics records these statistics on teen pregnancy rates in Northern Virginia during 1988: 199

	Alexandria	Arlington	Fairfax	Falls Church
Number of girls aged 10 to 19	4,801	6,501	46,604	394
Total pregnancies	436	326	1,578	22
Births 160	146	508	4	
Abortions 256	165	1,035	16	
Fetal deaths	17	15	35	2

In response to these staggering statistics, Ms. Tamara Ballou, coordinator of the Falls Church Family Life Education curriculum, said: "[FLE] has an effect on the knowledge level and the attitude. But when it comes down to behavior, it's kind of like math. You can teach people to add and subtract, but you can't make them balance their checkbook." 199/4A

Another *Richmond Times-Dispatch* editorial argued that the "line of reasoning is seriously flawed" that wants to prescribe standardized curriculum for the sex education program. The writer contends that if the curriculum is fixed, there is no room for local school boards to tailor the program to their needs. The editorial points out that no other putting undue emphasis on sex over against other more important issues like math and reading. In fact, the editorial sarcastically quips: **"The new four R's: reading, 'riting, 'rithmetic and reproduction—but the greatest of these is reproduction?"** Here the priorities of education are all out of whack. 326

On October 4, 1989, the *Alexandria Gazette* carried the headline: "Teen Pregnancies Rise 23%; Abortions Up 45%" The story reported:

> "It's an enormous rise. I had hoped for a fall," said Dr. Anne Albertson, health director for Alexandria.
>
> The increase in the number of abortions was almost the same as the increase in the number of pregnancies. There were 160 live births to teen-aged females in 1988—exactly the same as in 1987. But abortions increased more than 44 percent, from 177 to 258.
>
> The city's teen pregnancy rate—number of pregnancies per 1,000 girls aged 15 through 19—jumped from 134.1 to 166.3. The rate was 82.1 in Northern Virginia and 87.4 in the state as a whole in 1988, according to the department's Center for Health Statistics. Alexandria's ranking among Virginia jurisdictions was not available.
>
> The new Alexandria figure suggests that over 16 percent of females aged 15 through 19 became pregnant in 1988. There were clear increases across the board—in pregnancies among girls under 15, girls 15 through 17, and women 18 and 19.
>
> Albertson said one of the things that particularly concerns her is the increase in the number of pregnant girls under 15. 200/1

Mary Ann Heil, the nurse at Alexandria's T.C. Williams School, confessed that "the education and services Alexandria is providing seem to do more to discourage pregnant girls from having babies than to discourage girls from becoming pregnant in the first place." 200/11

In a well-written, lengthy letter to the *Richmond News Leader*, former teacher Anne Marie Morgan pointedly asked:

> Has the State Board of Education no consideration for those parents who are trying to inculcate different, higher standards than the lowest common denominator? . . . The frustration of at least some Virginia teens with explicit instruction is summed in the following: "It took away our excuse to say no." 328

Morgan focuses on two important issues which are almost always overlooked in sex education: the fact that *the program ignores or is hostile to parents,* and that no real values in regard to abstinence are ever communicated.

The FLE mandate, by design, does not tell students what is right or wrong, legal or illegal. It is non-directive. For example, in Fairfax County, the law declaring sexual intercourse or involvement outside of marriage to be illegal is not taught until the twelfth grade, and then it is taught in the Virginia Government class—several years *after* students are taught all the various sexual behaviors.

The week-long sex education teacher-training seminars conducted by the Virginia Department of Education instruct teachers not to tell students that abstinence before marriage is right behavior for them. Abstinence is presented only as a form of birth control.

♦ Political Objections to FLE

The response to Virginia's FLE program has also been vigorous on the political front, as the following testimonies reveal.

In responding to a joint subcommittee study on teenage pregnancy prevention which recommended FLE, Delegate S. Vance Wilkins contended that the program had a "fatal flaw: lack of parental involvement." Wilkins said in his report:

> Parental involvement is essential to the success of any FLE program. Yet, in the State-mandated program, there is no mechanism, no means, no instructional material and no text that involves the parents in the teaching of family life education to their children. . . . Why do we mandate a program that does not include the one factor which we have concluded is essential to the success of any program? . . .
>
> Another serious problem is the fact that the State Department of Health, via its local health departments, is also procuring abortions for teenagers without parental knowledge or permission. This became legal in Virginia in 1973, and our teenage pregnancy rate continued to increase. . . .
>
> Teen pregnancy rates skyrocketed in Virginia after 1972 when the Virginia Code was amended to permit minors to receive birth control without parental consent or notification. . . .
>
> I recommend that statistics be kept by the State Department of Health on teenage pregnancy rates to allow comparison of programs implemented in different localities as to their effectiveness in reducing the teenage pregnancy rate. There is no need to mandate a program if we're not going to monitor it to see if it works. In effect, if we mandate the State Board of Education program, we're mandating a program which is very similar to programs which have been proven not to work. . . .
>
> I do not concur with the requesting of additional funds for programs which have proven to be of dubious value. . . .
>
> I further recommend that in future studies of teen pregnancy we study those states such as Utah, whose pregnancy rates are less than half that of Virginia. The subcommittee instead studied only states such as Maryland, where a safe-sex program like that recommended by our State Board of Education is already in effect, and where their teen pregnancy rate is one-and-one-half times that of Virginia. We did not study a state that had a different program from our State-mandated plan, or a state with documented success in lowering the rate of teen pregnancies, which is our goal. 418/2-4

The *Richmond News Leader* printed part of the text of an address given by staff member Mrs. Gribben of the U.S. House Select Committee on Children, Youth and Families. Her comments were delivered to a hearing of the Virginia General Assembly's Joint Committee on Adolescent Pregnancy on September 5, 1986:

> In December 1985, the Select Committee on Children, Youth, and Families of the U.S. House of Representatives published a report on teen pregnancy in the United States. The majority members of the Committee focused their study primarily on programs which serve pregnant and parenting adolescents, while the minority members looked primarily at efforts to prevent adolescent pregnancy. They also studied the results of those efforts. . . .
>
> *They found that oral contraceptive use among unmarried sexually active teens almost doubled* between 1971 and 1976, and then declined slightly thereafter, but *this made no difference in the percentage of unmarried teens who became pregnant* . . .
>
> Here is the basic figure: three out of ten. In 1971, three out of ten sexually active, unmarried adolescent women had become pregnant. In 1976, three out of ten sexually active, unmarried adolescent women had become pregnant. In 1979, again, three out of ten; and in 1982, again, three out of ten. Nothing changed.
>
> Except there was one change, and it was a significant one; indeed, it was the most significant change to occur during all the years studied. Between 1971 and 1982, the percentage of all adolescent women who were sexually active increased more than 50 percent. As a consequence, the percentage of all adolescents who had ever become pregnant also increased more than 50 percent.
>
> To summarize the point, there are two major variables in the adolescent pregnancy rates: (1) the percentage of unmarried teens who are sexually active, and (2) the percentage of sexually active teens who become pregnant. Thus far our nation has tried to affect only the second variable, and has failed completely. In the meantime, the first variable, the percentage who are sexually active, has caused all the increase in the problem of teen pregnancy. There ought to be a lesson in this somewhere. . . .
>
> They have examined fertility rates (births) and then extrapolated their results to estimate effects on pregnancy rates. Olsen and Weed, using the same basic method of these other studies, examined both fertility and pregnancy directly. Their analysis showed, similar to previous studies, about thirty fewer births to adolescents for every 1,000 teenage clients served by organized family planning programs. But it also showed an increase of 120 pregnancies for every 1,000 teen clients. . . .
>
> That increased pregnancy rates should occur in conjunction with decreased birth rates is not difficult to explain. Increases in abortion have caused decreases in births nationwide, despite increases in pregnancies. The difficulty with these findings, rather, is that *family planning programs seem to cause increases in teen pregnancies* [emphasis mine]. 212/13-14

♦ Major Objections to FLE

Most of the following are specific legal objections to the proposed FLE mandate in Virginia. Some, however, are only quasi-legal in nature—they specifically object to the statute which, opponents believe, violates the civil rights of the students and parents involved. The first is one example.

1. *FLE does not work.* It neither reduces teen pregnancy, abortions and STDs, nor enhances a student's performance in school.
2. *FLE has no stated behavioral or academic goals and no measurable objectives.* Without goals or objectives, any program can be put in place with no way to measure its progress or its lack of progress.
3. *FLE risks disrupting normal childhood development.* This is especially true of the elementary years. Psychologists and child development experts are deeply divided on the appropriate age at which the topic of human sexuality should be introduced in the classroom, if at all. They are also at odds about who should do the teaching: parents, school, or both.

   Substantial psychiatric clinical evidence shows three negatives often occur from exposure to non-parental sex education during latency: (1) When a child this age (6-12) is made prematurely wise sexually, the natural eagerness to learn in school is diminished; 329/3 (2) the normal development of compassion is dangerously jeopardized by non-parental sex education during latency. The results are best seen in later anti-social behavior; 330 and (3) a higher incidence of turning later to promiscuity, drugs and perversion is observed. 331
4. *FLE fails to address critical questions publicly.* Some of these questions are: (a) Since the curriculum uses the present total hours available, what subjects in the current curriculum will be eliminated to make room for FLE? (b) Who will decide which subjects are least valuable and will be eliminated? What about public input where all sides are expressed and changes made in accordance with that input? (c) How many hours will FLE require per semester per grade? Will PPFA guidelines be used here? (d) Will the FLE curriculum be taught as separate subjects or integrated into the core curriculum? If sex education is integrated, parents and students will be unable to opt in or opt out. (e) Why are topics not to be covered not listed? Controversial topics to be omitted must be stipulated. Such topics include homosexuality as an alternative lifestyle (which is virtually part of all sex education classes endorsed by PPFA), lesbianism, incest, masturbation and abortion. (f) What standards will be

used of those who will teach the teachers? What about public input on this issue? There are no published moral standards or guidelines used in the selection of sex education teachers. I have heard personally from several parents who are vitally concerned about this issue, since teachers, whether intentionally or not, tend to teach what they believe and promote what they practice.

5. *FLE violated current guidelines specifying sex-separate classes for explicit human sexuality instruction.* Presently, the law specifies that children must be separated by sex for instruction which includes verbal and visual descriptions of topics such as penis, testicles, scrotum, vagina, vulva, ovaries, breast development, menstruation, nocturnal emissions, wet dreams, erections and masturbation. When children are not sex-separated for these discussions, their sense of natural modesty and protection is damaged.

   Here's a key point. Can you imagine a mixed group of men and women teachers sitting around their lunchroom table discussing the breast development of the female teachers? If the male teachers participated, they would be slapped with a sexual harassment suit so fast it would make their heads spin. Teachers don't have these kinds of discussions because they're embarrassing and inappropriate. Why should we expect our young people to participate when they are even much more vulnerable and modest? The current guidelines leave the decision of separate sex classes up to the local school board.

6. *FLE lacks safeguards against the invasion of privacy or moral and religious conviction.* The proposal provides no safeguards against abuse. There are no restrictions against an invasion of the students' privacy. In accordance with the Supreme Court rulings on the matter, programs must state that they will avoid teaching or promoting to public school children personal sexuality behaviors, practices and alternatives which are contrary to those taught or held as religious convictions by the parents or students, or which are contrary to law.

   If a subject cannot be taught without violating convictions or countervailing the law, a statement to that effect must be made and the students must be referred to their parents or guardians for further information. 417

7. *FLE lacks safeguards against the use of improper extracurricular materials (videos, films, literature, guest speakers).* Programs such as the Virginia's Family Life Education open the door for all kinds of literature. The following information was distributed to a mixed eighth-grade "Family Life Planning" class at the Azalea Gardens Middle School in Norfolk, Virginia,

in February 1988. The pamphlet, "Proper Use of Condoms," was provided by the Norfolk Department of Public Health.

WARNING: The following instruction information will be offensive to you. It is to me. Yet you need to be accurately informed as to what some schoolchildren are receiving.

When properly used, latex rubbers create a strong protective barrier. Research has shown that condoms prevent the transmission of HIV (the virus that causes AIDS). They also help prevent the spread of other opportunistic infections such as cytomegalovirus (CMV) and Epstein Barr Virus (EBV) as well as herpes, gonorrhea and syphilis.

Instructions for using a condom are simple but must be followed carefully. The main reason rubbers fail is incorrect usage. They seldom leak or break due to faulty manufacture.

(1) Keep a convenient supply of condoms in a cool, dry place for "every-time" use.

(2) Do not test rubbers by inflating or stretching them (and then use them with a partner).

(3) Use condoms every time you have sex, even for oral sex.

(4) Open the package carefully. Tearing it open can damage the rubber, especially if one's nails are long and jagged.

(5) Gently press air out of the receptacle tip before putting on the condom; air bubbles cause condoms to break. Plain-ended rubbers require about a half inch free at the tip to catch the sperm. A dab of waterbase lubricant in the tip will solve the air problem and greatly increase sensation.

(6) Unroll the condom so that it covers the entire erect penis. If the penis is uncircumcised, pull back the foreskin before covering the head with the condom. Fitting an erect penis with a condom insures the best fit, but if the penis is soft, be sure to unroll the entire condom down to the base as the organ hardens. Eliminate any air bubbles.

(7) Use plenty of water-soluble lubricant on the outside of the condom and on the anus or vagina

before entry. Cavities that are too dry can pull condoms off and tear them as well. Oil- and petroleum-based lubricants like Crisco and Vaseline cause rubbers to deteriorate quickly.

(8) Hold on to the base of the rubber when you need to so that it won't slip off. If the penis is getting soft, or if the opening is very tight, the condom may tend to slip.

(9) After climax, hold on to the condom around the base to avoid spilling the ejaculate or losing the rubber inside a partner. Withdraw gently.

(10) Throw used rubbers away. Condoms should never be used more than once. Never go from one person to another without cleaning yourself well and changing rubbers.

For more information here are some phone numbers you can call: U.S. Public Health Service, 1-800-342-AIDS (recorded message); National Gay Task Force (New York), 80 Fifth Avenue, Suite 1601, New York, NY 10011, 1-800-221-7044 (3-9 P.M.); Gay Men's Health Crisis, Box 274, 132 West 24th Street, New York, NY 10011, (212) 807-6655; Virginia AIDS Hotline (General Information and Counseling Resources), 1-800-533-4148 (Mon.-Fri., 8:30 A.M.–5 P.M.); Tidewater AIDS Crisis Taskforce (TACT), 814 West 41st Street, Norfolk, VA 23508, (804) 423-5859; MCV Healthline, (804) 786-1000.

Then in bold letters the pamphlet proclaims, "Protect your lover; wear a rubber."

When there are no safeguards against extracurricular materials in a sex education program, the teacher is free to bring in anything or anyone which promotes his or her moral values without prior approval by parents. This is why Mary Lee Tatum, one of the designers and promoters of the Virginia FLE program, tells sex education teachers that it is best not to use a textbook. She advocates using resources that are hard for parents to get their hands on. 56

8. *FLE lacks basic provisions for parental responsibility and involvement.* Virginians for Family Values report two pertinent guidelines which preclude parents in the education and protection of their children in a possible life-and-death situation. PPFA would like to see all these parental restrictions in every state. The Legislative Briefing Packet points out this legal

quandry in Virginia which precludes parental involvement: 423/1,3

> (1) A minor child can undergo an abortion, and/or receive contraceptive devices in Virginia, without her parents' permission, or even their knowledge. . . .
>
> The Virginia Legislature has refused to strike down a law prohibiting parents from being notified or giving their permission for abortion or contraception, despite the fact that a vast majority of Virginia parents want a parental notification law.
>
> (2) A child could be diagnosed as having the fatal disease AIDS, as well as other sexually transmitted diseases, and by law the doctor cannot notify a parent without the minor child's permission.

* * *

After reading the above, you probably wonder, *Who is the parent in Virginia?*

Nationwide, the taxpayer-subsidized Planned Parenthood has used millions of dollars and every resource possible–education, legislative lobbying, and the courts–to lobby against parents being able to be notified before their minor child is going to have an abortion. So far, due to a lack of citizen awareness and organization, they have been extremely effective.

♦ Outside Influences on FLE

Two of the most effective outside influences on local and statewide sex education are Planned Parenthood Federation of America (PPFA) and the Sex Information and Education Council of the United States (SIECUS). They are also the two organizations most strongly aligned against traditional values. This description is not necessarily true of every individual who is in some way associated with these groups, but overall, I believe it is an accurate statement of the groups as a whole.

PPFA has targeted every state for a comprehensive K-12 sex education curriculum mandate. Their aims include not only initiating sex education but also instituting school-based clinics and indoctrinating parents with their sexual values. PPFA proudly takes credit for the programs they have implemented. One PPFA publication reports:

> Two states–Virginia and Iowa–passed comprehensive K-12 sexuality education mandates during their 1988 legislative sessions. The Virginia legislature appropriated $5.5 million for teacher training and resource materials to help school districts establish family life education curricula.

Both states participated in the 1988 Sexuality Education Project developed by PPFA's Public Affairs Division. . . .

Ohio, Iowa, Connecticut, Illinois, and Texas have been selected as "targets" for the 1988 Sexuality Education Project. The project is designed to help reach PPFA's goal of having fifteen states with kindergarten-through-twelfth-grade (K-12) sexuality education mandates by 1990. 373/1,3

Your minor child cannot have her ears pierced, or even take an aspirin in school, without parental permission—*but Virginia law allows her to leave school grounds to get contraceptives . . . or an abortion . . . without parental permission or knowledge.* And school officials are prohibited from telling the child's parents.

In a related article in the *Insider,* PPFA amplifies its concept of state participation in its goals:

States were selected according to their ability to: (1) establish a broad-based grass-roots coalition committed to achieving a statewide K-12 sexuality education mandate; (2) gain state office and affiliate board of director's approval for staffing and financing the project; (3) plan a collaborative effort between state public affairs and education staffs; (4) provide models for different geographic regions of the country; (5) develop a statewide PURPOSE (Parents United for Responsible Policies on Sexuality Education) Campaign [these are key components of their targeted state education departments]. . . .

Further, PPC (Planned Parenthood of Connecticut) will work with a state university to design and implement a model sexuality education program in a *private* school [emphasis mine]. . . .

Arizona, Georgia, Vermont, Virginia, Washington and Wisconsin were selected as Tier II states, those pursuing a sexuality education initiative but unable to meet all the necessary requirements mapped out above. They, too, will receive technical assistance and will be encouraged to move into targeted status in 1989. 373

PPFA's objectives are clear. It wants sex education programs like FLE in every state, not only in the public schools but also in the private schools. PPFA has different levels of involvement of states in the program, and its personnel will aid wherever and whomever they can to help states meet the goals.

As you, a school board member, begin to evaluate programs for Julian Unified School District, please examine all material and curriculum in light of the above analysis of the Virginia Family Life model.

The comparison by the Educational Guidance Institute, Inc. (used by permission and appearing on the next three pages) can be particularly helpful in analyzing and evaluating both directive and non-directive approaches to Family Life Education programs.

Two Models of Family Life Education A Comparative Analysis

By: Educational Guidance Institute, Inc.
927 South Walter Reed Drive, Suite 1
Arlington, VA 22204

Which model of Family Life Education meets the needs of children and youth?

Guiding Assumptions

DIRECTIVE	NON-DIRECTIVE
Abstinence-based FLE Model	Contraceptive-based FLE Model
1. Basis for Sexual Rights and Responsibilities	
Sexual rights and responsibilities are not merely personal; they are linked to society's needs and a moral code. Every known human society has regulated sex and marriage, and in our society the basis for sexual conduct has been the Judeo-Christian ethic.	Sexual rights and responsibilities are grounded in the right of the supposed "autonomous" individual to choose those actions that are right for him or her based on personally chosen values.
2. Primary Educational Goals	
Supporting the institutions in which individuals thrive. Recognizing the complementary roles of family, school, church and community.	Building up the individual's sense of autonomy.
3. Core Values	
In a pluralistic society core values like honesty and respect should preclude teaching youth how to use and obtain contraceptives to perform illegal, unhealthy and, many believe, immoral actions.	Core values like honesty and respect provide sufficient framework to justify teaching contraception in the public school classroom.

DIRECTIVE continued	NON-DIRECTIVE continued
(Abstinence-based)	(Contraceptive-based)
Marriage and family recognized as foundation for society and indispensable framework for public school Family Life Education.	Society's values today do not include sufficient agreement on priority value of marriage and the family to justify their clear defense in public classroom.
4. Parent's Role	
Primary: Parental guidance is essential and irreplaceable in sex education. Research shows parental role to be critical factor in positive behavioral outcomes for youth. Primary role of parents as the sex educators of their children must be supported and encouraged in FLE programs.	Limited: Only minority of parents are willing to guide their children effectively. Therefore school must take primary role in sex education.
5. Presentation of Premarital Abstinence	
Premarital abstinence is defined as a positive lifestyle for adolescents that promotes self-control, character and self-esteem. The only recommended option for children and adolescents.	Premarital abstinence is defined in the context of contraceptive options; presented as most effective choice for children and adolescents but not the only option.
6. Educational Rationale for Models	
Adult guidance and consistent message of premarital abstinence essential to outweigh media and peer pressures for all children and youth.	Contraceptive information is essential for all children and youth to learn in the public school classroom.
Contraceptive information is not value-neutral. Can undermine the decisions of abstaining students.	Contraceptive information will only be used by students likely to be sexually active.
Contraceptive information taught in classroom reinforces youth perception that adults assume they will be sexually active.	Contraceptive information given in the classroom will not negatively impact abstaining students.
7. Priority Needs of Children and Youth	
All children and youth, especially those at risk, need positive rationale for premarital abstinence and high expectations from adults.	Children and youth at risk are becoming sexually active earlier and nothing can be done to prevent this.

DIRECTIVE continued	NON-DIRECTIVE continued
(Abstinence-based)	(Contraceptive-based)
Research shows youth, especially high risk youth, are not developmentally able to use contraception effectively.	Contraception can be effectively learned and utilized by children and youth.

8. Teacher's Role

DIRECTIVE	NON-DIRECTIVE
Role model and leader: provides clear principles and guidance as well as information.	Facilitator: provides information and teaches decision-making skills.

9. How Decision-Making Is Taught

DIRECTIVE	NON-DIRECTIVE
Sexual decisions of students must include social and ethical considerations that go beyond individual self interest.	Sexual decision-making is based on: a learned process, information, and personal values of a child.
Students mature and make decisions in context of family, community and moral values.	Student seen as autonomous decision-maker.

CHAPTER 21

➧ A **key section** for busy parents.

Resource 2

28 Positive Reasons to Teach Abstinence

It must be kept in mind that effective abstinence-based programs don't stop with "Just say no!" There's more to abstinence education than that. The "just say no" campaign wouldn't be very effective in dealing with the adolescent sexual crisis if all we did was teach kids, "Don't do it!"

Family planning advocates seem to ridicule and mock the "just say no" stance as being naive and out of touch – fantasizing. One example is a statement by free-lance writer Beverly Walth, in the opinion section of the *Dallas Times Herald:* "Sexual abstinence is a fantasy solution." Walth emphatically states that advocates of abstinence "put forth the view that the solution to the problem of teen sex is merely to tell them not to do it." Walth continues, "What irritates me most about this manner of thinking – if indeed there is any thought buried in there at all – is that abstinence is a fantasy solution to these very real problems." 325

Please realize that neither I nor other abstinence education advocates are endorsing or promoting a simplistic "just say no" approach to the teenage sexual crisis. What I desperately want to convey about teaching abstinence can be summed up in five brief statements:

1. Teens need to know that it's not only okay to say no, it's also *right* to say no.
2. Teens need to know *why* to say no.

3. Teens need to know *how* to say no.
4. Teens need to know the *benefits* of saying no.
5. Teens need authority figures who will *model* for them that abstinence is not only acceptable but also right.

This chapter deals primarily with the fourth statement. The following are just 28 of the multitude of positive reasons for teens to practice chastity. For a more in-depth look at these reasons see the book *Why Wait? What You Need to Know About the Teen Sexuality Crisis* written by Dick Day and myself. 375

♦ Medical Benefits of Abstinence

1. Abstinence protects you from both the fear of and the consequences of sexually transmitted diseases (STDs).

During the late '60s everyone was raving about the pill. Women were finally liberated from the fear of pregnancy, and now sex could be natural and unencumbered. **What they didn't know about the sexual revolution is that pill-inspired casual sex would usher in one of the greatest epidemics of sexually transmitted diseases in history.**

Today everyone is extolling the condom as the solution to the STD problem, and many people view it as a free ticket to promiscuity. But as earlier chapters have documented, condoms are not the answer any more than the pill was. Sexually transmitted diseases are raging through the population like a firestorm. The only 100-percent effective way to avoid the fear and consequences of STDs is abstinence.

"Abstinence-based sex education," writes pediatrician Dr. S. DuBose Ravenal, "is free of harmful side effects, while the birth control approach, if the proven association with increased rates of sexual activity is causal, is replete with dangerous effects. These include an increase in sexually transmitted diseases, including AIDS, increased pregnancies, various complications of early use of oral contraceptives, and the increased risk of cervical cancer with early onset of sexual activity." 287

Dr. Joe S. McIlhaney, a gynecologist, explains, "If sex is avoided until marriage and then engaged in only in marriage, all these sexually transmitted diseases would be of no importance at all because they could not enter into a closed circle relationship between husband and wife. Such an approach is [neither naive nor "moralizing," but it *is*] now necessary." 297/28-30

Even PPFA's own Lou Harris Poll showed:

In evaluating arguments for delaying sex, teenagers say that the danger of catching sexually transmitted diseases and the danger of a pregnancy ruining one's life are two messages that are most likely to influence their peers. Sixty-five percent think that telling teenagers to worry about catching diseases like AIDS and herpes would be likely to influence them to wait to have sexual intercourse. Sixty-two percent think that telling them how a pregnancy could ruin their life would be effective. 27/9

Abstinence is a health issue. There are fifty-two sexually transmitted diseases, and that gives you fifty-two good, positive, medical reasons to abstain. For an understanding of sexually transmitted diseases, see chapter 14—Strategy 2: "Teach the Consequences of Promiscuity."

2. Abstinence frees you from the fear and consequences of pregnancy.

Abstinence is the only method of birth control that is 100-percent effective and 100-percent free of side effects. The U.S. Centers for Disease Control reports that 50 percent of women 15-19 years old who obtained an abortion in 1976 had been using a birth control method when their pregnancy occurred. 309 PPFA reports on the percentage of single women under 18 who had an unwanted pregnancy within the first twelve months of using contraceptives: diaphragm, 31.6 percent; condom, 18.4 percent; pill, 11 percent. 298

There is an emotional trauma in pregnancy for a teen. It is best described by a girl who wrote: "I used to think, ten years from now I'll be a woman of 24. Now I think, I'll be 24—and my child will be 10." To have a child at such an early age limits for many years to come what a young mother is able to do—and the father too, if they choose to get married. Many of their early dreams will go unfulfilled.

The National Academy of Science, in the report, "Legalized Abortion and the Public Health," points out: "There probably is no psychologically painless way to cope with an unwanted pregnancy whether it is voluntarily interrupted or carried to term." 427/98

3. Abstinence frees you from the dangers of various birth control methods.

Some IUDs can be harmful, and the pill should be closely monitored, especially when used by teens—but these precautions are seldom considered. Even PPFA president Faye Wattleton admits, "All contraceptive methods currently in use have serious drawbacks in their efficacy, safety and acceptability. The most effective methods, the pill and IUD, [both] have side effects." 419

4. Abstinence frees you from the trauma of abortion.

The responsibilities of pregnancy are often overlooked in the heat of passion. For a teenager, raising a child is a heavy financial and social burden. Giving the child up for adoption can leave a painful emotional scar. But perhaps the most terrible anguish associated with unwanted pregnancy is the trauma of abortion.

Abortion can solve the unwanted pregnancy situation for the moment, but it never resolves the guilt or breaks the bond between a mother and her baby. Dr. Anne Speckhard studied the emotional impact of abortion on the aborting mother. Although the women she studied came from diverse backgrounds, the reactions were almost identical:

81% reported preoccupation with the aborted child;
73% reported flashbacks of the abortion experience;
69% reported feelings of "craziness" after the abortion;
54% recalled nightmares related to the abortion;
35% had perceived visitations from the aborted child;
23% reported hallucinations related to the abortion.

In Dr. Speckhard's findings, 72 percent of the subjects said they held no religious beliefs at the time of their abortions, and 96 percent, in retrospect, regarded abortion as the taking of life or as murder. 299/69

The report, "Legalized Abortions and the Public Health," by the National Academy of Science, points out:

> Certain trends emerge from a review of the scientific literature on the mental health effects of abortion. Emotional stress and pain are involved in the decision to obtain an abortion, and these are strong emotions that surround the entire procedure. . . . Medical complications associated with legal abortion may occur at the time of abortion (immediate), within thirty days following the procedure (delayed), or at some later time (late). 420/88-98

Abortion is a painful procedure. Complications may develop and the emotional fallout can be overwhelming. M. Uchtman, Ohio director of Suiciders Anonymous, told the Cincinnati City Council on September 1, 1981: "Suiciders Anonymous, in a 35-month period, reported counseling 5,620 members in the Cincinnati, Ohio, area. The members had attempted or were considering suicide. Of these, 1,800 had had abortions, of whom 1,400 were between 15 and 24 years old."

The Alan Guttmacher Institute, the research arm of PPFA, admitted: "The health, social and economic consequences of teenage pregnancy are almost all adverse. Pregnancies that end in abortion or miscarriage are, at the least, upsetting and sometimes traumatic to the pregnant woman." 300/28

Hall and Zissok, in their study, "Psychological Distress Following Therapeutic Abortion," found that "the trauma of abortion may have significant emotional sequelae [consequences]." 301/34 Kumar and Robson report in *Psychological Medicine* that "eight of twenty-one women who had obtained a past abortion were found to be clinically depressed and anxious. In contrast, only eight of ninety-eight who had not had abortions were depressed." 302/711-715

Dr. Bulfin, in the article "A New Problem in Adolescent Gynecology" in the *Southern Medical Journal,* explains that some teenagers have significant post-abortion complications:

> As more abortions are being done in teenage girls than ever before, an unusually large number of complications are being seen by some private practitioners. Because many of these adolescent patients in whom complications develop do not return to the physicians who did the abortions, accurate data on the incidence of abortion complications are difficult to obtain. . . . The diversity of complications that can occur in teenage girls after legal abortion is startling. 303

Dr. Bulfin reports the wide range of traumas among women who suffer with complications from abortions:

Trauma	Experienced by those with complications
Damage to reproductive organs	42.6%
Uterine rupture or perforation	5.6
Endometritis	13.0
Salpingitis, pyosalpinx	13.0
Cervical lacerations	11.0
Severe emotional and psychiatric [problems]	16.1
Hemorrhage, intractable	13.0
Pelvic pain and dyspareunia	11.1
Infertility and repeated miscarriage	7.4
Incomplete operations; subsequent passage of fetal parts and tissue	74.0
Bowel resection with colostomy	1.9

Dr. Bulfin also related some sad case studies of abortion trauma:

- A 17-year-old girl, nine weeks pregnant, had a suction abortion at a local clinic. Fever, chills and pelvic pain became progressively worse. . . . She was hospitalized when a pelvic mass failed to respond to antibiotic therapy, and laparotomy on the eighth day after abortion revealed a perforated uterus with massive pyosalpinx and pelvic abscesses, necessitating total hysterectomy. . . .
- A 17-year-old girl . . . suffered cervical lacerations and severe hemorrhage after a clinic abortion. . . . She suffered prolonged

disability, remorse and guilt, and regretted very much having had the procedure. In the four years since the operation she has been unable to become pregnant. . . .

- A 16-year-old girl was seen the day after a suction curettage abortion. . . . She had been bleeding. . . . She evidently had had acute gonorrhea when the abortion was done, and . . . pelvic pain, tenderness and dyspareunia persisted for many months afterwards.
- None of them felt they had been afforded any meaningful information about the potential dangers of the abortion operation. Incongruously, some had actually stopped the birth control pill because they had read it was "too dangerous," believing that since abortion was legal, it must be safe. . . .

Serious complications and even deaths may go unreported for the following reasons: (1) There is no mandatory reporting of legal abortions and their sequelae in most states; (2) often the physician who does the abortion never knows of his complication; (3) vital facts may be omitted from death certificates; and (4) the average physician will not report the complication because of the paperwork involved.

The teenager, frightened and mentally and physically traumatized by her abortion, will often not seek help until she is almost moribund. Her parents may be the last to know. . . .

More teenagers are having abortions in the United States than in any other country in the world. 303

One of the great benefits of abstinence is that all of the tragic physical and emotional traumas of abortion are completely avoided.

♦ Emotional Benefits of Abstinence

5. Abstinence protects you from sexual addiction.

Psychologists and counselors will tell you that sexual addictions are a fast-growing problem in society, and counseling sex addicts is an increasing trend. Whether sexual addiction is strictly psychological or a combination of psychological and physical problems, no one can say for sure at the moment; but it is a real addiction. Like compulsive eating, bulimia or anorexia, sexual addiction may be caused by mental trauma or personality disorders in the person's life.

Pornography is proving to be just as addicting for many people as drugs, alcohol or food. Premarital sex also can become addicting. Constant sexual stimulation causes chemical changes in the body just as other addictions. You need to have a physical relationship with someone in order to survive. Communication begins to disappear.

Petting becomes a pattern, and it's hard to go back to holding hands. Other areas of your relationship also become obscured by the physical. One girl who was heavily into drugs wrote, "Sex is like drugs. You keep wanting bigger highs. In fact, I think it made me do more drugs. I'd get high, and then I'd do some weird, kinky stuff. Regular sex wasn't enough. I'd do things I felt horrible about. Then I would do more drugs to take away the pain. It was a vicious circle."

The only reward from sex outside a loving, trusting relationship is the physical high. **When the sexual high becomes the goal, you become addicted to the high.** The high serves as a form of denial of reality, denial of the pain, and denial of the need for love and understanding and the intimacy that is sought in the relationship. The pain of coping with the drugs and the sex is easier than the pain of coping with a lonely life.

"Sexual addiction," reports *USA Today*, "is more apt to elicit snickers than concern. But addicts say it's no joke. And mental health professionals, increasingly concerned about the estimated 13 million sex addicts in the United States, are determined to bring the compulsion out of the closet. Sexual addiction can lead to destruction." **305/5D**

The first forum on sex addiction took place in Los Angeles in 1989. The National Association on Sexual Addiction Problems reports:

> "We live in a quick-fix society prone to using things like drinking, eating and sex as solutions to anxiety," says Patrick Carnes, architect of the USA's first inpatient program for sex addicts – the Sexual Dependency Unit at the Golden Valley (Minnesota) Institute for Behavioral Medicine. "We are a very addictive culture."
>
> Although sex addicts can be news-making criminals, most aren't fringe characters.
>
> "People have a picture of a sex addict in their minds," says Golden Valley's Robin Anderson. "The truth is most of the people are professionals with a devastating illness."
>
> A recent survey of fifty-four Golden Valley patients showed 42 percent earned more than $30,000 a year; 58 percent were college graduates. Equally revealing: As children, 74 percent had been sexually abused; 91 percent emotionally abused.
>
> "The more abused you were as a child, the more addictions you will tend to have as an adult," says Carnes.
>
> Sexual addiction – whose symptoms can range from excessive masturbation to incest – can be as destructive as alcohol or drug addictions, often ruining careers and marriages.
>
> Sex addicts often:
>
> - Live a secret sexual life steeped in lies and shame;
> - Find controlling urges nearly impossible;

- Pursue sexual interests obsessively despite personal and financial risks. 305/5D

The obsessions have a way of staying underground.

"Our society likes to deny its sexuality and doesn't like hearing about sex offenders," says Richard Salmon, executive director of the NASAP, Boulder, CO. 305/5D

6. Abstinence frees you from the pressure to get married before you are ready.

Premarital sex adds a sense of urgency to a relationship which is often vaguely expressed by one or both partners as a desire for greater commitment. Be it spoken or unspoken, the pressure for marriage is still there.

Physical intimacy cries out for emotional closeness and commitment. Yet those qualities are seldom present in a physically charged relationship. Indeed, they cannot be forthcoming without a lifetime commitment.

7. Abstinence frees you from being put on a performance basis.

Teens today are often put on a sexual performance basis; they must put out sexually if they are to be accepted. A performance-based relationship is one in which you are accepted for what you do, not for who you are.

When the physical performance becomes the standard for acceptance or rejection, fear is built into the relationship. Without the committed bonds of marriage, sex is inherently a selfish act done for personal gain. For a relationship based on performance to continue, the sex partners must continue to be pleasing to each other. As soon as one partner no longer lives up to what the other wants, the relationship is in trouble. Or if someone else comes along who has more of what the other is looking for in bed, the relationship takes a dive. The relationship is really one of mutual exploitation.

If your cute face and large breasts are what attracted him to you, when someone comes along with a cuter face or larger breasts you will be rejected. **Performance partners keep each other in a state of perpetual insecurity, a state that symbolizes much of what true love is not.** Couples in these circumstances experience an unspoken element of fear: the fear of rejection.

8. Abstinence protects you from comparison later in marriage.

The famous psychologist Abraham Maslow once described sex as the peak of human emotions. The powerful emotions and memories of an illicit sexual encounter are forces a person may have to deal with for years after the actual event. I have counseled people who can describe the details of a number of sexual encounters, but they don't even remember their sex partners' names. Such is the influence sex has on our emotions and memories.

If you become involved with someone in an intimate physical relationship so you know her physical qualities and points of sexual arousal, you will later compare your future wife to her. One woman wrote to me, "My two friends must also deal with the problem of comparing their husbands to the men of their past relationships. Although guilt makes them feel hesitant or inhibited, they also fight the attitude of scorn or rejection for their husbands, who always seem to fall short, not measuring up to idealized memories of previous sexual encounters."

A female student at the University of Chicago said to me, "I've decided that I don't want to marry a virgin. I want to marry an experienced man, someone who knows what he's doing in bed."

"You've got to be nuts, lady," I replied. "You're telling me that you want an experienced man who will know how to arouse you because that's how he aroused some other woman. **He'll be comparing your breasts to her breasts, your thighs to her thighs, your ecstatic experience to her ecstatic experience.** He'll be trying positions on you some other woman enjoyed."

She immediately responded, "I don't want that!"

If you marry an experienced man, you will miss the joy of discovery and the bonding that takes place when you learn love-making together. **You will always be just one of many.**

The first time you make love is to be remembered. It is to be a wonderful time, something to look back upon as a symbol of your fidelity to one another. Sadly, if you choose not to remain a virgin, that first time with someone else will also always live in your memory.

9. Abstinence protects your most delicate sex organ: your mind.

Your most important sex organ is your mind. How does your mind relate to your loins? In this way. In the New Testament is one of the most profound verses ever written about marriage and sex: "Let marriage be held in honor among all. Let the marriage bed be undefiled [pure]" (Hebrews 13:4). "In honor" means in high esteem. The words "marriage bed" in the Greek language literally mean "sexual coitus." The verse is saying, "Let sexual coitus [intercourse] be pure, undefiled and unadulterated in the context of the marriage bed."

What does it mean to be sexually pure? The word pure means "no foreign element." For example, an unopened bottle of aspirin is 100 percent aspirin–it's pure aspirin. But if someone comes along and injects arsenic into the bottle, the aspirin becomes impure, defiled or adulterated. Why? A foreign element entered the pure substance. The above passage says, "Don't let any foreign element enter sexual coitus in your marriage bed."

Guys will say, "What does my mind have to do with sex?"

A lot. Your mind is your most powerful and most sensitive sex organ. Sex begins in the mind. Disconnect your mind and try to get aroused!

How does it work–sex and the mind? Have you ever wondered why you remember certain things and don't remember other things? Let's say somebody really embarrassed you a year ago. You can probably recall the face, the place and the event. But you probably can't remember who you had lunch with that day.

There are a number of explanations for our experiences with "selective remembering." One is that it's a biochemical reaction. Research shows that when you have an intense emotional experience involving the five senses, a chemical is released which implants that experience in your mind for recall. This biochemical reaction allows you to remember the significant events over the insignificant, the important over the unimportant.

Nothing triggers us biochemically quite like sex, starting with pornography. There are many men who are hooked on pornography. They can't go through a day without looking at it. In fact, most can't even close their eyes without picturing it. Many can't even look at a woman without recalling pornographic images. Some distraught women have confessed that their husbands can't make love to them or have an orgasm without a picture of a nude woman on the pillow. Why? Because of the way these men have programmed their main sex organ–their mind.

Not only does pornography lodge in the memory, but past sexual experiences can too. A 32-year-old man I've known for a number of years came to me in tears one day. "What's wrong?" I asked.

He said, "Josh, I need your help. You know that I've been married for eight years. I love my wife. There's nobody in the world as beautiful and sensitive as she. But in eight years of marriage, we've never been alone in bed."

I knew what was coming, but I asked, "What do you mean?"

He went on to say that in high school he had played around a lot sexually with a number of women. His behavior carried over into the university where it got out of control. During his junior year he met his wife-to-be. They fell in love and got married a year after college.

At this point he was crying as hard as anyone I've ever seen cry. "Starting on our wedding night," he continued, "I began to experience 'reruns in the theatre of my mind.' I can't even have sex with my own wife without thinking of other women. I picture other women when I look at my wife. It's destroying the intimacy in our marriage."

"Reruns in the theatre of my mind"—that says it all! Our mind is like a piece of film—it records everything. He couldn't control the flashbacks and it was tearing his life and marriage apart.

One 26-year-old woman who had been married three years wrote me, "Josh, how do I get rid of the ghosts of relationships past?" You see, you can date someone, become sexually involved and then break up. You can send back the class ring, you can cut his or her picture into a thousand pieces, and you can burn all the mementos, but you can't send back the memories. Men and women don't forget sexual experiences—even when they want to.

10. Abstinence protects from misleading feelings.

One solid reason for waiting is that sexual involvement, especially for teens, can produce confusion between sex and love. Premarital sex can terribly confuse a person who actually may have had a legitimate understanding of love. One writer said sexual encounters outside marriage give an illusion of intimacy which can be mistaken for the lasting commitment that ultimately makes marriage work.

Often when sex enters into a relationship, the physical becomes its all-consuming element. The intellectual, emotional, social and spiritual all take a back seat to sex (no pun intended!). All the couple wants to do is spend time alone engaging in physical activity, and they mistake sex for love. Sadly and ironically, when one partner breaks off the relationship, he or she often can't stand to be near or talk to the other because the guilt feelings over the sexual activity are too strong. The guilt quickly washes away the false feelings of love.

Sex before marriage turns relationships upside down and mixes emotions to the point where a person can misinterpret feelings. A couple often becomes sexually involved and then misinterprets the act of sex and their own feelings. They think they "know" the other person better than they really do. They think the relationship is deeper than it really is. They mistake their feelings for love and say "I do." But the marriage is probably doomed.

Don Smedley writes:

> When we mix sex and love, we confuse the simple concepts of giving and taking. Love always gives and always seeks the best interests of the other person. Premarital sex usually takes. Each individual has his or her own goal in having sex before marriage, but each is in it for personal reasons. The problem is that taking can sometimes look like the giving.
>
> A girl may give her boyfriend "what he wants," thus making it look as though she is giving to him in love. But she does it from a personal motive. She may want the security he provides. She may want to achieve popularity by being his girlfriend. She may have one of a dozen other reasons, but her "giving" is actually a form of taking. She is manipulating him for her own ends. She is being misled by her emotions.

Sex always changes the dynamics of a relationship.

11. Abstinence protects you from sustaining "bad" relationships.

Breaking up from dating relationships or meaningful relationships can tear teens apart emotionally. We all have experienced the sadness of breaking off a relationship with someone we cared about but could no longer get along with. But when you add physical involvement, breaking emotional ties is even harder. **Abstinence reduces the pain of breaking up.**

So many people have said to me, "When I walked away from that relationship, I left a part of myself behind." Sex forms a bond that can exist no matter what the rest of the relationship is like. Even if communication has broken down and emotions are strained, sex forms an almost unexplainable bond. It locks people into relationships. The longer it goes on, the harder it is to break it off and then leave it behind.

12. Abstinence frees you from the trauma of having to give up your baby for adoption.

One of the hardest decisions an unwed couple must make is giving up their out-of-wedlock child for adoption. Often, however, this is their only option. The financial responsibilities of parenthood make it almost impossible for teenagers to raise children, but the emotional tug, especially between mother and child, is very strong.

13. Abstinence helps you avoid deep scars.

"Love you forever" feelings, which convince couples to think that premarital sex is okay, don't last forever. When they engage in sex, they give a special part of themselves to each other. When they break up, that part which was given is lost—never to be regained. This type of emotional scarring can be very difficult to overcome.

14. Abstinence provides a basis of trust.

One of the most powerful factors for a fulfilled love and sex relationship inside marriage is trust. Any marriage counselor will tell you that trust is one of the most vital factors, if not *the* most vital one, in a fulfilled love, sex and marriage relationship. Abstinence protects you from suspicion and distrust, and provides the trust you need for fulfilling love and sex in a marriage relationship.

In a study of students at Virginia Tech, one of the questions asked was, "What is the number one thing you want in a relationship?" Do you know what came out? Trust, far above anything else. At San Jose State University, fifty men and women did an article called, "Sexual Liberation: Is It Worth the Hassle?" for a major women's magazine. These students concluded that sex wasn't worth the hassle without two basic ingredients: love and trust. 421

Where do suspicion and mistrust come from? They are often built into the relationship before marriage. **If a person was sexually active before marriage, there is nothing to guarantee he or she won't be promiscuous after marriage.** Your commitment might change at the altar, but your personality doesn't change. As the years go by, many who had roving eyes before marriage find their eyes roving again. The seeds of suspicion and mistrust, which were hidden and unspoken all along, begin to sprout. Once trust is gone, so is the marriage.

After two, three or four years of marriage, your mind starts playing tricks on you. You think, *If she slept with someone before, will she now? If he played around before, can I trust him now?* And when there's distrust in the relationship, you can never allow yourself to be vulnerable. How can you open yourself up to somebody you don't trust 100 percent? And if you can't be vulnerable, you can't be transparent. And if you can't be transparent, you can't be real—and intimacy goes right out the window. Please realize that fulfilling love and sex in marriage starts with trust.

I never dreamed that the way I treated a woman on dates some twenty years ago would affect my marriage today, but it does. As a graduate student I dated a young lady named Paula for more than three years. We almost got married, and then we realized we weren't in love. We didn't have the kind of love needed on which to build a lasting, deep, intimate, marriage-sex-family relationship. We just liked each other and had a good time together. But you don't get married on that.

So we broke off our relationship. It was one of the hardest things I've ever done in my life. I felt when I walked away from Paula, I was walking away from everything I'd ever dreamed of in a woman. I thank God now, but it was hard then. It tore me apart. Paula and I did remain friends, and to this day she is one of my dearest, closest friends.

Several years later I met Dottie, and she became my wife. Dottie then met Paula. They became friends, really hit it off, and started to spend time together. One morning Dottie came home from having breakfast with Paula and said, "Honey, I'm so glad you behaved yourself for those three and a half years."

I said, "What do you mean?"

"Paula shared with me this morning that there were times when she was so in love with you she would have done anything, and you never once took advantage of her."

I breathed a sigh of relief and was extremely thankful.

You cannot imagine what it meant to my wife to know: "I can trust my husband." I never realized that the way I treated a woman on a date would contribute one of the most positive factors in my marriage to Dottie. My wife trusts me, and trust is one of the greatest motivations for fidelity and faithfulness in marriage.

15. Abstinence helps develop respect for life.

When you realize that you will never need to have an abortion, your commitment to abstinence will help produce a new respect for the dignity of human life. When an unmarried girl is pregnant and considering abortion, she is under the binding pressure of thinking about the life of her child. By saying no to premarital sex, you won't ever have to rationalize your thoughts in order to justify an abortion.

16. Abstinence frees you to focus your energy on establishing and realizing life goals.

If you become a teenage mother or father, your life dreams and ambitions, for all intents and purposes, must be put on hold indefinitely if not forever. Of course for some, motherhood and fatherhood is a way of escape from a lonely existence. The sad fact is that the adulation they may receive after the baby comes is short-lived, because the reality of raising the child sets in. It can be all the more troubling if their friends move away or go on to other things.

A teenager told me recently that her friend had a baby, and that she never has time for herself. She can't go places she would normally go and her evenings are always spoken for.

As you follow abstinence and stay away from premarital sex, you can focus your drives and energy on your dreams and aspirations. Every student, every athlete and every businessman or woman who ever made it had dreams and goals.

17. Abstinence gives freedom from guilt.

Guilt is a consequence of premarital sex that can haunt a person for a very long time, and perhaps offers the best reason to wait until marriage. The emotional and psychological distress is very real, and a crippling guilt with little joy can be the result.

Whatever people may say about guilt, it is real. As psychologist Erich Fromm said, "It is indeed amazing that, in as fundamentally irreligious a culture as ours, the sense of guilt should be so widespread and deep-rooted."[423]

Why does guilt follow promiscuity? True guilt comes from the awareness of having transgressed a standard of right and wrong. If waiting on sex until marriage is God's standard, you will experience guilt when you violate it, even if only for a short time, because you refuse to face the issue and admit the guilt.

False guilt comes from outside influences, such as other people who try to make you feel guilty when there is no reason for you to feel that way. For example, friends may make you feel guilty for missing their party when you chose to do something else that you needed to do. Going to the party would have violated what you felt was right. If you had given in to your friends and not listened to your own conscience, your guilt would have been valid.

Unless guilt is dealt with, it can be a heavy burden. Only through a personal relationship with Christ can true guilt be dealt with and false guilt be avoided.

Feelings of guilt and hurting consciences are two of the most common results of premarital sex teens talk about in their letters. One girl told me that the guilt from a few minutes of sexual pleasure destroyed a year's worth of fun, happy times and good memories.

Manhattan sex therapist Shirley Zussman comments about the inner hurt which results from premarital sex: "Being part of a meat market is appalling in terms of self-esteem." Dr. Elizabeth Whelan, in her book *Sex and Sensibility,* cites a study of unmarried women which showed that 85 percent of those under psychiatric care were sexually active.[424]

A faculty member at the University of Wisconsin (Madison) explained to me that a study showed 86 percent of psychologists' patients who were interviewed had engaged in premarital sex. Their main problem was guilt caused by those acts.

A man in Tucson speaks frequently to health and family classes at the University of Arizona. In 1970, 1975 and 1980 he surveyed hundreds of students in his seminars. He asked them, "If you have had sexual intercourse outside of marriage, what were the results?" The answers showed: 425

	Male	Female	Total
Tremendous guilt	50%	63%	57%
Led to break up	50	26	38
Created intense desire for more	44	26	35
Increased sexual frustration and pressure	33	26	30
Felt used	17	42	30

It seems obvious that premarital sex and emotional instability are related.

18. Abstinence helps develop unselfish sensitivity.

When a person is not operating under guilt, he is free to give to others. By avoiding premarital sex, you are able to focus more on others and their needs. You are not forced into trying to meet needs that you cannot possibly fulfill this side of marriage.

♦ Relational Benefits of Abstinence

19. Abstinence enhances true communication in a relationship.

Not only does premarital sex cloud the issue of true love, but it also tends to thwart the communication process. Most of us by nature gravitate toward what comes easily and is pleasurable. Therefore, sex offers an easy out to those who have never learned to communicate intimately apart from the physical. Many people believe that sex produces intimacy, but William McCready of the School of Social Work at the University of Chicago points out, "Sexual activity only celebrates what's there. Sex cannot deliver what doesn't already exist."

Hunger for an intimate relationship is built into each of us. We all want to love and be loved. Sex is merely the physical expression of that intimate love we seek, not the source of it. That is why premature sex will shortcut an immature relationship. It tries to express something that isn't there yet.

In the 1979 *Redbook* survey of more than 700 sex therapists and counselors, 85 percent said that the number-one complaint they hear is lack of communication in their relationships. Of the 30,000 women who took this survey, most said they had chosen their husbands based on sex appeal. But 80 percent said if they had to do it over again, they would choose a husband based on his ability to communicate. **306/66-67**

Immature lovers (which everyone is at the beginning) get confused about the difference between the sex act and real communication. They think they are the same. (This is a pattern often begun early in their relationship when they confuse sex with love.) But true sharing between two people is much, much more than just sex. Outside of marriage, the genuine communication upon which a mature relationship should grow is lost while the couple concentrates on a shallow substitute.

20. Abstinence helps build patience and self-control.

Patience and self-control are major building blocks in a maximum love, marriage and sexual relationship. The media says "hurry up" to everything, especially sex. I say "wait," and in so doing you build the discipline of patience and concern. If you are guided by lust and the inability to wait, you will be crippled in your marriage. In marriage there are many times you must have patience, especially in the sexual area. Your partner may be ill, and you must wait for sex until he or she feels better. If you have a job that requires you to travel, patience and self-control build in a tremendous trust factor with your spouse. If you fail to develop patience and self-control before marriage, impatience and lack of control will carry over into every aspect of your life, especially your marriage.

21. Abstinence helps to enhance a special relationship found only in marriage.

The unique oneness, the joy of fidelity and the bond of love and trust found in a marriage where each waited on sex until he or she was married is a case where "the whole is much greater than the sum of the parts." It is indeed a special relationship. Waiting to be physically intimate until you are married doesn't guarantee a great marriage—but if you wait, the joys you will know, the pleasures you will enjoy and the trust you will build will surpass anything you could possibly imagine.

Sexual promiscuity does not exclude you from a fulfilled love, marriage and sexual relationship. However, premarital sex can add many negative factors that will be difficult to overcome. You will not miss out on anything if you wait, but if you don't wait, you can miss out on something wonderful.

22. Abstinence helps develop positive principles of relational growth.

Abstinence encourages growth in the areas of discovering who each person is and what each personality is like and in developing a real friendship. These areas are far more important than sex to a successful, life-long relationship. In fact, they are the real basis for great sex in marriage. Abstinence creates and encourages more time for talking, building mutual interests and spending time with other friends. Through abstinence you can develop an intimacy that is more than physical.

23. Abstinence provides freedom to enjoy being a teenager.

This is one of the most important reasons for abstinence. Staying uninvolved sexually allows you to enjoy a healthy and fun-loving time as a teen. The pressure of premarital sex is not healthy. It can add undue pressure and frustration.

24. Abstinence provides one of the greatest gifts of true love: virginity.

One of the greatest gifts you can give your future mate is your own sexual fidelity. I have never heard anyone complain because he (or she) waited to have sex with the person he married. No one! Yet I know countless heartbroken teens who wished they had waited. What a contrast!

Many of those who didn't wait felt they needed the practice, needed to get the technique down. Nothing could be further from the truth–the plumbing almost always works. More important, the sexual patterns you build with someone other than your mate can infect your marriage later on and come between you and your spouse. Learning about sex together provides a bonding that ultimately can be enjoyed and appreciated only in a faithful marriage.

Some of you already have lost your physical virginity and it can never be recovered. But you can start over again right where you are and practice "secondary virginity." Most of the "plus factors" of abstinence can be true in your life again. And if you haven't lost your virginity, remember, it's something that cannot be recovered. There is only one "first time," and it's meant to be with the one you marry.

A while back I received the following letter:

> *I'm a 17-year-old virgin. I'm a high school senior. My friends make jokes about my virginity. They often make remarks about my "lack of experience." The pressure gets pretty great.*

So last Tuesday, when I had lunch at school with five of my girlfriends, I said, "Look, I don't want any more pressure about me becoming sexually involved. I don't want any more jokes about my virginity. Each of you needs to realize that, **whenever I want to, I can become like you, but you can never again become like me** [emphasis mine]."

That's a powerful way for a teenager to cope with sexual peer pressure.

♦ Personal Benefits of Abstinence

25. Abstinence helps increase self-esteem.

Michael Carrera, health sciences professor at Hunter College, concentrates on the contraceptive effect "of enhancing young people's self-esteem as their weapon to fight teen pregnancy: There is nothing like being loyal to the royal within. Education should promote discipline, thus plant dreams, raise hopes and open doors." 307

People are not really seeking sex today—they're seeking intimacy. They look to sex as a means to gain that closeness, but it doesn't work. It can't work outside a committed marriage relationship. Why? Because sex as it should be in marriage is based on security. There is a need for total love, companionship and freedom in giving to each other sexually. The marriage is designed to be a permanent commitment in which the partners are completely secure. There is no need to prove anything, no need for ego-boosts, no cause for insecurity. The relationship provides mutual trust and unconditional love and thus an atmosphere of understanding, acceptance and intimacy.

When this intimacy is attempted in a relationship without the marriage commitment, it is usually doomed to fail. No lasting trust can be forged without commitment. Yet many people try, and in doing so only further damage their sense of self-worth. If they get into a relationship looking for intimacy and then fail to achieve it, which is often the case, their already low self-esteem spirals even lower. They feel incapable of being loved and incapable of truly loving anyone. **They seek emotional intimacy through physical intimacy—and they never achieve it.**

The modus operandi becomes, "It's easier to bare your bottom than to bare your soul." Then, in the words of family, child and marriage counselor Dick Day, "Your body becomes a psychological barrier."

26. Abstinence can be a good "test" of love.

In response to the cheap, self-centered pressure line, "If you really love me, you will," you can say, "If you really love me, you'll wait."

Abstinence lets you test your feelings beyond the first attraction, whether physical or emotional.

27. Abstinence can make you a better lover.

It encourages you to explore a greater variety of ways to express love and your sexual desires.

28. Abstinence can be an expression of emotional integrity.

So many give in to sexual pressure when they don't want to be involved sexually. It requires strong personal integrity to be able to resist someone you like and possibly love. Personal integrity is needed to make decisions that are compatible with your own convictions and values.

Abstinence makes a lot of sense to a lot of teenagers. A high school health education teacher asked his three health classes to come up with reasons teens should say no to sex. The following 41 reasons were mailed to me by the instructor.

♦ Students' Reasons for Saying No to Sex

1. To avoid teen pregnancy.
2. To avoid STDs.
3. I don't want to feel guilty.
4. I don't want a reputation where dates expect sex and date me only for that reason.
5. I would disappoint my parents and would lose their trust and respect.
6. I might lose respect for the other person, they might lose respect for me, and I might lose respect for myself.
7. Sex is better in a secure, loving relationship like marriage.
8. The thought of having an abortion scares me to death.
9. Sex gets in the way of real intimate communication.
10. Sexual relationships are a lot harder to break up even when you know you should.
11. It may ruin a good relationship rather than make it better.
12. There are better ways to get someone to like you.
13. You won't have to worry about birth control side effects.
14. I'm not emotionally ready for that intense a relationship.
15. I could become scared of my partner.

16. I don't want to hurt someone I really care about.
17. Sex could become the central focus of the relationship, like an addiction. At that point it's no longer a meaningful relationship, but you are using each other to satisfy sexual desires.
18. You begin to compare sexual experiences leading to lots of disappointments.
19. I don't want to make myself vulnerable to being used or abused sexually.
20. If I'm hurt too many times, I might miss out on something great because I'm so afraid of being hurt again.
21. I like my freedom too much. Sexual relationships are too binding.
22. I'm only 16!
23. I'm proud of my virginity and I want it to stay that way. (This was shared by a boy and a girl.)
24. Building a relationship in other ways is more important.
25. I don't want to risk becoming someone's sex object.
26. I want my first experience to be a good one with someone who won't laugh at me, reject me, tell lies about me, and who I know will always be there tomorrow.
27. It's possible to enjoy ourselves physically without going all the way.
28. Why rush something that could be lousy or mediocre now, when it could be great later.
29. I don't want sex to lose its meaning and value so I feel "sexually bankrupt."
30. I am afraid that at this age it might not meet up to my expectations and I may be seriously disappointed.
31. I don't want to risk ending a relationship and hating each other because of it.
32. I might find it painful and the other person rough and uncaring.
33. It may only serve for the boy to brag about scoring with you.
34. It's the safest way not to become pregnant.
35. You may feel invaded and you can't take it back after it's happened to you.
36. You may have to grow up too fast and too soon.
37. Sex may become the only thing that keeps the relationship together.
38. You may have sex too early to really enjoy or understand it.

39. You lose the chance to experience the "first time" with someone who really cares for you.
40. I want my most intimate physical relationship to be with the one I marry.
41. Sex brings feelings of jealousy, envy, and possessiveness. Every relationship changes.

While I was speaking in Portland, Oregon, a group of teenagers approached me after a Why Wait? talk at the fairgrounds. They enthusiastically explained that they were part of an organization of teens that speaks in schools on the advantages of abstinence. They shared that the Why Wait? campaign and book had helped them prepare their presentations.

Then they gave me one of their handouts listing just some of the advantages they see in premarital abstinence. They defined chastity as "a virtue including sexual control or using one's sexual powers according to one's state in life. A virtue is a good habit."

Their list of advantages for abstinence included:

1. Free from pregnancy and disease.
2. Free from the bother and danger of the pill and other contraceptives.
3. Free from the pressure to get married before you are ready.
4. Free from abortion.
5. Free from the trauma of giving your baby up for adoption.
6. Free from exploitation by others.
7. Free from guilt, doubt, disappointment, worry and rejection.
8. Free to experience fuller communication in dating relationships.
9. Free to be in control of your life.
10. Free to focus energy on establishing and realizing life goals.
11. Free to develop a respect for life.
12. Free to develop unselfish sensitivity.
13. Free to have greater trust in marriage.
14. Free to enjoy being a teenager. 426

As you think about the importance of teaching abstinence in our schools, it is good to recall these comments made by teens:

"Whenever I want to, I can become like you, but you can never again become like me";

"Thank you for telling me it's okay to wait";

"I am 17 years old and have waited this long—I'm not going to stop waiting now."

CHAPTER 22

♦ A **key section** for busy parents.

Resource 3

How to Approach Schools About Sex Education

An article by Linus Wright
(used with permission)

When reading this chapter, remember that parents will find most school boards and administrators conscientious and helpful. They are in those positions because they care about kids. This has been one of the joys of living in Julian, California. Both the school board and junior and senior high school administrators welcome parental inquiry. This year they invited the parents in to look at the sex education material and to interact with the teacher and principal. Afterward they invited constructive input, and, as a parent, I deeply appreciated that.

Since school administrators and board members get books and training on how to deal with parents, I thought it appropriate to include an article for parents on how to approach board members and administrators in a positive manner.

Linus Wright was nominated by President Reagan as Under Secretary for the U.S. Department of Education on October 15, 1987, confirmed by the Senate on November 20, 1987, and sworn in on November 24, 1987.

Under Secretary Wright advised the Secretary of Education on all major program and management issues. As the agency's second-highest official, he oversaw the daily operations of the Education Department's 4,500 employees.

From August 15, 1978 to 1987, Linus Wright served as superintendent of the Dallas Independent School District–one of the nation's largest, with 130,000 students, 184 schools and 14,000 employees. Mr. Wright had a reputation in Dallas as a consensus builder with an ability to get along with all segments of the community, as well as one of the premier experts on school finance in Texas.

While he was superintendent in Dallas, Mr. Wright improved student test scores, involved 15,000 volunteers and more than 2,000 groups in school programs and partnerships, provided state leadership in school finance and program reform, gained citizen support for the largest school construction bond issue ever approved in Dallas, and initiated an expanded employee-relations program in the Dallas School District.

Mr. Wright was superintendent for administration for the Houston school system from 1974 to 1978 and chief financial officer from 1971 to 1974.

Mr. Wright has received numerous awards for his work in civic affairs and was named by *Executive Educator* magazine as one of the nation's "Top 100 Educators." He also served on the 32-member Urban Superintendents Network of the U.S. Department of Education and has served as a member of the Governor's Advisory Committee on Education in Texas.

* * *

Sex Education: How Parents Can Intelligently Approach Their School Board, Administration or Teacher

by Linus Wright

Any parent who is not worried about the problem of sexual promiscuity among young people is either naive or insensitive. More than one million teenage girls become pregnant each year; and of these, more than 400,000 have abortions and another 250,000 give birth out of wedlock.

Those statistics only begin to hint at the suffering, the sorrow, the ruined lives that are the inevitable by-product of an increasingly permissive society. For every unmarried teenage couple "in trouble," there are usually two sets of parents, grandparents, and brothers and sisters who are potential co-sufferers, as well as family friends and school mates. There are also the children of such liaisons, surely the greatest sufferers of all and the most blameless.

But pregnancy is no longer the only worry among those concerned about teenage promiscuity. Sexually transmitted diseases increasingly pose a threat to the health and lives of all who engage in irresponsible sexual behavior, and young people are increasingly at risk. The permissiveness of American society over the past twenty years has exposed a generation of teenagers to a variety of medical dangers that were known in an earlier time only to the most jaded and irresponsible of adults. And there is no reason to believe that things are improving significantly. Indeed some medical authorities predict that promiscuous conduct among young people will be even more dangerous in two years than it is today.

Changing Values

It is understandable that in the wake of such social devastation educators are attempting to devise ways in which the schools can help the family in this area—and the result has been a renewed push for required sex education in the classroom. In fact, legislatures in more than thirty states have mandated such courses as part of AIDS-prevention programs; and in some cases these courses are prescribed for kindergarten through the twelfth grade.

The idea of such courses has upset a number of people who believe in traditional moral and social values, and while I am a life-long believer in public schools, I sympathize with those parents who are reluctant to see the educational system assume the burden of sex education at this particular moment in our history. I have no objections to schools offering sex education of a certain sort. Indeed, I think such courses can perform a useful service to the community. For example, I see no reason why young people of 13 or 14 should not receive basic instruction on human sexuality in their biology classes. Taught in the same way that other systems of the body are taught, these classes can teach young people all they need to know about the physiological aspects of this subject. Such information is useful and can be presented objectively and scientifically.

Unfortunately, many high school courses go far beyond the proper limits of biology in exploring this subject—and they do so at the urging of organizations that are philosophically committed to values that run counter to those held by more traditionally minded people.

Many of these courses stress the idea that young people have a "right" to be "sexually active" if they want to, that society has no legitimate role in prescribing sexual conduct for its members. Sometimes the courses contain explicit and detailed instructions in erotic behavior. A few are obscene by most people's standards. I am convinced that such programs are very damaging to young people and have contributed to the permissive atmosphere that exists in our society today.

Excluding Parents

I am also concerned about the failure of many schools to share their plans for sex education with parents. Several nationally prominent programs begin with statements that warn against parental involvement or suggest that the inclusion of parents would be ill-advised. For example, in one widely used curriculum the following note appears in the opening section, "How to Begin the Program": "Caution: Participants should not be given extra copies of the form to show to their parents or friends. Many of the materials of this program, shown to people outside the context of the program itself, can evoke misunderstanding and difficulties." 645

This popular program includes highly explicit color slides of both heterosexual and homosexual intercourse, as well as audiocassettes of homosexual males and lesbians who talk about the pleasure and satisfaction they derive from their deviant behavior. One of the stated purposes of this program is "To make clear that sexual relationships with the same sex during youth are normal and do not necessarily indicate one's future sexual orientation as an adult." 645

Small wonder the author warns that these materials, shown to parents, "can evoke . . . difficulties." 645

Other texts are similarly cautionary in their instructions to teachers. Some even suggest that the very purpose of the program would be subverted were parents to be informed about course contents, since, as a recent program puts it: "One of the primary developmental tasks for teens is to separate from their parents." 646 If "to separate from their parents" means to adopt a different set of moral values, then I believe the public school system has no business deliberately encouraging students to do such a thing.

Fortunately, most public school officials are respectful of what the community believes and go out of their way to make sex education curricula compatible with family values. If, however, you should live in one of those communities where the schools have initiated programs at variance with your religious or moral beliefs, then you may need to take one of several steps to make certain that your children are not subjected to potentially unhealthy indoctrination.

Examine the Contents

The first step in determining the nature of your children's sex education program is to examine the contents.

If you don't feel competent to judge the quality or bias of the materials, then ask for help from someone whose opinion you value. For example, you might enlist your pastor, since clergy usually have the training and critical judgment to assess the meaning of the written word. If you know other parents who share your concern, then ask one or more of them to join you in this evaluation.

When you have decided who is to accompany you, then call and make an appointment with the teacher or school nurse in charge of the program. Be as polite and as specific as possible. Tell the instructor you are interested in what kind of sex education your child is receiving and would like to look over the materials used. Ask if your child can bring home a copy of the materials before your meeting so that you can review everything at your leisure. Be sure to ask for videocassettes and audiotapes as well, since they are often the most vivid and provocative materials used.

If the instructor agrees to furnish these materials and gives you everything you ask for, then chances are you have little to worry about. Most of the genuinely destructive programs warn the teacher to keep texts and tapes from parents at all costs. However, when you receive the materials, examine them carefully, noting questionable or objectionable segments.

In so doing, don't be too picky. Chances are that even the instructor doesn't think the program is perfect; and if you quibble over minor points, you may forfeit your credibility when you address major points.

If the instructor refuses to send the materials home, then ask that they be assembled for you when you have your meeting. Be sure to reserve at least an hour so you will have time enough to review everything used in the course. Ask if there are copying facilities available in case you want to reproduce a page for closer scrutiny.

Ask Questions of the Teacher

In evaluating materials in your discussions with the instructor you should ask the following questions:

A. *Does the program encourage young people to engage in sexual intercourse or does it send a clear message of abstinence and self-restraint?*

Many bad programs mention abstinence in an initial sentence or two, then devote the balance of their presentation to a discussion of erotic behavior in explicit detail. Balance and proportion are important elements to consider in evaluating the total impact of sex education materials.

B. *Does the program violate community standards of taste and decency?*

This is a difficult question to answer objectively, and you should not make the mistake of assuming that what you find indelicate or insensitive would necessarily offend a substantial portion of the community. So you might want to seek help from a cross-section of your friends. Ask others what they think. Listen carefully to their answers. Write them down. In discussing this criterion with instructors or administrators it is much better to say, "Ten people I questioned found this passage objectionable," than to say, "This passage offended me."

C. *Does the program present traditional viewpoints toward sexuality as well as those of more permissive individuals and organizations? If so, does it present them in comparable detail and with the same degree of objectivity or sympathy?*

Again, these are difficult questions to answer, and you should be careful to use criteria that are as logical and unbiased as possible: amount of space (or time) devoted to each point of view, the use of "weighted" language, the presentation of all available evidence. For example, in examining programs that touch on the subject of birth control devices, you should make certain that negative as well as positive statistics appear. According to generally accepted studies, the failure rate of condoms to prevent pregnancy is 10 percent overall and 18 percent for women in their middle and late teens. And there is reason to believe the failure rate in the prevention of diseases such as AIDS may be the higher of these two figures. These studies should be cited in discussing such an important issue as birth control and disease prevention.

D. *What selection process was used in choosing this particular program?*

It is important to find out whether or not other programs were considered. If they were, you might want to see if any were "abstinence programs." Ask for specific names of curricula that were rejected. Then ask for the criteria used in making a final decision. If other options were not explored, you should ask why they weren't.

Also, you should ask who was involved in the selection process. Were outside "experts" consulted, and if so, who were they and how were they chosen?

If you feel the process has been unfair, you might want to give the instructor or principal information concerning programs that emphasize abstinence. These have increased in popularity over the past few years, largely because of their measurable success. For example, Teen-Aid, an abstinence program used at San Marcos (California) Junior High School, reports a reduction of pregnancies from 147 in the 1984-85 school year to 20 in 1986-87.[647] When asked, "Are you now more willing to say 'No' to sex before marriage?" 69 percent of students completing the Sex Respect program answered affirmatively, as opposed to 16 percent at the beginning of the program.[648]

E. *What is the purpose of the program now in place?*

There are many possible answers to this question and in some cases several of them could apply. One answer might be, "To teach teenagers the biological facts of reproduction." Another might be, "To teach young people to abstain from sexual intercourse until maturity and marriage." Still another might be, "To teach students to minimize the dangers of pregnancy and disease while engaging in premarital intercourse." One of the common answers given to explain the more destructive programs goes something like this, "To teach young people to clarify their own values concerning sexuality so they can make intelligent decisions regarding their own conduct." Such an approach—the so-called "values-clarification" approach—is deceptive in its appeal to fairness and objectivity. In fact, values-clarification curricula usually tell young people that they can do anything they want to with little or no regard for parental or societal inhibitions.

One of the pioneers of this approach, educational psychologist W. R. Coulson, has termed such education a failure and has said of the student exposed to it: "The outcome (confirmed in the research) is that he's become more likely to give in to what before he would have regarded as temptation to be resisted. Now he sees it as a developmental task, a 'risk of further growth.' " [649] In dealing with such programs, you should ask instructors and administrators whether or not they would apply the same "even-handed approach" to such issues as murder and racism.

Teenage sexuality is a major problem in America today largely because too many young people think they have the right to make decisions for themselves, even though they are in no position to bear the financial and emotional costs of pregnancy or a sexually transmitted disease such as AIDS. To suggest they are mature enough to decide about such questions independent of community codes and norms is to fly in the face of all the statistics [which have been collected in recent years] on pregnancy and disease.

Be sure that the stated purpose of the program is comprehensive enough to explain those parts you find most objectionable. If the offical purpose of the program is "to teach young people the basic biological facts about human reproduction" then it is justifiable to ask why entire segments are devoted to such subjects as homosexual conduct and petting.

The Principal

If the instructor refuses to show you the program or if you have questions that remain unanswered, then you probably need to talk to the principal of the school. Some principals keep a close watch on the classroom activity of their teachers while others try to give instructors a freer rein. There are arguments in favor of both approaches. However, every good principal should be concerned when parents believe something is going on in the school that undermines the values of the community. If you have such a complaint, in all likelihood the principal would prefer that you voice it directly rather than repeat it throughout the community. So when you call for an appointment, you should again specify exactly what is bothering you and give an account of your efforts to resolve your doubts about the program.

In setting up the appointment **remember that your best approach will be in the role of a parent seeking information rather than as someone who already has all the answers and wants to pick a fight**. If you come to the principal as a calm and reasonable person, then your own position on these matters will seem more credible.

At the same time, you should make your own position clear from the outset and give the distinct impression that you are interested in all the facts before you decide what to do about the problem. Perhaps the principal is likewise worried about this particular course or instructor. Perhaps your testimony is precisely what is needed to generate some action. Don't assume that the principal will necessarily prove to be an adversary, but be prepared for anything. A good principal will back up an experienced teacher until given sufficient reason to do otherwise.

If you have not been granted access to the materials used in the class then request that the principal obtain the texts and tapes for you. Explain that you are simply trying to determine what is going on in that particular class or unit, that the subject matter includes sensitive materials about which any responsible parent should be concerned.

Legal Aspects and Actions

If the principal refuses to intervene in your behalf to obtain the materials, then you have a right to know why. He may reply that the instructor is merely exercising his or her academic freedom in choosing materials without interference from parents. Such an argument may or may not be legally defensible. While teachers usually have some leeway to choose course materials, in many cases the state prescribes certain approaches and publishes a list of approved texts, particularly in the field of sex education. Several state legislatures (e.g., Oklahoma, California) have passed bills defining precisely what should and should not be taught in the classroom. Others (Alabama, North Carolina) have developed their own authorized texts to be used in every school. You might write or call your state board of education to find out what laws and procedures are in force in your state.

In addition, you might want to check with a lawyer to determine if your state has a "Freedom of Information Act" and if it applies to textbooks and other materials used in the public schools. In many states the law specifies that all documents and materials used by public agencies must be made available to the public upon request, with the single exception of personnel files, which may contain information of a highly personal and confidential nature. Many parents throughout the country have obtained classroom materials by invoking a Freedom of Information Act, though sometimes they have had to take the matter to court.

I would advise you to avoid this kind of confrontation if at all possible. Most teachers and principals are reasonable when faced with a strong and unswerving will; and I am willing to bet that if you continue to go through channels, you will eventually get what you want without threats or legal action. Principals are more likely to be pragmatic and accommodating than teachers, though such is not always the case.

The Superintendent of Schools

If your principal is adamant and confrontational, then you may want to talk with your superintendent of schools. The superintendent is responsible for what happens in the entire district, and all principals report to him or her. A superintendent is sometimes elected and sometimes appointed, so you may be dealing for the first time with someone directly responsible to the voters of the community and hence more sensitive to widespread dissatisfaction among parents and other adult groups.

Most superintendents have come up through the system, been teachers and principals, and therefore have a certain sympathy for those under their jurisdiction. On the other hand, superintendents are usually more experienced and therefore more likely to know the limits to which a classroom teacher is entitled to go in the use of questionable materials and in the encouragement of values contrary to those of parents.

If you have followed the chain of command, then you should be able to gain an appointment with your superintendent (or with a key staff member) and to make the source of your dissatisfaction clear. The superintendent can assess the validity of your case, then interview the principal and make whatever recommendations seem appropriate under the circumstances.

As a former superintendent, I can say that when parents came to me, the first thing I did was to make certain they had talked with both teacher and principal first. Certainly it would never have occurred to me to refuse an interview to anyone who had followed proper procedures before seeking my intervention.

The School Board

However, if you don't get anywhere with your superintendent, you should consider visiting a member of the school board. If you live in a small town, you may know one of these people personally; but if you don't know any member or if you live in a larger city, you should make inquiries and find out who on the board is most traditional in opinion and in voting habits. Then call and make an appointment.

Remember, however, that it is not ordinarily the function of a school board member to intervene in the day-to-day operations of the school. The board's responsibility is to set general policy and to oversee the management of the school district. Its chief duties are financial in nature, and most board members would deny their competence to judge classroom materials.

However, they are responsible for the establishment of policies and procedures within the district, and if the state's Freedom of Information Act or policy on sex education is being abused, then they are a legitimate avenue of appeal. Do not, however, make your case exclusively on the merits of the materials. Say that you have come to a board member because broad policies are being ignored or violated and you have received no satisfaction from the instructor or principal or superintendent. If state laws are being violated, then point out precisely how. If you have yet to see the materials used in the course, then request the board member to get them for you. Such a request–particularly where state law forbids the withholding of such documents–is reasonable and should be entertained with some sympathy.

At the same time, be advised that many school board members have received briefings from staff members on such subjects as sex education and that they may therefore be predisposed to dismiss your request as coming from an annoying and potentially dangerous crank. It is a sad fact that a number of well-financed organizations support permissive sex education programs and in their literature provide ammunition to school administrators and board members, telling them how to deal with parents who come to meetings to complain about specific approaches and objectionable materials.

Board members quickly learn to tell parents they are too inexperienced to speak on the subject of education, that all the experts oppose their point of view, that scientific evidence proves them wrong, that they are trying to impose their morals on others, and that they are the only people in the community who have raised such complaints.

When parents have attempted to combat these charges by bringing in experts of their own, board members are sometimes advised to say that these people are outside agitators, brought in to stir up trouble. Of course *most boards would never mistreat members of the community who appeared before them, either in public or in private.* Yet some parents around the country have reported such experiences to my office. For this reason, I offer the following replies to such attacks [as these]:

1. *"Parents don't know enough about education to speak with any authority. Only professional educators have enough experience to make decisions on curricular matters."*

The question of what kind of sex education to offer in schools is a matter of great concern to all citizens, since it involves the basic values of the community rather than such purely academic considerations as teaching methodology. It's one thing to argue that schools should teach biology or sex education, and quite another to maintain that young people should be taught that sexual intercourse prior to marriage is a matter of "personal choice" and that homosexuality is a "normal and even desirable lifestyle."

In order to clarify this point, let's take an example in another area—that of racial prejudice. It is one thing for schools to decide that a course in race relations should be taught, quite another to argue for an approach that stresses the right of each student to his own opinion on the question of bigotry, or which suggests that Martin Luther King and Hitler represent two equally valid "alternate lifestyles."

The truth is, racism is bad for society. It causes terrible problems and eventually costs human lives. It goes against the basic tenets of our religious heritage, as summarized in the Golden Rule. But even if there were no religious principles involved, racism would still be destructive to the community and therefore a bad attitude to condone.

Likewise, sexual license is bad for society. It causes terrible problems and eventually costs human lives (thousands are now dead of AIDS). It goes against the basic tenets of our religious faith. But even if there were no religious principles involved, sexual promiscuity would still be destructive to the community and therefore a bad attitude to condone.

Parents know just as much about what is and isn't good for society as teachers do; and while parents can't prescribe teaching methods or particular textbooks, they can certainly give expert testimony on what teenagers should believe and how the wrong kind of sex education can undermine family values.

You also might want to remind the board that they too are not trained experts, yet sit in judgment on everything that happens in a school system, including classroom activities. They, like parents, must judge the larger consequences of what's being taught in the schools; so they, least of all, have the right to impugn the qualifications of those parents who intelligently question what's going on.

All the experts agree that explicit and "non-judgmental" sex education courses are the best and most effective means of preventing unwanted pregnancies and sexually transmitted diseases.

There is virtually no educational issue of any consequence on which all the experts agree—and certainly not this one. A number of experts are highly critical of programs that tell young people sexual promiscuity is a valid option for them and that all they need to do is take certain precautionary measures to avoid "undesirable consequences."

- After examining a number of alternatives, a team of researchers at the U.S. Department of Education recommended abstinence programs as the best means of combatting AIDS among young people. 650

- Dr. Melvin Anchell, psychiatrist and author of several books on human sexuality, has written: "Some educators have a compulsion to teach sex, beginning with the three-year-old and continuing until high school graduation. Paradoxically, the effects of their schooling produce the very abnormalities that parents, and, perhaps, some well-meaning sex educators, wish to prevent." 651

  Devoid of real clinical experience and, in some cases, sexual maturity, sex educators can cause severe maladjustments by undue meddling. 651

  Psychoanalysis has established that the period in a child's life between ages of six and twelve is asexual; that is, a period during which sensual pleasures are normally repressed. . . . The period is well-recognized by psychiatrists throughout the world and has been designated as the "latency period." . . . During latency, the first stirring of compassionate feelings arises from the human mind. . . . This valuable instinct is dangerously jeopardized by sexually stimulating children in latency. Such interferences can prevent the "capability" to feel compassion. The results can be increasingly noted in the antisocial behavior of sexually "overstuffed" youths. 651

  In natural development, preteen children derive sexual pleasure from sensual excitements caused by sexual fantasies. Sex educators who catapult the child into a world of authoritative sexual knowledge shatter these normal fantasy satisfactions. . . . Later in life, drugs and pornography are used as adjuncts to help recapture the pleasures from thwarted childhood fantasies that had not been allowed to resolve naturally. 651

  By their loyalty, normal parents teach children that sex is a one-woman/one-man affair. The sex educator's advice, "Sex is for fun," desecrates the affectionate and monogamous nature of human sexuality. 651

- William R. Coulson, noted psychologist, has said:

  Society ought to be paying more attention to parental perspective right now, not waiting for the backlash. Science supports mothers and fathers in wanting their children spared the trials of sexual precocity, AIDS or not. And it supports the children in asking not to be underestimated. Self-discipline isn't beyond them, if they're told the truth. . . . The truth is summed up in six words: "Abstinence before marriage, fidelity within it." . . . Our children and grandchildren don't deserve to be judged sexually insatiable. 652

These are but three examples of a growing body of opinion that supports not only the possibility but the appropriateness of sex education based on traditional morality. These experts, whatever their religious backgrounds, are speaking as professional educators (or therapists) who base their conclusions on scientific data as well as years of experience in their respective fields. They are distinguished by any objective standards, yet they voice the same concerns about permissive sex education that traditional-minded parents have been expressing. And there are many other educators and psychologists who share these views.

Of course, those who defend such education usually try to discount such authorities by saying that they are "not respectable," that "nobody takes them seriously," that "their methodology is flawed." If you are met by such a response, you can reply either by demanding that they prove such a statement right there on the spot, or by pointing out that this is precisely what your authorities say about their authorities—that no side has a monopoly on the experts. Therefore, the question must be decided on other than "scientific" grounds. At this point you can begin to talk about the rights of parents to teach a morality at home that is not systematically contradicted at school.

2. *"Anyone who opposes 'explicit, non-judgmental sex education' in school is a right-wing extremist."*

If you have to deal with such name-calling then you are in for a very difficult time. This kind of argument is neither fair-minded nor intelligent. Usually it reveals a loss of patience or else an inability to continue the debate on an intellectual level. Phrases like "right-wing extremist," "bigot," and "moralist" indicate no more than animosity. They don't answer legitimate arguments or counter persuasive evidence, and you must make that point to the person who tries to avoid a discussion of the issues by calling you names. You might want to point out that when people in the 1950s used similar words and phrases against liberal opponents they were called "McCarthyites." Ask politely but firmly that the discussion be confined to the issues and that everyone avoid personal attacks, not only because they are rude and uncivil but because they are illogical–examples of the fallacy called "ignoring the question."

3. *"You are the only parents who have raised any complaints about this program."*

Of course, it's possible that you are; but what does that prove? It may simply mean that other parents don't know what is going on in the classroom. You might want to ask the board if they have any objections to your sending a copy of the materials to all the parents in your child's class and ask them for comments. If the board says "no objections," then do it. If they say "we object," then you have a right to question their suggestion that you constitute an insignificant minority of parents.

You might also ask them if they believe the majority is always right. If they say "no," then thank them for conceding your point. If they say "yes," then ask them if they will be willing to decide the fate of this program by a vote of all concerned parents, with a majority deciding the issue.

However, it is much better to answer this objection by making certain that you are not the only person present at the board meeting. You should try to persuade as many people as possible to join you in voicing their objections. In the first place, there is nothing so intimidating to members of an elected (or appointed) board as a large delegation prepared to protest board actions or school policy. Numbers suggest not only widespread concern but also a certain intensity of commitment, since it takes a lot to move people to come before a public body and express themselves.

Also, many school boards restrict each speaker to a time limit, usually three minutes; so the more people you have with you, the more time your side will have to state its case. You should definitely coordinate your presentations so that each person makes a different point, or at least makes the same point in a different way, though once your entire case is on the table, it is quite all right for succeeding speakers to say, "I just want to second what's been said," or "I don't like this program either and would like to see it removed from our schools."

If you bring enough people to the meeting and present your case in a reasonable and persuasive manner, you will make it difficult for the board to treat you with disrespect or to ignore completely the points you make.

Summary

In the final analysis, whether or not you can motivate the teacher, principal, superintendent, or school board to abandon an objectionable sex education program will probably depend on your ability to convince whoever makes the decision that the program is either severely deficient or else offensive to the sensibilities of a number of intelligent people.

It may be some consolation for you to know that a number of parents throughout the nation have been disturbed by the same kinds of materials and have been willing to voice their objections to teachers and other school authorities. While many have been disappointed in the response, more and more are reporting that they have been able to make significant changes both at the local and at the state levels. In fact, there are several national organizations that are deeply involved in the fight for decent and traditional approaches to sex education. Among these are: Focus on the Family, the American Family Association, Concerned Women of America, the American Life League, the Eagle Forum, and Parents' Roundtable.

If you have problems that are not covered in this brief discussion, you may want to contact one or more of these groups. They will be happy to give you the benefit of their experience in supporting approaches to human sexuality that are more compatible with traditional family values.

Conclusion

The verdict is in: Teenage promiscuity, pregnancies, abortions and out-of-wedlock births are all on an unprecedented increase. This is doubly alarming in light of the massive government programs aimed at reducing those rates. So far, comprehensive sex education has been able to lower the adolescent birth rate only through a sharp increase in abortions.

The Family Policy, a publication of the Family Research Council, strongly admonishes, "For the sake of the next generation of American children, it is time for a generous dose of domestic 'new thinking' about one of the nation's most intractable social problems." 341/8

As a concerned parent, I beg you to exercise new thinking in regard to the type of sex education you introduce into our school system. It is quite ironic that just when our children need adult guidance and moral restitution, so many school boards, educators and legislators abdicate moral responsibility. Please don't let this happen in Julian.

Thank you for reading this letter. Dottie and I appreciate all the effort you put into making our school more effective in the lives of our children. If I can ever be of any help to you, please do call on me immediately.

A concerned parent,
Josh D. McDowell

Documentation

1. Elias, Marilyn. "With guidance, a child can control negative traits." *USA Today,* August 9, 1989, p. 4D.
2. Chairman of the House Select Committee on Children, Youth and Families as quoted in *St. Paul Pioneer Press Dispatch,* February 10, 1986.
3. Beyette, Beverly. "Teen Sex-Education Campaign Launched." *Los Angeles Times,* October 17, 1986.
4. Vobejda, Barbara. "Koop and Bennett Issue Joint Advice on AIDS." *Washington Post,* January 31, 1987.
5. Gordon, Sol, and Everly, Kathleen. "Increasing Self-Esteem in Vulnerable Students . . . A Tool for Reducing Pregnancy Among Teenagers." Reprinted from *Impact '85,* 2:Article 41:9-17. Publication of Institute for Family Research and Education, 760 Ostrom Avenue, Syracuse, NY 13210-2999.
6. Mosbacker, Barrett. "Teen Pregnancy and School-Based Health Clinics." *Vision,* October/November 1986.
7. *Issues,* January 1982.
8. *Associated Press,* January 23, 1984 (PM cycle).
9. *Newsweek,* October 13, 1986.
10. "Can We Save Our Teenagers From Pregnancy?" *Washington Star,* July 3, 1977.
11. "TV's Getting Sexier . . . How Far Will it Go?" *TV Guide,* January 7, 1989.
12. Towarnicky, Carol. "Positive Images Needed to Combat Teenage Pregnancy." *Houston Chronicle,* January 12, 1986.
13. Simon, Roger. "Casual Sex on TV Part of the Problem." *Los Angeles Times,* January 4, 1987.
14. "The Teen Environment." Based on A Study of Growth Strategies for Junior Achievement. The Robert Johnston Company, Inc., 1980.
15. Fletcher, Sheila. "Experts Seek Answers About Teen Pregnancy." *Oklahoman,* February 2, 1984.
16. Liebert, Sprafkin, and Davidson. "The Early Window: Effects of Television on Children and Youth," 1982.
17. Gaylin, Jody. "What Girls Really Look for in Boys." *Seventeen,* March 1978.
18. *Broadcasting,* February 15, 1988.
19. *TV Guide,* January 7, 1989.
20. *Parade,* August 21, 1989.
21. "A Thumbs Down for Music Videos." *USA Today,* November 14, 1988.
22. Parker, Suzy. "No rush for remarriage." *USA Today,* April 24, 1987, p. 1A.
23. Lord, Lewis J. "Sex With Care." *U.S. News & World Report,* June 2, 1986.
24. Curry, Jack. "Free love gives way to responsibility." *USA Today,* April 23, 1987.
25. Towarnicky, Carol. "Positive images needed to combat teenage pregnancy." *Houston Chronicle,* January 12, 1986.
26. Simon, Roger. "Casual Sex on TV Part of the Problem." *Los Angeles Times,* January 4, 1987.
27. "American Teens Speak: Sex, Myth, TV, and Birth Control." The Planned Parenthood Poll. Louise Harris and Associates, Inc., September/October 1986.
28. Alcorn, Randy C. *Christians in the Wake of the Sexual Revolution.* Portland, OR: Multnomah Press, 1985.
29. *Ad Age,* May 14, 1984.
30. Sanderson, Jim. "The Importance of Thanking Dad." *Los Angeles Times,* June 4, 1986.
31. Koop, Everett J. Personal interview. February 2, 1987.
32. Painter, Virginia. "Kids' drug pressure: Crack, wine coolers." *USA Today,* April 24-26, 1987.
33. Bibby, Reginald W., and Posterski, Donald C. *The Emerging Generation – An Inside Look at Canada's Teenagers.* Toronto: Irwin Publishing, 1985.
34. Powell, Stewart. "What Entertainers Are Doing to Our Kids." *U.S. News & World Report,* October 28, 1985.
35. *Focus on the Family Bulletin,* 1989.
36. Harris, Myron, and Norman, Jane. *The Private Life of the American Teenager.* New York: Rawson, Wade Publishers, Inc., 1981.
37. Bennett, William J., United States Secretary of Education. "Our Children." Address to the National School Board of Education, January 22, 1987.
38. Klucoff, Carol. "Teens: Speaking Their Minds." *Washington Post,* February 3, 1982.
39. Coulson, W. R. "Founder of 'value-free' education says he owes parents an apology." *American Family Association Journal,* April 1989, pp. 20-21.
40. *The Memorandum on Sex Education in the Schools of the German Austrian Citizens' Initiative.* Translated by E. C. Freiling, Ph.D. Emphasis in the original. N.d., n.pub.
41. Leithart, Peter J. "Modern Sex-Speak." Chalcedon Report:270 (January 1988).

42. "Universities Have Fallen Down on the Job of Teaching Values." *Newsweek,* October 1, 1984.
43. "Morals Mine Field." *Newsweek,* October 13, 1986.
44. Mark, Alexandra, and Mark, Vernon H. *The Pied Pipers of Sex.* Plainfield, NJ: Haven Books, a division of Logos International, 1981.
45. Ellis, Tottie. "Most 'advice' on sex promotes promiscuity." *USA Today,* March 20, 1985.
46. Woody, Dr. Degar J. "Teenage Morality–Another Look." *Journal of the Medical Association of Georgia* 68 (May 1979).
47. *USA Today,* August 15, 1988.
48. "Drugs, AIDS and Babies." *AIDS Protection,* February 1989.
49. Stewart, Sally Ann. "Sex is casual, despite new concerns." *USA Today,* May 15, 1986, p. 5D.
50. Kasun, Jacqueline R. "Turning Your Children Into Sex Experts." A position paper. Department of Economics, Humboldt State University, Arcata, CA (October 1979).
51. Pomeroy, Wardell B. *Boys and Sex.* New York: Delacorte Press, 1968. Revised edition, New York: Dell Publishing, 1981.
52. Pomeroy, Wardell B. *Girls and Sex.* New York: Delacorte Press, 1969. Revised edition, New York: Dell Publishing, 1981.
53. Bell, Dr. Ruth. *Changing Bodies, Changing Lives.* New York: Random House, 1980.
54. *The New Our Bodies, Ourselves.* New York: Simon & Schuster, 1984. Recommended highly for teens by Planned Parenthood in their San Diego Clinics for teenagers 13-19 years old.
55. *You've Changed the Combination.* A pamphlet published by Rocky Mountain Planned Parenthood, Denver, CO. It is frequently passed out for adolescent boys in the San Diego Planned Parenthood Clinics.
56. Weed, Stan, et al. "The Teen-Aid Family Life Education Project." Second Year Evaluation Report prepared for the Office of Adolescent Pregnancy Programs (OAPP), by the Institute for Research and Evaluation, December 31, 1989.
57. Lorand, Rhoda L. "The Betrayal of Youth." *Educational Update* 3:3 (Summer 1979).
58. Fossedal, Gregory A. "Dartmouth's 'safe sex kit' is far from morally neutral." *Orange County Register,* February 10, 1987.
59. Carmody, Deirdre. "Increasing Rapes on Campus Spur Colleges to Fight Back." *New York Times,* January 1, 1989.
60. *Parade,* September 27, 1987.
61. Lubbock, Texas, *Avalanche-Journal,* December 20, 1987.
62. "Scientific Evidence Shows Pornography Is Harmful." *Focus on the Family Citizen,* June 1989.
63. *New York Times,* February 28, 1989.
64. *Dallas Morning News,* July 17, 1989.
65. Howard, John A. "AIDS Grew in a Hothouse of Permissiveness." *Orange County Register,* February 10, 1987.
66. Report of the House Select Committee on Children, Youth and Families. "Teen Pregnancy: What Is Being Done? A State-by-State Look." December 1985.
67. Raspberry, William. *Washington Post,* 1986.
68. *National Review,* July 3, 1987.
69. Curry, Jack. "A Life Lost in Confusion and Crisis." *USA Today,* April 6, 1984.
70. Popenoe, Paul. "Do Your Children Know You Love Them?" *Parents and Better Homemaking* 40 (December 1965).
71. Toth, Ronald S. "Teen Pregnancy." *Plain Truth,* September 1986.
72. Arrington, Carl. "Animal Magnetism." *People,* December 19, 1983.
73. "Teenagers Cresting New Values for the Future." Based on a Gallup/AP youth survey. *Emerging Trends.* Princeton Religious Research Center, October, 1985.
74. *Psychology Today,* January/February 1989.
75. Stanton, Greta W. "Parental Divorce and Remarriage Seen as Leading Cause of Problems for Today's Teens." *Children and Teens Today,* 6:11:1-2 (July 1986).
76. Lawson, Annette. "Experts: Adultery Hurts Children." *New York Times,* March 9, 1989.
77. Akpim, Akpom and Davis. "Prior Sexual Behavior of Teenagers Attending Rap Sessions for the First Time." *Family Planning Perspectives,* July/August 1976.
78. Martin, Yvonne M. "Lack of Parental Closeness Seen as Teen Sex Cause." *Orange County Register,* May 6-7, 1981.
79. Zorn, Eric. "Is Virginity Finding an Unwanted Ally?" *Denver Post,* 1981.
80. Painter, Kim. "What Women Want Most: Intimacy." *USA Today,* October 14, 1986.
81. "Reaching Out for Inner-Awarenesss–An Interview With Dr. Rollo May." Author of "Love and Will." *Nutshell,* 1973-74 school year edition.
82. *Newsweek,* September 1, 1980.
83. "Teen Pregnancy: 16.6 Billion." *Chicago Tribune,* February 19, 1986.
84. "HTLV-III/LAV Antibody and Immune Status of Household Contacts and Sexual Partners of Persons With Hemophilia." *Journal of the American Medical Association,* January 10, 1986.
85. Fineberg, Dr. Harvey V., Dean, Harvard School of Public Health. "Prevention Better Than Cure." *AIDS Protection*

3:1 (May 1989).

86. Chilton, David. *Power in the Blood—A Response to AIDS*. Brentwood, TN: Wolgemuth & Hyatt, 1987.
87. *U.S. Newsweek Review*, June 15, 1987.
88. "The Impact of AIDS on Benefit Plans." *The Nation's Business*, March 1989.
89. Zamichow, Nora. *Times Herald*.
90. *Time*, June 15, 1987.
91. Seligmann, Jean. "A Nasty New Epidemic." *Newsweek*, February 4, 1985.
92. *The Common Appeal*, November 7, 1988.
93. "Drugs, AIDS & Babies." *AIDS Protection*, February 1989.
94. Lubbock, Texas, *Avalanche Journal*, March 3, 1988.
95. *The Island Packet*, June 15, 1988.
96. *AIDS Prevention*, May 1989. Newsletter put out by National AIDS Prevention Institute, P. O. Box 2500, Culpeper, VA 22701, (703) 825-4040.
97. Painter, Kim. "AIDS plague hits teen heterosexuals." *USA Today*, July 20, 1989, p. 1D.
98. Painter, Kim. "AIDS preys on the underclass." *USA Today*, March 23, 1989, p. 2D.
99. *U.S. Newsweek Review*, April 24, 1989.
100. Crenshaw, Dr. Theresa L., M.D. "Teen AIDS Myths Answered." *AIDS Protection*, September 1989.
101. Sorokin, Pitirim. *American Sex Revolution*. New York: Porter Sargent, 1956.
102. Alcorn, Randy C. *Christians in the Wake of the Sexual Revolution*. Portland, OR: Multnomah Press, 1985.
103. Unwin, J. D. Cited in Lunn, Arnold, and Lean, Garth. *The New Morality*. London: Blanford Press, 1964, p. 25. Cf. Unwin, J. D., *Sex and Culture*, London: Oxford University Press, 1934.
104. Lewis, C. S. *God in the Dock*. Grand Rapids: Wm. B. Eerdmans Publishing Co., 1970.
105. "The Revolution Is Over." *Time*, April 9, 1984.
106. "Reassuring News About AIDS: A Doctor Tells Why You May Not Be at Risk." *Cosmopolitan*, June 1988.
107. Ventura, S. J.; Taffel, S.; and Mosher, W. D. "Estimates of Pregnancies and Pregnancy Rates for the United States, 1976-1981." *Public Health Reports* 100:1, table 1 (January/February 1985).
108. Kasun, Jacqueline R., Ph.D. "Teenage Pregnancy: Media Effects Versus Facts." *American Life Education and Research Trust*, 1984.
109. Richard, Dinah, Ph.D. "Has Sex Education Failed Our Teenagers? A Research Report." Pomona, CA: Focus on the Family Publications, 1990.
110. Zelnik, Melvin, and Kantner, John F. "Contraceptive Patterns and Premarital Pregnancy Among Women Aged 15-19 in 1976." *Family Planning Perspectives* 10:3, table 3 (May/June 1978).
111. Congressional Budget Office. Pregnancy and abortion data from the Alan Guttmacher Institute, unpublished data. Birth data from National Center for Health Statistics, *Advance Report of Final Nationality Statistics* 33:6, 1982 Supplement. September 28, 1984, p. 16. Cited in Committee Report, p. 398.
112. Rowe, Dr. H. E., President, National AIDS Prevention Institute. "Knowing the AIDS Virus and Avoiding Infection." *AIDS Prevention*, March 1987.
113. *U.S. News & World Report*, October 19, 1987.
114. Gotzsche, Peter, and Hording, Merete. *Scandinavian Journal of Infectious Disease*. From the Department of Infectious Diseases. Rigshospitalet, Copenhagemn, Denmark, 20:233-234, 52, 1988.
115. *NBC News*, February 24, 1988.
116. Fischl, M. A. "Evaluation of Heterosexual Partners, Children, and Household Contact of Adults With AIDS." *Journal of the American Medical Association* 257 (February 6, 1987), pp. 640-44; and Susan Okie, *Washington Post*, February 6, 1987.
117. ALPH 78:1 (January 1988).
118. International Conference on AIDS, June 1-5, 1987. Washington, D.C. Abstracts volume.
119. *Consumer Reports*, March 1989.
120. "AIDS & Blacks." *Parade*, October 9, 1988.
121. *AIDS Protection* 3:2 (September 1989).
122. Hayward, Mark D, and Yogi, Jonichi. "Contraceptive Failure in the United States: Estimates From the 1982 National Survey of Family Growth." *Family Planning Perspectives* 18:5 (September/October 1986). See also Zelnik, Melvin; Koenig, Michael A. K.; and Young, Kim. "Sources of Prescription Contraceptives and Subsequent Pregnancy Among Young Women." *Family Planning Perspectives*, January/February 1984.
123. Kenney, Asta. "School-Based Clinics: A National Conference." *Family Planning Perspectives* 18:1 (January/February 1986).
124. *Boston Herald*, July 13, 1989.
125. Painter, Kim. " 'Disturbing' data on birth control failure." *USA Today*, July 13, 1989, p. 1D.
126. Cline, Victor B., Ph.D. "Correlating Adolescent and Adult Exposure to Sexually Explicit Material and Sexual Behavior." University of Utah Dept. of Psychology, National Conference on HIV: Human Immunodeficiency Virus.
127. *Family Planning Perspectives*, March/April 1981.
128. Zelnik, Melvin, and Kantner, John F. "First Pregnancies to Women Aged 15 to 19; 1976 and 1971." *Family Planning*

Perspectives. January/February 1978.

129. *Tuscon Citizen,* September 12, 1989.
130. *Consumer Reports,* March 1989.
131. Goedert, James, J., M.D. "What Is Safe Sex? Suggested Standards Linked to Testing for Human Immunodeficiency Virus." *The New England Journal of Medicine* 316:21 (May 21, 1987).
132. Fischl, Dickinson, Segal, Flanagan, and Rodriguez, University of Miami. "Heterosexual Transmission of Human Immunodeficiency Virus. HIV, Relationship of Sexual Practices to Seroconversion." International Conference on AIDS, June 1-5, 1987, Washington, D.C. Abstract volume.
133. "Condoms for Prevention of Sexually Transmitted Diseases." *Journal of the American Medical Association* 259:13 (April 1, 1988).
134. Kasun, Jacqueline R. "The Economics of Sex Education." A position paper. Department of Economics, Humboldt State University, Arcata, CA (1986).
135. Source: Minnesota, Department of Health, *Minneapolis Star* and *Tribune,* April 20, 1984.
136. United Families of America. Press release. March 8, 1983. Based on data from the Utah Department of Health.
137. "Fewer Girls Under 16 Have Abortions." *London Daily Telegraph,* September 27, 1985.
138. *American Teens Speak: Sex, Myths, TV, and Birth Control.* The Planned Parenthood Poll, Louis Harris & Assoc., 1986.
139. "School-Based Clinics." *Pro-Life Advocate* 1:3 (1989).
140. Marsiglio, Wm., and Mott, Frank L. "The Impact of Sex Education on Sexual Activity, Contraceptive Use and Premarital Pregnancy Among American Teenagers." *Family Planning Perspectives* 18:4 (July/August 1986).
141. Dawson, Deborah Anne. "The Effects of Sex Education on Adolescent Behavior." *Family Planning Perspectives* 18:4 (July/August 1986).
142. Conant, Jennet, with Springen, Karen. "How to Talk About Sex." *Newsweek,* February 16, 1987, p. 68.
143. *Dallas Morning News,* January 3, 1989.
144. Princeton Religion Research Center. "Emerging Trends," October 1988.
145. Weed, Stan E., and Olsen, Joseph A. "Effects of Family Planning Programs for Teenagers on Adolescent Birth and Pregnancy Rates." 20:3 (1986).
146. Weed, Stan E. "Curbing Births, Not Pregnancies." *Wall Street Journal,* October 14, 1986.
147. Plagenz, George. "Sex Ed Conflict." Lubbock, Texas, *Avalanche Journal,* January 18, 1987.
148. Bell, Reed, M.D. Position paper, October 23, 1985.
149. Zelnik, Melvin, and Kantner, John F. "Contraceptive Patterns," p. 138, Table 8.
150. Ryder, Norman B. "Contraceptive Failure in the United States." *Family Planning Perspectives* 5:3 (Summer 1973).
151. Ford, James F., M.D., and Schwartz, Michael. "Birth Control for Teenagers: Diagram for Disaster." *Linacre Quarterly,* February 1979.
152. "Does Contraception Prevent Abortion?" Human Life Center, 1983.
153. Zelnik, Melvin, and Kantner, John F. "Sexual Activity, Contraceptive Use, and Pregnancy Among Metropolitan-Area Teens: 1971-1979." *Family Planning Perspectives* 12 (1980).
154. *Family Planning Perspectives* 12:5:229 (September/October 1980).
155. "Muskegon Heights School-Based Clinic—A Survey." Muskegon Heights Area Planned Parenthood, September 1984—June 1985.
156. Kirby, J. Report issued by the Support Center for School-Based Clinics, a subdivision of the Center for Population Options, Washington, D.C., n.d.
157. Weatherly, Richard, et al. "Comprehensive Programs for Pregnant Teenagers and Teenage Parents: How Successful Have They Been?" *Family Planning Perspectives* 18:2:77 (March/April 1986).
158. McManus, Michael J., ed. *Final Report of the Attorney General's Commission on Pornography.* New York: Rutledge Hill Press, 1986.
159. "A Teen-Pregnancy Epidemic." *Newsweek,* March 25, 1985.
160. Scott, David, ed. "Proceedings of the Symposium on Media Violence and Pornography." Toronto: Media Action Group, February 1984.
161. O'Reilly, Sean, M.D., professor, School of Medicine and Health Sciences. "Sex Education in the Schools." Thaxton, VA 24174: George Washington University, *Sun Life,* 1978.
162. Tottie, Dr. Malcolm, of Sweden's National Board of Health. Quoted in Linner, Birgitta. *Sex and Society in Sweden.* New York: Pantheon, 1967.
163. Linner, Birgitta. "Sexual Morality and Sexual Reality—The Scandinavian Approach." *American Journal of Orthopsychiatry* 36:4 (July 1966).
164. Linner, Birgitta. *Sex and Society in Sweden.* New York: Pantheon, 1967, Appendix K.
165. Elliott, Neil. *Sensuality in Scandinavia.* New York: Weybright and Talley, 1970.
166. Sundstrom, Kajsa. "Young People's Sexual Habits in Today's Swedish Society." *Current Sweden* 125. Swedish Institute (July 1976).
167. Davis, Kingsley. "The American Family, Relation to Demographic Change." *Research Reports.* U.S. Commission on Population Growth and the American Future 1. Demographic and Social Aspects of Population Growth. Robert Parker, Jr. and Charles F. Westoff, eds. Washington D.C.: U.S. Government Printing Office, 1972.

168. *Action Line* X:4 (May 12, 1986).
169. Cutright, Phillips. "Illegitimacy in the United States: 1920-1968." *Research Reports.* U.S. Commission on Population Growth and the American Future 1. Demographic and Social Aspects on Population Growth. Robert Parker, Jr., and Charles F. Westoff, eds. Washington, D.C.: U.S. Government Printing Office, 1972.
170. *Family Planning Perspectives* 12:5 (September/October 1980).
171. *Archives of Sexual Behavior* 10 (November 1981).
172. Kirby, Douglas, Director of Research of the Center for Population Options. "Effectiveness of School-Based Clinics." At the 16th Annual Family Planning and Reproductive Health Assoc., March 2, 1988, in Washington, D.C. Tape recording and transcription by Richard Glasow, quoted in *School-Based Clinics.*
173. Muroskin, L. D. "Sex Education Mandates: Are They the Answer?—Commentary." *Family Planning Perspective* 18 (1986).
174. *New York Times,* March 16,1989.
175. Ravenel, J. DuBose. "On the Other Hand." *North Carolina Medical Journal* 49:7 (July 1988).
176. Kasun, Jacqueline R. "Teenage Pregnancy: What Comparisons Among States and Countries Show." A position paper. Department of Economics, Humboldt State University, Arcata, CA 1986.
177. Thomas, Cal. "What Did Teen Sex Study Prove?" *Inside Washington,* March 30, 1985.
178. "Teens, Sex and Values." *AIDS Protection,* September 1989.
179. Hogan, Dennis P., and Kitagawa, Evelyn M. "The Impact of Social Status, Family Structure, and Neigborhood on the Fertility of Black Adolescents." *American Journal of Sociology,* January 1985 (included in #662).
180. Frech, Frances. "Update of Teen Pregnancies." *Heartbeat Quarterly,* Summer 1980.
181. Olsen, Joseph, and Weed, Stan. "Effects of Family Planning Programs on Teenage Pregnancy—Replication and Extension." *Family Perspective* 20:3 (1986).
182. *Family Practice News,* December 15, 1977.
183. *New York Times,* June 12, 1981.
184. Reichelt, P. A. "Changes in Sexual Behavior Among Unmarried Teenage Women Utilizing Oral Contraception." *Journal of Population* 1 (1987).
185. Reichelt, P. A. "Changes in Sexual Behavior Among Unmarried Teenage Women Utilizing Oral Contraception." *Journal of Population* 1:57 (1987).
186. National Research Council. "Risking the Future—Adolescent Sexuality, Pregnancy, and Childbearing." Washington, D.C.: National Academy Press, 1987.
187. Cutright, Philip, M.D. "Illegitimacy in the United States: 1920-1968." *Research Reports.* United States Commission on Population Growth and the American Future. N.d.
188. Peitropino, A. "Survey on Contraception Analysis." *Medical Aspects of Human Sexuality,* May 1987.
189. "American Teens and Birth Control." *North Carolina Medical Journal* 48:11 (November 1987).
190. Figures for 1970-1978 from Susan Roylance testimony before U.S. Senate Committee on Labor and Human Resources, Washington, D.C., 1986.
191. Kasun, Jacqueline R. "The Economics of Sex Education" 20. *Christian Economics.* New South Wales, Australia (October 1987).
192. Figures are derived from a personal letter to Jerry Blackmon, Board of County Commissioners/County Board of Health from Basil Delta, M.D., M.P.H. Health Director, April 8, 1986.
193. Mosbacher, Barrett. "Teen Pregnancy and School-Based Health Clinics." *Family Research Council.* Washington, D.C., n.d.
194. Kasun, Jacqueline R., Ph.D. "Teenage Pregnancy: What Comparisons Among States and Countries Show." Arcata, CA: Humboldt State University, 1986, p. 6. Cutright, Phillips. "Illegitimacy in the United States: 1920-1968." *Research Reports.* U.S. Commission of Population Growth and the American Future 1. "Demographic and Social Aspects of Population Growth." Robert Parker, Jr., and Charles F. Westoff, eds. Washington, D.C.: U.S. Government Printing Office.
195. Mosbacker, Barrett L., ed. *School-Based Clinics.* Westchester, IL: Crossway Books, 1987.
196. Olsen, Joseph A., and Weed, Stan E. "Effects of Family-Planning Programs for Teenagers on Adolescent Birth and Pregnancy Rates." *Family Perspective,* 20:3 (1986).
197. Mullis, Ronald L. "Family Influences on Sexual Attitudes and Knowledge as Reported by College Students." *Adolescence* 23:92 (Winter 1988).
198. Morgan, Anne Marie. "Comprehensive Sex-Ed: Ten Fatal Flaws." Virginians for Family Values, n.d.
199. Toups, Catherine. "Pregnancies rising among North Virginia teens." The Legislators Briefing Packet. Prepared by Virginia Concerned Citizens Council, 1989. *Fairfax Journal,* October 10, 1989.
200. Frisk, David. "Teen pregnancies rise 23%, abortions up 45%." *Alexendria Gazette,* October 4, 1989.
201. Kasun, Jacqueline R. "Sex Education: The Hidden Agenda." *The World & I.* A publication of The Washington Times Corporation, © September 1989.
202. Mast, Coleen. "Sex and the Sanctity of Love—Beyond Biology." *The World & I.* A publication of The Washington Times Corporation, © September 1989. Used by permission.
203. Kava, Brad. "Stanford Study Puts Focus on Forced Sex." *San Jose Mercury News,* May 19, 1989.
204. Kirby, Douglas. "Sex Education Programs and Their Effects." *The World & I.* A publication of The Washington Times Corporation, © September 1989.

205. *Proper Use of Condoms*, Norfolk, VA: Department of Public Health, n.d.
206. Richard, Dinah. "Exemplary abstinence-based sex education programs." *The World & I*. A publication of The Washington Times Corporation, © September 1989.
207. Hayes, C. D. "Risking the Future: Adolescent Sexuality, Pregnancy, and Childbearing." Washington, D.C.: National Research Council, The National Academy of Science, 1987.
208. Kirby, Douglas. *Sexuality Education: An Evaluation of Programs and Their Effects*. Santa Cruz, CA: Network Publications, 1984.
209. Wright, Linus. *Sex Education – How to Respond*. Washington, D.C.: The Department of Education, n.d.. Used with permission.
210. *The Challenge Curriculum*. The Educational Guidance Institute, 927 S. Walter Reed Dr., Suite 4, Arlington VA.
211. Beach, Paul Cole, and Likoudis, James. "Sex Education: The New Manicheanism." *Triumph*, October/November 1969.
212. Gribbin, Anne M. "Sex Ed Doesn't Reduce Pregnancy" (an editorial). *Richmond News Leader*, September 29, 1986.
213. "Sex and the Education of Our Children" address to the National School Board Association, January 22, 1987.
214. Whitley, B., and Schofield, J. "Meta-Analysis of Research on Adolescents' Contraceptives Use." *Population and Environment* 8:3 & 4 (Fall/Winter 1985-86), 173-203.
215. Brann, Edward A., et al. "Strategies for the Prevention of Pregnancy in Adolescents." Reprinted by the U.S. Department of Health, Education and Welfare, Public Health Service, from Advances in Planned Parenthood 14:2 (1979).
216. Schwartz, Michael. "Lies, Damned Lies, and Statistics." *American Education Report*, March 1986.
217. "An Emerging Approach to Improving Adolescent Health and Addressing Teenage Pregnancy." N. pub., April 1985.
218. Dietz, Marie. "St. Paul In-School Sex Clinics." Unpublished paper, n.d.
219. Zabin, Laurie S. "Evaluation of a Pregnancy Prevention Program for Urban Teenagers." *Family Planning Perspectives* 18:3.
220. Demsko, Tobin W. "School-Based Health Clinics: An Analysis of the Johns Hopkins Study." Washington, D.C.: Family Research Council, n.d.
221. "Muskegon Heights School-Based Teen Clinic – A Survey." Muskegon Heights Area Planned Parenthood, September 1984 – June 1985.
222. Weatherley, Richard, et al. "Comprehensive Programs for Pregnant Teenagers and Teenage Parents: How Successful Have They Been?" *Family Planning Perspectives* 18:2 (March/April 1986).
223. Kirby, Douglas. Speaking at the Sixteenth Annual Meeting of the National Family Planning and Reproductive Health Association, March 2, 1988, Washington, D.C., session on "Education." Audio tape recording and transcription by Richard D. Glasow. The final report promised by Kirby had not yet been published.
224. *Minneapolis Star and Tribune*, April 20, 1984.
225. "Will 'Safe Sex' Education Effectively Combat AIDS?" This informal paper has been developed by staff in the Department of Education in response to questions and comments on the "safe sex" approach to educating young people about AIDS prevention. The paper summarizes research and other information relevant to this subject (January 22, 1987).
226. Ulene, Art. *Safe Sex in a Dangerous World*, 1987.
227. Quackenbush, Marcia, and Sargent, Pamela. *Teaching AIDS: A Resource Guide on Acquired Immune Deficiency Syndrome*, 1986, p. 24. In a chapter on teaching plans, a section addresses the question, "How can we help change people's beliefs and behaviors about safe sex?" and gives this advice: "1. Educate everyone about safe sex. 2. Educate everyone about condom use, including how and where to get them, how to use them, and how to talk about condom use with partners. 3. Tell young people about family planning or health clinics where they can get condoms free or at cost. 4. Educate about how to make condom use part of the intimate sharing of sexuality. 5. Educate sexually active youth to always have condoms available in situations where they might need them, so that spontaneity is not affected" (p. 33). In another place the book says: "By not sharing IV needles. or preferably, not using IV drugs at all, and having safe sexual contacts, or not having sex, young people can prevent exposure to AIDS" (p. 6). Not having sex seems no more preferable than using condoms.
228. *AIDS and Adolescents: The Time for Prevention Is Now*. Washington, D.C.: Center for Population Options, 1987.
229. "Safer Sex Is for Everyone." Published by the Gay Men's Health Crisis organization, 1987.
230. Advertisement in the *New York Times*, September 4, 1987.
231. Raspberry, William. "Aren't They Just Battling for Basic Decency?" *Washington Post*, November 7, 1986, p. A27.
232. Unsigned article. *American Medical News* (December 4, 1987), pp. 11-12; Leslie Dutton, telephone interview (December 17, 1987).
233. Eunice Kennedy Shriver, *Growing Up Caring: A Guide for Teachers, Staff and Parents*, pp. i-ii; "Characteristics and Statistics for a Community of Caring." The Joseph P. Kennedy, Jr., Foundation, p. 1; letter from Nabers Cabiniss, Director, Office of Adolescent Pregnancy, U.S. Department of Health and Human Services (March 26, 1987), p. 4.
234. *AIDS and the Education of Our Children*, U.S. Department of Education (1987), p. 14. Quotation from draft copy of "Character Education," a minority report of the House Committee on Children, Youth and Families (1987).
235. Anchell, Melvin. "Psychoanalysis vs. Sex Education." *National Review* (June 20, 1986), p. 33. Otherwise, in Dr. Anchell's view, sex education courses can become "almost perfect recipes for production personality problems and even perversions later in life"; they can "continuously downgrade the affectionate, monogamous nature of human sexuality"; and they can "desensitize students to the spiritual qualities of human sexuality." Ibid.

236. *Risking the Future: Adolescent Sexuality, Pregnancy, and Childbearing.* The National Research Council, p. 17. The text cites several studies to support such a generalization, including one which found that young women 15-19 who said religion was/is important to them and went to church were less likely to have sexual intercourse.

237. Kinsey, Alfred, et al. *Sexual Behavior in the Human Male* (1948), pp. 469, 474, 480-81. On p. 469 Kinsey writes: "Considering the frequency of total sexual outlet (Table 125), the sexually least active individuals in any age and educational group are the Orthodox Jews, who are the least active of all, the devout Catholics, and the active Protestants, in that order. Conversely, the sexually most active individuals are the no-church-going Catholics, with the inactive Protestants and the inactive Jewish males intermediate in the system."

238. "Adolescent Pregnancy and Childbearing—Rates, Trends, and Research Findings, CPR, NICHD." National Technical Information Service, August 1986.

239. "Update on Condoms—Products, Protection, Promotion." *Population Reports,* September/October 1982.

240. Grady, William; Hayward, Mark; and Yagi, Junichi. "Contraceptive Failure in the United States: Estimates From the 1982 National Survey of Family Growth." *Family Planning Perspectives,* September/October 1986.

241. Fischl, Margaret A., et. al. "Heterosexual Transmission of Human Immunodeficiency virus. HIV: Relationship of Sexual Practices to Seroconversion." III International Conference on AIDS, June 1-5, 1987. *Abstracts volume.*

242. Voeller, Bruce, and Potts, Malcolm. *British Medical Journal* (October 26, 1985), p. 1196; and UPI story: "Condoms may not prevent AIDS transfer, expert says." *San Francisco Examiner,* November 7, 1985.

243. Fiumara, Nicholas J. "Effectiveness of Condoms in Preventing V.D." *New England Journal of Medicine,* October 21, 1971.

244. Wigersma, Lode, and Oud, Ron. "Safety and acceptability of condoms for use by homosexual men as a prophylactic against transmission of HIV during anogenital sexual intercourse." *British Medical Journal* (July 11, 1987), p. 94; personal correspondence, Dr. Wigersma (October 14, 1987).

245. Valdiserri, Ronald; Lyter, O. D.; Callahan, C.; Kingsley, L.; and Rinaldo, C. "Condom Use in a Cohort of Gay and Bisexual Men." III International Conference on AIDS, Washington, D.C., June 1-5, 1987. *Abstracts volume.*

246. Poarachini, Allan. "Koop Warns on Risk of AIDS in Condom Use." *Los Angeles Times,* September 22, 1987.

247. Koop, C. Everett, interview. *USA Today,* September 18, 1987.

248. *FDA Medical Devices Bulletin,* September 1987.

249. *Insight,* June 22, 1987.

250. "Condoms: Experts Fear False Sense of Security." *New York Times,* August 18, 1987.

251. Goedert, James J. "What Is Safe Sex?" *New England Journal of Medicine,* May 21, 1987.

252. Crenshaw, Theresa, M.D. "Condom Advertising." Testimony before the House Subcommittee on Health and the Environment, February 10, 1987.

253. "Condoms: Experts Fear False Sense of Security." *New York Times,* August 18, 1987.

254. Telephone interview with staff of the Department of Education. Washington, D.C., September 1, 1987.

255. "Koch Orders New AIDS Ads Stressing Sexual Abstinence." *New York Times,* June 8, 1987.

256. "AIDS Study to Test Condoms, Spermicides." *Los Angeles Times,* January 16, 1987. The same newspaper reported ("Condom Industry Seeking Limits on U.S. Study," August 28, 1987) that the condom industry is attempting to obstruct this study into the effectiveness of condoms against AIDS. "The condom industry has launched an intensive campaign to weaken, delay or possibly shut down" the project, according to the paper. "Among other things, the [condom industry] association has insisted to federal funding officials that the research rely solely on testing standards established by condom makers, that condom companies be allowed to supply all prophylactics to be tested, and that only products currently sold in the United States be studied."

The paper reported that "the attempt to force major modifications in the condom study was apparently motivated by industry concerns that the research might conclude that no American-made condom is currently able to consistenly prevent the spread of HIV."

The *Times* also reported that the condom manufacturers contended that the study should rely upon the current standards, which are drawn up by the industry and accepted by the FDA, and be prohibited from using a more rigorous standard of the International Standards Organization. If the study was allowed to use the tougher ISO standard, condom makers wanted to be permitted to "provide special batches of condoms 'screened specifically for this,'" according to the paper. The report said the industry group wanted condoms tested only by the water leakage method now used by the FDA, rather than the inflation and electrical resistance measures which "are seen by researchers as more accurate than the comparatively crude water leakage evaluation."

257. *The Facts About AIDS: A Special Guide for NEA Members.* National Education Association, 1987.

258. "Students haven't changed behavior despite AIDS fear." *Washington Times,* September 3, 1987. Vicki S. Freimuth, Timothy Edgar, and Sharon L. Hammond, "College Students Awareness and Interpretation of the AIDS Risk." *Science, Technology and Human Values,* December 1987.

259. Edgar, Timothy; Freimuth, Vicki S.; and Hammond, Sharon L. "Communicating the Risk to College Students: The Problem of Motivating Change." *Health Education Research: Theory and Practice,* December 1987.

260. "The Big Chill: Fear of AIDS." *Time,* February 16, 1987.

261. The story of "Patient Zero" (Gaetan Dugas) is recounted in Randy Shilts, *And the Band Played On.* New York: St. Martin Press, 1987.

262. Calabrese, Leonard H.; Harris, Buck; and Easley, Kirk. "Analysis of Variables Impacting on Safe Sexual Behavior Among Homosexual Men in an Area of Low Incidence for AIDS." III International Conference on AIDS, *Abstracts volume,* June 1987.

263. Sheer, Lorraine, and Green, John. "Evaluation of Health Education in Britain." III International Conference on AIDS, *Abstracts volume,* p. 56. Cited in "Agressive Prevention Efforts Proliferate." *Washington Post,* June 5, 1987.

264. Fox, Robin; Ostrow, D.; Valdisseri, R.; Van Raden, M.; Visscher, B.; and Polk, B. F. "Changes in Sexual Activities Among Participants in the Multicenter AIDS Cohort Study." III International Conference on AIDS, *Abstracts volume,* June 1987.

265. "AIDS Risk Looms Over Gays Ignoring Advice, Experts Say." *Washington Post,* November 22, 1987.

266. Curran, James W.; Morgan, W. Meade; Hardy, Ann M.; Jaffe, Harold W.; Darrow, William W.; and Dowdle, Walter R. "The Epidemiology of AIDS: Current Status and Future Prosects." *Science* (September 27, 1985), pp. 1354, 1356. Dr. Vernon Mark comments on these findings in his testimony before the Select Committee on Children, Youth and Families, in "A Prescription for the AIDS Epidemic" (June 18, 1987).

267. The acceptable quality level is 0.4%, or four leaky condoms per thousand. "The industry standard requires, roughly, that no more than four condoms out of 1,000 leak. The condoms are tested by pouring 10 ounces of water in each and looking for leakage." HHS News, (June 19, 1987). See also FDA, *Compliance Policy Guidelines,* chapter 24, guide 7124.21 (April 10, 1987), p. 1, which also notes: "The sampling inspection plan used by the FDA also emphasizes adequate protection against FDA rejecting lots where the percent defective is less that [sic] or equal to 0.4%."

268. Koop, Everett C., interview. *USA Today,* September 18, 1987.

269. *AIDS and the Education of our children: A Guide for Parents and Teachers.* U.S. Department of Education, October 6, 1987.

270. From joint statement on AIDS education, William J. Bennett, Secretary of Education, and C. Everett Koop, Surgeon General, January 30, 1987.

271. "Officials say some intercourse too risky, even with condoms." *Dallas Times Herald,* February 18, 1989.

272. "Toronto High Schools to Get Condoms." *Chicago Sun Times,* September 22, 1989.

273. Flax, Ellen. "Explosive Data Confirm Prediction: AIDS Is Spreading Among Teenagers." *Education Week* IX:8 (October 25, 1989).

274. Koop, C. Everett. Comments at 1987 Congressional Hearings. *Education Week,* June 24, 1987.

275. Hines, William. "Other sex diseases dwarf AIDS." *Chicago Sun Times,* May 21, 1989.

276. Parachini, Allan. "Koop Warns on Risk of AIDS in Condom Use." *Los Angeles Times,* September 22, 1987, part I, p. 16.

277. Report to the President. The Family: Preserving America's Future, 1986.

278. Hatcher, Robert A., M.D., et al. *Contraceptive Technology,* 1986-1987, 13th revised edition. New York: Irvington Publishers, Inc., 1986.

279. *AIDS and the Education of Our Children, A Guide for Parents and Teachers.* U.S. Department of Education, October 1987.

281. "One Million Americans Treated for PID Each Year." *Family Practice Medicine,* December 1-14, 1983.

282. Dobson, James C., Ph.D. "Understanding Sexuality." Pomona, CA: Focus on the Family, 1982.

283. U.S. House Select Committee, p. 386.

284. Furstenberg, Frank, et al. *Teenage Sexuality, Pregnancy and Childbearing.* Philadelphia: University of Pennsylvania Press, 1981.

285. Vincent, M. L.; Clearie, A.F.; and Schluchter, J. "Reducing adolescent pregnancy through school and community-based education." *Journal of the American Medical Association* 257 (June 1987).

286. Ford, James H., M.D. *Rx: Adolescent Abstinence* (cited by 109).

287. Ravenel, S. DuBose, M.D. "Birth Control Doesn't Curb Teen Pregnancies." *News and Observer* (Raleigh, N.C., June 28, 1989).

288. California Senate Bill no. 2394, Chapter 1337. An act to add Section 51551 to the Education Code, relating to education. Approved by Governor, 9/24/88. Filed with Secretary of State, 10/26/88.

289. "Illinois Legislature Passes Abstinance Law." *Education Reporter* 46 (November 1989).

290. *Weekly Messenger.* Prince Williams, Virginia, July 27, 1989.

291. Fury, Kathleen. "Sex and the American Teenager." *Ladies Home Journal,* March 1986.

292. Bauer, Ed. "Sex Education Program Must Have a Clear and Consistent Message." *Bulletin.* Albemarle County, Virginia, March 15, 1988.

293. "Currents in Modern Thought: Sex Education in the Public Schools." *The World & I.* A publication of The Washington Times Corporation, © September 1989.

294. Raspberry, William. "Sex Education and Morality." *Washington Post,* June 6, 1983.

295. Davis, Frances, M.D. "Troubled by Planned Parenthood Stand." *Los Angeles Times,* November 16, 1986.

296. Beyette, Beverly. "Teen Sex-Education Campaign Launched." *Los Angeles Times,* October 17, 1986, part V, p. 1.

297. McIlhaney, Joe S., M.D. *CMS Journal* XVIII:1 (Winter 1987).

298. *Family Planning Perspectives* 18:5 (September/October 1986).

299. Speckhard, Anne Catherine. "The Psycho-Social Aspects of Stress Following Abortion." A thesis submitted to the Faculty of the Graduate School of the University of Minnesota, May 1985.

300. "Teenage Pregnancy: The Problem That Hasn't Gone Away." From a report on a study done by the Alan Guttmacher Institute, Section 5. New York, 1981.

301. Hall C., and Zisook, S. "Psychological Distress Following Therapeutic Abortion." *The Female Patient* 8 (March 1983).

302. Kumar, R., and Robson, K. *Psychological Medicine* 8 (1978).

303. Bulfin, M., M.D. "A New Problem in Adolescent Gynecology." *Southern Medical Journal* 72:8 (August 1979).

304. Bulfin, M., M.D. "A New Problem in Adolescent Gynecology." *Southern Medical Journal* 72:8 (August 1979).

305. "Sexual Addiction Can Lead to Destruction." *USA Today,* February 2, 1989.

306. Sarrel, Lorna and Philip, eds. "The Redbook Report on Sexual Relationships: A Major New Survey of More Than 26,000 Women and Men." *Redbook,* October 1980.

307. *USA Today,* March 18, 1989.

308. *Webster's New Collegiate Dictionary.* Springfield, MA: G. & C. Merriam Co., 1980.

309. Frech, Frances. "Update of Teen Pregnancies." *Heartbeat Quarterly,* Summer 1980.

310. *Pediatric News* 20:1 (January 1986).

311. Stout, James, M.D., and Rivara, Frederick P., M.D. "Schools and Sex-Education: Does it work?" *Pediatrics* 83:3 (March 1989).

312. "Abating Teen Pregnancy." *Richmond Times Dispatch,* December 17, 1986.

313. Stout, James, M.D., and Rivara, Fredrick P., M.D. "Schools and Sex Education: Does it Work?" *Pediatrics* 83:3 (March 1989).

314. Firor, Nancy. "Family Life Classes now mandatory, but controversial." *Cincinnati Enquirer,* November 20, 1989.

315. Personal correspondence from Coleen Mast, developer of Sex Respect (February 10, 1990).

316. Bennet, William. "Sex and the Education of Our Children." Quoted in *School-Based Clinics.* Barrett L. Mosbacker, ed. Westchester, IL: Crossway Books, 1987.

317. Forrest, J. D., and Silverman, J. "What Public School Teachers Teach About Preventing Pregnancy, AIDS and Sexually Transmitted Diseases." *Family Planning Perspectives* 21:2 (March/April 1989).

318. Kirby, Douglas. *Sexuality Education: An Evaluation of Programs and Their Effects.* Santa Cruz, CA: Network Publication, 1984.

319. Vobejda, Barbara. "Right and Wrong and the Three R's – Consensus Supports a Return to Teaching Values in Public Schools." *Washington Post,* April 4, 1987.

320. "Fact Sheet on the Family and Adolescent Pregnancy." Office of Population Affairs, U.S. Dept. of Health and Human Services, n.d.

321. "Adolescent Pregnancy and Childbearing – Rates, Trends and Research Findings, CRR, NICHD." National Technical Information Service, August 1986.

322. Baumrind, Diana. "Authoritarian vs. Authoritative Parental Control." *Adolescence* 3:11 (Fall 1968).

323. Strommen, Merton P., and Strommen, Irene A. *Five Cries of Parents.* San Francisco: Harper and Row, 1985.

324. Olson, Terrance. "AANCHOR." U.S. Dept. of Health and Human Services Fact Sheet, Adolescent Pregnancy and Child Bearing.

325. Walth, Beverly. "Sexual abstinence is a fantasy solution." *Dallas Times Herald,* April 26, 1988.

326. "The Fourth 'R.' " *Richmond Times – Dispatch,* January 7, 1988.

327. Dash, Leon. *Washington Post,* February 9, 1986. Cf. Testimony Before the Joint Legislative Subcommittee on Teen Pregnancy, State of VA, July 23, 1986, by Rosemary Evans, Ettrick, VA.

328. "Sex-Ed Won't Deter Activity." *Richmond News Leader,* January 8, 1988. Letter to the editor by Anne Marie Morgan in their "Special to the Forum" section in the editorials.

329. Schwartz, Michael. *Our Sunday Visitor,* March 1987.

330. Cutwright, Phillip. *Family Planning Perspectives,* January 1971.

331. Anchell, Melvin, M.D. *Sex and Insanity.* Portland, OR: Halcyon House, 1983.

332. Leary, Warren E. *New York Times,* February 9, 1989.

333. "Teens Are Starting to Have Sex Earlier." *USA Today,* January 17, 1989.

334. Williams, Lena. "Teen-Age Sex: New Codes Amid the Old Anxiety." *New York Times,* February 27, 1989, p. B11.

335. Chassler, Sey. "What All Boys Think About Sex." *Parade,* December 18, 1988, p. 16.

336. Van Biema, David. "What you don't know about teen sex. How often they do it, how little they tell." *People,* April 13, 1987, pp. 110-21.

337. "Canada fights AIDS with clean needles, condom machines." *Atlanta Journal and Constitution,* December 31, 1989.

338. "Girls Having Sex at Younger Age." *San Diego Union,* February 6, 1990.

339. Bennett, William J. "Sex and the Education of our Children." U.S. Department of Education, January 22, 1987. Transcript of talk at the National School Board Association in Washington, D.C.

340. Carlin, David R., Jr. "Liberals, Conservatives and Sex Education." *America,* May 21, 1983.

341. "Family Policy." A publication of the Family Research Council, Washington, D.C., n.d.

342. Findlay, Steven, and Silberman, Joanne. "The Emerging Strategy to Contain AIDS." *U.S. News & World Review,* June 19, 1989.

343. Goldsmith, Marsha F. " 'Silent Epidemic' of 'Social Disease' Makes STD Experts Raise Their Voices." "Medical News and Perspectives" column. *Journal of the American Medical Association* 261:24 (June 23-30, 1989).

344. "Medical News and Perspectives" column. *Journal of the American Medical Association* 261:24 (June 23-30, 1989).

345. *U.S. News & World Report*, August 14, 1989.

346. "Who's Selling Sex in Public Schools?" *Focus on the Family Citizen* 3:12 (December 1989).

347. Dryfos, Jay. "School-Based Health Clinics: A New Approach to Preventing Adolescent Pregnancy?" *Family Planning Perspectives* 17:2 (March/April 1985).

348. Weatherly, Richard A.; Perlman, Sylvia B.; Levine, Michael H.; and Klerman, Lorraine V. "Comprehensive Programs for Pregnant Teenagers and Teenage Parents: How Successful Have They Been?" *Family Planning Perspectives* 18:2 (March/April 1986). Based on a report, "Patchwork Programs: Comprehensive Services for Pregnant and Parenting Adolescents." Available from the Center for Social Research, JH-30, University of Washington, Seattle, WA 98195.

349. Goldsmith, Marsha F. " 'Silent Epidemic' of 'Social Disease' Makes STD Experts Raise Thier Voices." "Medical News and Perspectives" column. *Journal of the American Medical Association*, 261:24:3509-10 (June 23-30, 1989).

350. Hines, William. "AIDS toll expected to soar in 90s." *Chicago Times*, December 3, 1989.

351. Tepper, Shari S. "The Problem With Puberty." Denver, CO: Rocky Mountain Planned Parenthood, 1975.

352. Tepper, Shari S. "The Great Orgasm Robbery." Denver, CO: Rocky Mountain Planned Parenthood, 1975.

353. Gordon, Sol. *The Heavy Facts About Sex*. Syracuse, NY: ED-U Press, 1975.

354. Webber, Robert. Taken from a taped presentation at Santa Maria High School, Santa Maria, CA. This class was given by the Director of Santa Barbara North County Planned Parenthood, November 16, 1983.

355. Tepper, Shari S. "The Perils of Puberty." Denver, CO: Rocky Mountain Planned Parenthood, 1974.

356. "Safety Dance." Brochure. Ithaca, NY: Planned Parenthood of Tompkins County, 1989. Suggested as homework by Vermont Dept. of Health.

357. Barth, Richard P. "Enhancing Skills to Prevent Pregnancy." Draft. Santa Cruz ETR Associates, 1988.

358. *Sex Education: Teacher's Guide and Resource Manual*. Planned Parenthood, Santa Cruz County, 1979.

359. Haney, Daniel Q. "Lies and sex make dishonest bedfellows." *San Diego Union*, March 15, 1990.

360. Gram, David. "Condoms Sought in School." *San Diego Union*, March 15, 1990.

361. Kasun, Jacqueline R., Ph.D. "Teenage Pregnancy: Media Effects Versus Facts." Arcata, CA: Humbolt State University, 1984, p. 3; 1985 figure from a speech by Fay Wattleton, president of the Planned Parenthood Federation of America, reprinted in *The Humanist*, July/August 1986.

362. Kenney, Asta. "School-Based Clinics: A National Conference." *Family Planning Perspectives* 18:1 (January/February 1986).

363. Bauer, Gary. "The Family: Preserving America's Future." A Report of the Working Group on the Family, November 1986.

364. Murray, Charles. *Losing Ground: American Social Policy 1950-1980*. New York: Basic Books, 1984, p. 127. It is important to note that the difference between the number of births to teenage mothers as reported by the National Research Council (470,000) and that reported by Charles Murray (272,000) results from the National Research Council's inclusion of births to married teenagers, whereas the figures reported by Charles Murray reflect births to unmarried teenagers. For additional information, see "Teen Pregnancy: What Is being Done? A State-by-State Look." Minority Report of the House Select Committee on Children, Youth and Families, December 1985.

365. Olsen, Joseph A., and Weed, Stan, Ph.D. "Effects of Family Planning Programs for Teenagers on Adolescent Birth and Pregnancy Rates." *Family Perspective* 20:3 (October 1986).

366. Kirby, Douglas. "Sexuality Education: A More Realistic View of Its Effects." *Journal of School Health* 55:10 (December 1985).

367. "Teenage Pregnancy: The Problem That Hasn't Gone Away." New York: The Alan Guttmacher Institute, 1981.

368. A speech by Fay Wattleton, president of the Planned Parenthood Federation of America. Reprinted in *The Humanist*, July/August 1986.

369. Kirby, Douglas, Ph.D. "School-Based Health Clinics: An Emerging Approach to Improving Adolescent Health and Addressing Teenage Pregnancy." Washington, D.C.: Center for Population Options, April 1985.

370. Pittman, Frank. *Private Lies*. New York: Norton Publishing Co., 1989

371. State of Illinois 85th General Assembly 1987-88, H.B. 1225; Indiana First Regular Session 105th General Assembly S.B. 72, and Indiana Second Regular Session 105th General Assembly H.B. 1067; State of Washington S.B. 6221, passed March 1988; California S.B. 2394, passed August 1988; Rhode Island General Assembly, January Session 1987, S.B. 182 and H.B. 6603; and Florida 1988 Committee Substitute H.B. 1519.

372. Testimony prepared for the Virginia General Assembly, February 1988, "Concerning Family Life Education Programs in Virginia."

373. *Insider*. Planned Parenthood Federation of America (PPFA), May 1988, pp. 1,3.

374. Hass, Aaron. *Teenage Sexuality—A Survey of Teenage Sexual Behavior*. New York: Macmillan Publishing Company, 1981.

375. McDowell, Josh, and Day, Dick. *Why Wait? What You Need to Know About the Teen Sexuality Crisis*. San Bernardino, CA: Here's Life Publishers, 1987.

376. McDowell, Josh. *Teens Speak Out: "What I Wish My Parents Knew About My Sexuality."* San Bernardino, CA: Here's Life Publishers, 1987.

377. St. Clair, Barry and Carol. *Talking With Your Kids About Love, Sex and Dating*. San Bernardino, CA: Here's Life Publishers, 1989.

378. McDowell, Josh, and Wakefield, Norm. *The Dad Difference: Creating an Environment for Your Child's Sexual Wholeness*. San Bernardino, CA: Here's Life Publishers, 1989.

379. Grady, Emory. "Postponing Sexual Involvement" (sex education program). Atlanta: Teen Service Program, 1985.
380. Personal correspondence from Dr. Jacqueline R. Kasun, Professor of Economics at Humboldt State University in Arcata, California, February 1987.
381. King, Wayne. "Teenagers on Sex: Confusion Is Clear." *New York Times*, June 21, 1978.
382. Greenberg, Bradley S.; Abelman, Robert; and Neuendorf, Kimberly. "Sex on the Soap Operas: Afternoon Delight." *Journal of Communication*, Summer 1981.
383. *Facets*, July, 1989.
384. Manning, Anita. "Teens and sex in the age of AIDS." *USA Today*, October 3, 1988, p. 2D.
385. Staimer, Marcia. "Where kids spend their time." *USA Today*, June 14, 1989, p. D1.
386. McDowell, Josh, and Day, Dick. *Why Wait? What You Need to Know About the Teen Sexuality Crisis*. San Bernardino, CA: Here's Life Publishers, 1987.
387. "Sharp Rise in Rare Sex-Related Diseases." *New York Times*, Health Section, July 14, 1988.
388. "Proper Use of a Condom." Brochure. Norfolk, VA: Norfolk, Virginia Health Department, n.d.
389. Goedert, James J., M.D. "What Is Safe Sex?" *New England Journal of Medicine* 316:21.
390. From the Rhode Island Department of Health, prepared by the Concerned Citizens Council, Lorton, Virginia, n.d.
391. *American Journal of Public Health*, 1986.
392. Virginian Vital Statistics, State Health Department, n.d.
393. "Teen Sex Survey in the Evangelical Church." Survey done by Barna Research Group, Glendale, California, for Josh McDowell Ministry, 1988.
394. Fox, Greer L. "The Family's Role in Adolescent Sexual Behavior." *Teenage Pregnancy in a Family Context*, Theodore Doms, ed. Philadelphia: Temple University Press, 1981.
395. Gordon, S., and Snyder, C. *Personal Issues in Human Sexuality*, Newton, MA: n. pub., 1986.
396. Darling, C. A., and Hicks, H. W. "Parental Influence on Adolescent Sexuality—Implications for Parents as Educators." *Journal of Youth and Adolescence*, 1982.
397. Keeney, A. M., and Orr, M. T. "Sex Education: An Overview of Current Programs, Policies and Research." Phi Delta Kappa. *KAPPA*, March 1984.
398. "Safe Sex." Pamphlet published by the Norfolk, VA Department of Public Health, n.d.
399. Heron, Ann, ed. *One Teenager in Ten: Writings by Gay and Lesbian Youth*. Promoted and sold by PPFA; part of "Project 10." Project 10 was prepared by the Office of Counseling and Guidance Services Branch, Los Angeles Unified School District, 6520 Newcastle Ave., Reseda, CA 91335.
400. "Teacher Training." The 1988 update of an article by Anne Marie Morgan, (a high school psychology and government teacher in Chesterfield, Virginia) relating to the Virginia Family Life Education, FLE/Sex Education Mandate.
401. Tepper, Shari S. "The Great Orgasm Robbery." Denver, CO: Rocky Mountain Planned Parenthood, 1975.
402. *Family Planning Perspectives*, January/February 1980.
403. Edwards, Laura, M.D., and Arnold, Kathleen, R.N., M.A. "Adolescent Pregnancy Prevention Services in High School Clinics: An Update." Unpublished report, 1983; and "St. Paul M.I.C. Adolescent Program—Progress Report," 1981 and 1983.
404. *Family Planning Perspectives* 18:3 (May/June 1986).
405. Kasun, Jacqueline R., Ph.D. "The Baltimore School Birth Control Study: A Comment." Arcata, CA: Humboldt State University, 1986.
406. Forrest, J. D. "Projected Reductions." From a report on a study by Alan Guttmacher Institute, New York, 1981.
407. Figures for 1970-1978 from Susan Reylance's testimony before U.S. Senate Committee on Labor and Human Resources (March 31, 1981). Based on data from National Center for Health Statistics, U.S. Department of Health and Human Services, U.S. Bureau of the Census, and the Alan Guttmacher Institute. Figures for 1979-1981 from the National Center for Health Statistics and the Alan Guttmacher Institute. The figures for family planning expenditures are estimates of certain categories of spending only. While they appear to be internally consistent, they are substantially smaller than other estimates of the same kinds of spending. In "Teenage Pregnancy, Media Effects vs. Facts." Jacqueline R. Kasun, Ph.D., 1984.
408. Huntford, Roland. *The New Totalitarian*. New York: Stein and Day, 1972.
409. Rate for American States computed from data on abortions from U.S. Centers for Disease Control. Rates for foreign countries from Jones, Elise F., et al. "Teenage Pregnancy in Developed Countries: Determinants and Policy Implications." *Family Planning Perspectives* 17:2 (March/April 1985), pp. 53-63.
410. "The Why Wait? Teen Sex Survey in the Evangelical Church," commissioned by the Josh McDowell Ministry with technical assistance by Barna Research Group of Glendale, California, June/August 1987.
411. *Young Adolescents and Their Parents*. Minneapolis, MN: Search Institute, 1984.
412. *Family Life Education*. Pamphlet. Published and prepared by the Virginia Department for Children's Committee on Youth and Family Life, n.d.
413. Joint Subcommittee on Teen Pregnancy, November 30, 1987.
414. Pennsylvania's Subcommittee on Teen Pregnancy, November 30, 1987.
415. The Legislators Briefing Packet. Prepared by Virginia Concerned Citizens Council, 1989.
416. American Academy of Pediatrics, September 1987, 1988 General Assembly Testimony. Compiled by The Virginian Concerned Citizens Council.

417. Zanga, Joseph E., M.D. Personal and professional letter, January 15, 1988, to Delegate Stephen H. Martin, Virginia House of Delegates, urging him to cast his vote in opposition to the Family Life Education Program proposed by the State Board of Education.
418. "Dissent in Part of Delegate S. Vance Wilkins, Jr., on the Report and Recommendations of the Joint Subcommittee Studying Teenage Pregnancy Prevention Pursuant to HJR 280." June 2, 1988.
419. Written testimony of Faye Wattleton before Jeremiah Denton. Title XX Hearings, March 31,1981.
420. "Legalized Abortion and the Public Health." Washington, D.C.: The Institute of Medicine, National Academy of Sciences, May 1975.
421. McDowell, Josh, and Lewis, Paul. *Givers, Takers and Other Kinds of Lovers.* Wheaton, IL: Tyndale House Pubs., 1980.
422. Fromm, Erich. *The Sane Society.* New York: Rinehart, 1955.
423. *Insider.* A PPFA pubiication, May 1988.
424. Whelan, Dr. Elizabeth. *Sex and Sensibility: A New Look at Being a Woman.* New York: McGraw-Hill Book Co., 1974.
425. Personal correspondence from Jerry Peyton, Tucson, Arizona, January 1990.
426. Northwest NFP Services, 4805 NE Glisan, Portland, OR 97213, (503) 230-6377.
427. "Legalized Abortion and the Public Health." Report of a study by the Institute of Medicine, National Academy of Sciences, Washington, D.C., May 1975.
428. Tatum, M. L. "Sex Education in the Public Schools." Brown, L., et al. *Sex Education in the Eighties, Toward a Healthy Sexual Evolution.* New York: Plenum Press, 1981.
429. Personal correspondence with Educational Guidance Institute, Inc., January 1990.
430. *London Daily Telegraph,* September 27, 1986.
431. Lord, Lewis J. with Thornton, Jeannye, and Carey, Joseph. "Sex, With Care." *U.S. News & World Report,* June 2, 1986, p. 53.
432. *New England Journal of Medicine,* July 6, 1989.
433. Painter, Kim. "Prudence tests could curb VD." *USA Today,* May 19, 1989, p. D1.
434. Goldsmith, M. F., Stockholm. Speakers on Adolescents and AIDS. Reports from the Fourth International Conference on AIDS. *Journal of the American Medical Association* 260:6 (August 12, 1988).
435. "Medical Aspects of Human Sexuality." *Contemporary Ob/Gyn.* September, 1972. (An expanded version appeared in the same publication, September 1974.)
436. *Journal of the American Medical Association,* February 17, 1962.
437. *Cancer Research,* April, 1967.
438. "Venereal Factors in Human Cervical Cancer." *Cancer* 39 (1977).
439. Barron, S. L. "Sexual Activity in Girls Under 18 Years of Age." *The British Journal of Obstetrics and Gynecology* 93 (1986).
440. "Sharp Rise Found in Syphilis in U.S." *New York Times,* October 4, 1987.
441. *All News,* July 28, 1989. Sources: *Journal of the American Medical Association,* June 23-30, 1989; *Washington Times,* June 12, 1989; *Washington Post,* Health Section, July 11, 1989.
442. Koop, C. Everett. "AIDS, What We All Need to Know." Presentation to the National Association of Elementary School Principals, San Francisco, California, April 19, 1988.
443. Kasun, Jacqueline R., Ph.D. "The State and Adolescent Sexual Behavior." *The American Family and the State.* Joseph R. Peden and Fred R. Glahe, eds. The Pacific Institute, n.d.
444. Kasun, Jacqueline R., Ph.D. *The War Against Population: The Economics and Ideology of Population Control.* Jameson Books, 1988. Imprint of Green Hills Pubs., New York.
445. "One Million Americans Treated for PID Each Year." *Family Practice News,* December 1-14, 1983.
446. Washington, A. Eugene, M.D.; Arno, Peter S., Ph.D.; and Brooks, Marie A., MBA. "The Economic Cost of Pelvic Inflammatory Disease." *Journal of the American Medical Association* 255:13 (April 4, 1986).
447. "PID Incidence in United States Placed at 1 Million Cases Yearly." *Family Practice News* 14:16 (August 15-31, 1984).
448. Gibbs, Ronald S., M.D. "Management of Pelvic Inflammatory Disease." *Sexual Medicine Today,* January 1985.
449. "PID – A major cause of abdominal pain." *Acute Care Medicine,* October 1984.
450. "Salpingitis." *The Merck Manual,* thirteenth edition. Merck, Sharp & Dohme Research Laboratories, 1977.
451. Roundtable. Moderator: Wiegart, H. T., M.D. Panel members: Hager, W. D., M.D.; Noble, R. C., M.D.; Schnel, E. R., M.D.; Turner, Rev. W.; Engelberg, J., Ph.D. "Consequences of Gonococcal Pelvic Inflammatory Disease." *Medical Aspects of Human Sexuality* 17:11 (November 1983).
452. Livengood, Charles H., III, M.D. "Management of Acute Pelvic Inflammatory Disease." *Continuing Education,* February 1985.
453. "OCs Do Not Appear to Prevent Recurrences of Chlamydia But May Mask It." *Infectious Diseases,* January 1986.
454. Druessner, Harold T., M.D.; Hansel, Nancy K., Dr., P.H.; and Griffith, Marilyn, M.D.; "Diagnosis and Treatment of Chlamydial Infections." *American Family Physician* 34:1 (July 1986).
455. Interview with Masood A. Khatamee, M.D. "Chlamydia Mycoplasma: What Are the Hidden Risks of These STDs?" *Modern Medicine,* February 1984.
456. "Asymptomatic Disease Can Cause Mechanical Sterility." *Sexually Transmitted Diseases Bulletin,* October 1982.

457. Wong. Edward, M.D., and Handsfield, Hunter, M.D. "Non-gonococcal Urethritis." *Medical Aspects of Human Sexuality* 17:8 (August 1983).

458. "Clindamycin Effective vs. M. Hominis and Chlamydia; Less so vs. U. urealyticum." *Infectious Diseases,* February/March 1985.

459. "Chlamydia Infection Blamed for Rupture of Fetal Membranes." *American Medical News,* April 11, 1986.

460. "GC Patient Should Be Treated for Chlamydia as Well." *Family Practice News,* July 1-14, 1983.

461. Schachter, Julius, Ph.D. "Perinatal Transmission of Chlamydia Trachomatis – High Incidence Warrants Preventive Measures." *Sexually Transmitted Diseases Bulletin* 7:1 (February 1987).

462. Rapoza, Peter, M.D.; Quinn, Thomas, M.D.; Kiessling, Lou Ann, M.D.; Green, W. Richard, M.D.; Taylor, Hugh, M.D. "Assessment of Neonatal Conjunctivitis With a Direct Immuno-fluorescent Monoclonal Antibody Stain for Chlamydia." *The Journal of the American Medical Association* 255:24 (June 27, 1986).

463. "Latent and Reactive Properties of Chlamydia Linked to Growing Number of STD Cases." *Sexually Transmitted Diseases Bulletin* 5:1 (February 1985).

464. Krieger, J. N. "Epididymitis, Orchitis, and Related Conditions." *Sexually Transmitted Diseases,* 1984, 11:173-81 as noted by Harold Pruessner, M.D.; Nancy Hansel, D.P.H.; and Marilyn Griffith, M.D. "Diagnosis and Treatment of Chlamydial Infections." *American Family Physician* 34:1 (July 1986).

465. Schachter, Julius, Ph.D. "Chlamydia Trachomatis Infections. *Medical Times* 110:12 (December 1982).

466. Pruessner, Harold, M.D.; Hansel, Nancy, D.P.H.; and Griffith, Marilyn, M.D. "Diagnosis and Treatment of Chlamydial Infections." *American Family Physician* 34:1 (July 1986).

467. "Selective Screening Detects Most Chlamydia Cases." *American Medical News,* April 4, 1986.

468. "Direct Test Better Than Cultures for Dx of Chlamydial Infection in Women." *Infectious Diseases,* January 1986.

469. Haglund, Keith. "Find High Rate of Chlamydia in Suburban Girls." *Medical Tribune,* June 18, 1986.

470. Collins, Patricia J. "New Tests, New Importance for Chlamydia." *Patient Care,* October 30, 1985.

471. National Institute of Allergy and Infectious Diseases: "Chlamydia and Nongonococcal Urethritis." In *Sexually Transmitted Diseases: 1980 Status Report.* Washington, D.C., 1981 (DHHS Publication No. 81-2213) as referred to by Julius Schachter, Ph.D., in "Chlamydia Trachomatis Infections." *Medical Times,* December 1982.

472. Spence, Michael, M.D. "PID: Detection and Treatment." *Patient Care,* June 30, 1983.

473. Klein, Aaron E. Adopted from a CME lecture by B. Frank Polk, M.D. "PID: How to track down its cause." *Patient Care,* June 30, 1983.

474. Roundtable: (moderator) H. Thomas Wiegert, M.D.; (panel members) W. David Hager, M.D.; Robert C. Noble, M.D.; Eileen R. Scherl, M.D.; Rev. William Turner; Joseph Engelberg, Ph.D. "Consequences of Gonococcal Pelvic Inflammatory Disease." *Medical Aspects of Human Sexuality* 17:11 (November 1983).

475. "PID – Longterm Physical and Emotional Effects Seen." *Sexually Transmitted Diseases Bulletin,* October 1982.

476. Chavkins, W. "The Rise in Ectopic Pregnancy: Exploration of Possible Reasons." Int. J. Gynaecol. Obstet., 1982, 20:341-50, as noted by David A. Grimes, M.D. "Deaths Due to Sexually Transmitted Diseases." *Journal of the American Medical Association* 255:13 (April 4, 1986).

477. "Official: High-risk Women Need to Visit STD Clinics." *American Medical News,* May 3, 1985.

478. Snyder, Jon R., M.D. "Defusing the Deadly Ectopic." *Emergency Medicine,* November 30, 1983.

479. "Ectopic Pregnancy." *Merck Manual.* Thirteenth edition. Merck, Sharp & Dohme Research Laboratory, 1977.

480. "Rate of Ectopic Pregnancy Has Doubled in U.S." *Family Practice News* 13:2 (January 15-31, 1985).

481. Horwitz, Nathan. "Ectopic Pregnancies Up, Now a Major Death Risk." *Medical Tribune,* January 26, 1983.

482. Kredentser, Jeremy, M.D.; and Schiff, Isaac, M.D. "Infertility: An Overview." *Medical Times,* July 1985.

483. Hunt, E., M.D. *Diseases Affecting the Vulva,* edition 4. London: Henry Kimpton, 1954, p. 195. As reported by Michael Jarratt, M.D. "Genital Herpes Simplex Infection." *Dermatologic Clinics* 1:1 (January 1983).

484. Klein, R. J., M.D.; Friedman-Kein, A. E., M.D.; and Hatcher, V. A., M.D. "Herpes Simplex Virus Infections: An Update (Part I)." *Hospital Medicine,* November 1983.

485. Driscoll, Charles E., M.D. "Genital Herpes." *Female Patient* 9 (December 1984).

486. "Herpes." *Sexual Medicine Today,* June 1983.

487. Larson, Trudy, M.D. "Genital Herpes: Natural History, Clinical Presentation, and Management." *Your Patient and Cancer,* May 1984.

488. Gunby, Phil. "Genital Herpes Research: Many Aim to Tame Maverick Virus." *Journal of the American Medical Association* 250:18 (November 11, 1983).

489. Greenwood, Vincent, Ph.D., and Bernstein, Robert, Ph.D. "Herpes: The Psychological Burden." *Sexual Medicine Today,* November 1983.

490. Horwitz, Nathan. "Herpes Hits the Suburbs." *Medical Tribune,* July 13, 1983.

491. "Woman receives settlement of $25,000 in herpes case." *American Medical News,* July 12, 1985.

492. "Oral Herpes Cases Increase." *American Medical News,* November 9, 1984.

493. Corey, Laurence, M.D. "The Diagnosis and Treatment of Genital Herpes." *Journal of the American Medical Association* 248:9 (September 3, 1982).

494. Prepared by Staff Editor Janet P. Crawhaw, based on individual interviews with Kenneth H. Fife, M.D., Ph.D.; Benjamin Raab, M.D.; and Stephen E. Straus, M.D. "New Options for Genital Herpes Dx/Rx." *Patient Care,* April 15, 1986.

495. Jarratt, Michael, M.D. "Genital Herpes Simplex Infections." *Dermatologic Clinics* 1:1 (January 1983).

496. Klein, R. J., M.D.; Friedman-Kien, A. E., M.D.; and Hatcher, V. A., M.D. "Herpes Simplex Virus Infections: An Update. Part 2." *Hospital Medicine,* December 1983.

497. Baker, Richard A., M.D. "Genital Herpes: A Review." *Family Practice Recertification* 6:4 (April 1984).

498. Reeves, W. C.; Corey, L.; Adams, H. G.; et al. "Risk of Reoccurrence After First Episode of Genital Herpes." *New Enqland Journal of Medicine* 305:315-19 (1981), noted by Richard A. Baker, M.D. "Genital Herpes: A Review." *Communicable Diseases* 6:4 (April 1984).

499. Schmidt, David D., M.D.; Zyzanski, Stephen, Ph.D.; Ellner, Jerrold, M.D.; Kumar, Mary Lou, M.D.; and Arno, Janet, M.D. "Stress as a Precipitating Factor in Subjects With Recurrent Herpes Labialis." *Journal of Family Practice* 20:4 (1985).

500. "Stress 'Acquited' as Herpes Trigger." *Medical World News,* September 23, 1985.

501. Brown, Z. A.; Kern, E. R.; Spruance, S. T.; et al. "Clinical and Virologic Course of Herpes Simplex Genitalis." *Western Journal of Medicine* 130:414-21 (1979). Noted by Richard A. Baker, M.D. "Genital Herpes: A Review." *Family Practice Recertification* 6:4 (April 1984).

502. Symposium: Nixon, S., M.D.; Alford, C., Jr., M.D.; Strous, S., M.D.; Larson, T., M.D.; Whitley, R., M.D.; Dolin, R., M.D.; "Questions and Answers on Genital Herpes." *Primary Care and Cancer,* October 1984.

503. Johnson, Roger S., Ph.D. "Coping With Herpes Stress." *Female Patient* 9 (January 1984).

504. "Herpes, Transmission of Genital Herpes by Asymptomatic Carriers." *Sexually Transmitted Diseases Bulletin* 7:1 (February 1987).

505. Scott, T. F. McNair, M.D.; Parish, Laurence Charles, M.D.; Witkowski, Joseph A., M.D. "Herpes Simplex Virus Infections. Part 2. Diagnosis and Treatment." *Drug Therapy,* October 1985.

506. Roundtable: (moderator) Felman, Yehudi M., M.D.; (panel members) Young, Alexander W., M.D.; Siegal, Frederick P., M.D.; Scham, Manuel, M.D. "Sex and Herpes." *Medical Aspects of Human Sexuality* 17:1 (January 1983).

507. Mertz, G. J., M.D.; Schmidt, O., Ph.D.; Jourden, J. L., B.A.; et al. *Sexually Transmitted Diseases Bulletin* 12:33-9 (January-March 1985). As reported in "Herpes Simplex: Asymptomatic Patients Transmit Most Cases." *Modern Medicine,* October 1985.

508. Rein, Michael F., M.D. "Condoms and STDs: Do the Former Prevent Transmission of the Latter?" *Medical Aspects of Human Sexuality* 19:6 (June 1985).

509. Symposium: Nixon, S., M.D.; Alford, C., Jr., M.D.; Strous, S., M.D.; Larson, T., M.D.; Whitley, R., M.D.; Dolin, R., M.D. "Questions and Answers on Genital Herpes." *Primary Care and Cancer,* October 1984.

510. Corey, L., M.D.; Mindel, A.; Fife, K. H., M.D.; et al. "Risk of recurrence after treatment of first episode of genital herpes with intravenous acyclovir." *Sex Transmitted Diseases* 12:215-8 (October-December 1985). Referred to in "Genital herpes: Rx aids healing but not recurrence rate." *Modern Medicine,* June 1985.

511. Katzenstein, David A., M.D. "The Sexual Transmission of Viral Infections." *Continuing Education,* January 1984.

512. Driscoll, Charles E., M.D. "Genital Herpes. Etiology, Diagnosis and Management." *Female Patient* 9 (December 1984).

513. International Medical News Service, "Herpes in Pregnancy: Protect Infants But Don't Overuse Caesarean." *Family Practice News,* August 1-14, 1984.

514. Kit, Saul, Ph.D. "Problems and Progress in the Development of Vaccines Against Genital Herpes. Part I: The Problems." *Infectious Diseases,* September 1982.

515. Jeffries, D. J. "Clinical Use of Acyclovir." *Continuing Education,* June 1985.

516. Giltman, Larry I., M.D., and Sanders, Steven A., M.S. "Herpes Simplex Encephalitis." *American Family Physicians,* September 1984.

517. "Cervical Cancer Linked With Papillomavirus." *Data Centrum* 4:1 (January/February 1987).

518. Scott, T. F. McNair, M.D.; Parish, Laurence C., M.D.; Witkowski, Joseph A., M.D. "Herpes Simplex Virus Infections. Part 1: Clinical Aspects." *Drug Therapy,* September 1985.

519. "Herpes – Truth and Consequences." *Sexual Medicine Today* 7:6 (June 1983).

520. Marzouk, Joseph B., M.D.; Dall, Lawrence, M.D.; Mills, John, M.D. "Genital Herpes: 1982." *Female Patient* 7 (September 1982).

521. Spector, Stephen A., M.D., and Michelotti, Valerie, M.D. "The Spectrum of Disease From Epstein-Barr Virus and Cytomegalovirus," *Diagnosis,* September 1985.

522. Drew, W. L.; Mintz, L.; Miner, R. C.; et al. "Prevalence of Cytomegalovirus Infection in Homosexual Men." *Journal of Infectious Disease* 143:188-92 (1982). Noted by David A. Katzenstein, M.D. "The Sexual Transmission of Viral Infections." *Continuing Education,* January 1984.

523. "10-20% of Babies With CMV Will Have Significant Handicaps." *Family Practice News* 13:7 (April 14, 1983).

524. "Undiagnosed Congenital CMV Major Cause of Pediatric Handicaps." *Family Practice News* 13:12 (June 15-31, 1983).

525. "CMV Vaccine Is on Horizon; Uses Cited." *Family Practice News,* November 15-30, 1983.

526. Howard, Rudolph G., M.D. (in consultation with editors of *Female Patient).* "Viral Infections in Pregnancy." *Female Patient* 8 (June 1983).

527. "10-20% of Babies With CMV Will Have Significant Handicaps." *Family Practice News* 13:12 (April 1-14, 1983).

528. Method of David H. Van Thiel, M. D. "How Hepatitis Affects Sexual Function." *Medical Aspects of Human Sexuality* 16:11 (November 1982).

529. Scheig, Robert, M.D. "Effects of Chronic Hepatitis: Protecting the Family." *Medical Aspects of Human Sexuality* 20:6 (June 1986).
530. Ismach, Judy M. "Hepatitis B Virus Infection." *Medical World News,* September 24, 1984.
531. "Says Hepatitis B Vaccine From Carrier Plasma Apparently Safe." *Family Practice News* 13:15 (August 1-14, 1983).
532. "Hepatitis B Vaccine Advised for Persons at Substantial Risk for Acquiring Disease." *Family Practice News,* August 15-31, 1985.
533. Romanowski, Barbara, M.D., FRCP(C) and Harris, J. R. W., MB, MRCP. "Sexually Transmitted Disease." *Clinical Symposia.* Ciba 36:1 (1984).
534. "Hepatitis B Vaccine Prevents Spread to Newborns." *Modern Medicine,* September 1984.
535. The editors of *Female Patient* in consultation with Rudolph G. Howard, M.D. "Viral Infections in Pregnancy." *Female Patient* 8 (June 1983).
536. "A Call to Combat Congenital Hep B." *Medical Tribune,* December 25, 1985.
537. "The Hepatitis B Vaccine: Should you get the shot?" *Modern Medicine,* September 1984.
538. "Experts Confer on AIDS Spread in Heterosexuals." *Medical Tribune,* July 23, 1986.
539. "AIDS risk spreading to heterosexuals." *Modern Medicine,* June 1986.
540. Selwyn, Peter A., M.D. "AIDS: What Is Now Known." *Hospital Practice,* June 15, 1986.
541. Francis, Donald P., M.D., DSc; Chin, James, M.D., MPH. "The Prevention of Acquired Immunodeficiency Syndrome in the United States." *Journal of the American Medical Association* 257:10 (March 13, 1987).
542. "MD's suggestions are invited in research on prevention of AIDS." *American Medical News,* May 4, 1984.
543. Macher, Abe M. "Acquired Immunodeficiency Syndrome." *American Family Physician,* December 1984.
544. Shepherd, F. A., M.D., FRCPC, et al. "A Guide to the Investigation and Treatment of Patients with AIDS and AIDS-Related Disorders." *Canadian Medical Association Journal* 134:999-1008, May 1, 1986. Noted in *Infectious Diseases,* April 1986.
545. Wallis, Claudia. Reported by Christine Gorman, J. Madeleine Nash and Dick Thompson. "Viruses." *Time,* November 3, 1986.
546. "Antigen Exposure May Hasten AIDS . . . and Trigger HTLV-III's Rapid-Fire Replication." *Medical World News,* March 24, 1986.
547. Selwyn, Peter A., M.D. "AIDS: What Is Now Known." *Hospital Practice,* May 15, 1986.
548. Gross, Ludwick, M.D. "The Role of Viruses in Cancer, Leukemia, and Malignant Lymphomas." *Medical Times,* September 1985.
549. Guroy, Mary Ellen, M.D., and Murray, Henry W., M.D. "Outpatient Evaluation of Patients at Risk for AIDS and ARC." *Emergency Decisions,* June 1986.
550. Ognibene, Frederick P., M.D. "Answers to Questions: Complications of AIDS." *Medical Aspects of Human Sexuality* 18:10 (October 1984).
551. Thomas, Patricia "Living With Dying on S. F. General's Ward S-B." *Medical Tribune,* July 3, 1985.
552. Guroy, Mary Ellen, M.D., and Murray, Henry W., M.D. "AIDS: Emergency Department Management." *Emergency Decisions,* May 1986.
553. "Antibiotics Failed AIDS Trial." *Medical Tribune,* May 7, 1986.
554. "Big Cities Report TB on the Rise." *Medical World News,* August 26, 1985.
555. Arno, Peter S., Ph.D.; Shenson, Douglas, M.D., MPH; Siegel, Naomi F., MSPH; Franks, Pat; Lee, Philip R., M.D. "Economic and Policy Implications of Early Intervention in HIV Disease." *Journal of the American Medical Association* 262:11 (September 15, 1989).
556. Sitz, Karl V., M.D.; Keppen, Michael, M.D.; Johnson, Dianne F., M.D. "Metastatic Based Cell Carcinoma in Acquired Immunodeficiency Syndrome-Related Complex." *Journal of the American Medical Association* 257:3 (January 16, 1987).
557. "Neurological Degeneration Linked to AIDS." *American Medical News,* May 10, 1985.
558. Levy, Jay A., M.D. "Human Immunodeficiency Viruses and the Pathogenesis of AIDS." *Journal of the American Medical Association* 261:20 (May 26, 1989).
559. "ARC Patients: In Need of Emotional Support." *Medical World News,* August 12, 1985.
560. "Ask U.S. Outlay of $2 Billion a Year for AIDS Research and Education." *Medical Tribune,* November 26, 1986.
561. Institute of Medicine, USA. "Confronting AIDS: Directions for Public Health, Health Care, and Research." Washington, D.C.: National Academy Press, 1986:91 as referred to by Donald S. Burke, M.D., et al. "Human Immunodeficiency Virus Infection Among Civilian Applicants for United States Military Service, October 1985 to March 1986." *New England Journal of Medicine* 317:3 (July 16, 1987).
562. "Wider AIDS Virus Testing Urged." *American Medical News,* March 13, 1987.
563. Wallis, Claudia. Reported by Dick Thompson/Washington, with other bureaus. "You Haven't Heard Anything Yet." *Time,* February 16, 1987.
564. "Close Sex Centers to Stop AIDS, Says AMA." *Medical World News,* July 28, 1986.
565. Corey, Lawrence, M.D.; Winkelstein, Warren, Jr., M.D.; Chaisson, Richard E., M.D. "AIDS Risk Rising Sharply in IV Drug Users and Their Sexual Partners." *Data Centrum* 4:4 (July/August 1987).
566. Bolognesi, Dani P., Ph.D. "Prospects for Prevention of and Early Intervention Against HIV." *Journal of the American Medical Association* 261:20 (May 26, 1989).

567. "AIDS: Can the Nation Cope?" *Medical World News,* August 26, 1985.

568. Ostrow, David G., M.D., Ph.D. "AIDS: How to Calm Your Patients' Fears." *Drug Therapy,* July 1986.

569. "FPs Should Become Familiar with AIDS Presentation." *Family Practice News* 16:7 (April 1-14, 1986).

570. Valle, S. L.; Saxingen, C.; Ranki, A.; et al. "Diversity of Clinical Spectrum of HTLV-III Infection." Lancet, 1985, 1:301-4 as referred to by William Lang, M.D.; Robert E. Anderson, M.D.; Herbert Perkins, M.D.; Robert M. Grant; David Lyman, M.D., MPH; Warren Winkelstein, Jr., M.D., MPH; Rachel Royce, MPH; and Jay A. Levy, M.D.; in "Clinical Immunologic and Serologic Findings in Men at Risk for Acquired Immunodeficiency Syndrome." *Journal of the American Medical Association* 257:3 (January 16, 1987).

571. Quarterly Report to the Domestic Policy Council on the Prevalence and Rate of Spread of HIV and AIDS—United States MMWR, 1988, 37:551-54,559. *Journal of the American Medical Association* 260:13 (October 7, 1988).

572. Andrulis, Dennis P., MPH, Ph.D.; Weslowski, Virginia Beers, MPA; Gage, Larry S., JD. "The 1987 US Hospital AIDS Survey." *Journal of the American Medical Association* 262:6 (August 11, 1989).

573. "AIDS Called 'Potentially Catastrophic' for Insurers." *American Medical News,* September 6, 1985.

574. Hardy, Ann M., DPH; Rauch, Kathryn; Echenberg, Dean, M.D., Ph.D.; Morgan, W. Meade, Ph.D.; Curran, James W., M.D., MPH. "The Economic Impact of the First 10,000 Cases of Acquired Immunodeficiency Syndrome in the United States." *Journal of the American Medical Association* 255:2 (January 10, 1986).

575. Goedert, James J., M.D., "What Is Safe Sex?" *New England Journal of Medicine* 316:21 (May 21, 1987).

576. Thomas, Patricia. "Does Safe Sex Exist at All in AIDS Era?" *Family Practice News* 15:18 (September 15-30, 1985).

577. Goldsmith, Marsha F. "Sex in the Age of AIDS Calls for Common Sense and 'Condom Sense.' " *Journal of the American Medical Association* 257:17 (May 1, 1987).

578. Morganthau, Tom; Hager, Mary; Cohn, Bob; Raine, George; Reese, Michael; Anderson, Monroe; and Ernsberger, Richard, Jr. "Future Shock." *Newsweek,* November 24, 1986.

579. "Is AIDS really spreading among heterosexuals?" *Patient Care,* April 30, 1989.

580. Marwick, Charles. "AZT. Zidovudine Just a Step Away from FDA Approval for AIDS Therapy." *Journal of the American Medical Association* 257:10 (March 13, 1987).

581. Yarchoan, Robert, M.D., and Broder, Samuel, M.D. "Development of Antiretroviral Therapy for the Acquired Immunodeficiency Syndrome and Related Disorders." *New England Journal of Medicine* 316:9 (February 26, 1987).

582. Fischl, Margaret A., M.D.; Richman, Douglas D., M.D.; Causey, Dennis M., M.D.; Grieco, Michael H., M.D., JD; Bryson, Yvonne, M.D.; Mildvan, Donna, M.D.; Laskin, Oscar L., M.D.; Groopman, Jerome E., M.D.; Volberding, Paul A., M.D.; Schooley, Robert T., M.D.; Jackson, George G., M.D.; Durack, David T., M.D.; Phil, D. ; Andrews, John C., Ph.D.; Nusinoff-Lehrman, Sandra, M.D.; Barry, David W., M.D.; and the AZT Collaborative Working Group. "Prolonged Zidovudine Therapy in Patients With AIDS and Advanced AIDS-Related Complex." *Journal of the American Medical Association* 262:17 (November 3, 1989).

583. McAuliffe, Kathleen; with Carey, Joseph; Wells, Stacey; Quick, Barbara E.; and Doffin, Muriel, in San Francisco and the magazine's domestic bureaus. "AIDS: At the Dawn of Fear." *U.S. News & World Report,* January 12, 1987.

584. "Variability of AIDS Virus Said to Complicate Vaccine Development." *Family Practice News,* February 1-14, 1986.

585. "Various Approaches to AIDS Vaccines Begin to 'Pierce the Armor' of Virus." *Journal of the American Medical Association* 262:1 (July 7, 1989).

586. Micha, John Paul, M.D. "Genital Warts: Treatable Warning of Cancer?" *Female Patient* 9 (October 1984).

587. Lamb, Carolyn. Based on interviews with George A. Farber, M.D.; Lafayette G. Owen, M.D.; and Theodore A. Tromovitch, M.D. "Help for the patient with venereal warts." *Patient Care,* September 30, 1984.

588. Micha, John P., M.D., and Silva, Paul D., M.D. "Condyloma Acuminata and Related HPV Infections." *Female Patient* 11 (August 1986).

589. Reid, Richard I., M.D., and Greenburg, Mitchell D., M.D. "Genital Warts and Cervical Cancer." *Medical Aspects of Human Sexuality* 19:10 (October 1985).

590. Micha, John Paul, M.D. "Genital Warts: Treatable Warning of Cancer?" *Female Patient* 9 (October 1984).

591. Oriel, J. D., M.D. "Genital Warts: What Kind of Association With Cervical Cancer?" *Sexually Transmitted Diseases Bulletin* 4:1 (February 1984).

592. Oriel, J. D., M.D. "Condylomata Acuminata as a Sexually Transmitted Disease." *Dermatologic Clinics* 1:1 (January 1983).

593. Farber, George A., M.D.; Owen, Lafayette G., M.D.; Tromovitch, Theodore A., M.D. "Help for the patient with venereal warts." *Patient Care,* September 30, 1984.

594. "Cancer Risk Said to Warrant Treatment of Condyloma Patients." *Family Practice News* 15:5 (March 1-14, 1985).

595. Oriel, J. D., M.D. "Genital Warts." *Medical Aspects of Human Sexuality* 18:5 (May 1984).

596. "Condylomas Said to Place Fetus, Neonate at Risk." *Family Practice News* 14:8 (April 15-30, 1984).

597. Lechky, Olga. "Does Condyloma Infect the Baby?" *Medical Tribune,* March 5, 1986.

598. "Condyloma Acuminatum Therapies Sadly Deficient." *Family Practice News* 14:17 (September 1-14, 1984).

599. Felman, Yehudi M., M.D., and Nikitas, James A., M.A., F.R.S.H. "Genital Molluscum Contagiosum, Cutis," 26:2-32, 1980. As referred to by Yehudi M. Felman, M.D., and James A. Nikitas, M.A., F.R.S.H. "Sexually Transmitted Molluscum Contagiosum." *Dermatologic Clinic* 1:1 (January 1983).

600. "Molluscum contagiosum infections have increased over past 18 years." *Sexually Transmitted Diseases Bulletin* 7:2 (April 1987).

601. Felman, Yehudi M., M.D., and Nikitas, James A., M.A., F.R.S.H. "Sexually Transmitted Molluscum Contagiosum."

Dermatologic Clinics 1:1 (January 1983).

602. "Cervical neoplasia caused by Condyloma virus." *Medical Aspects of Human Sexuality* 19:10 (October 1985).
603. Horwitz, Nathan. "Point to Cervical Cancer as STD, Papilloma Virus Culprit." *Medical Tribune,* June 15, 1983.
604. "Several types considered genital cancer risks." *Sexually Transmitted Diseases Bulletin* 6:5 (October, 1986).
605. "Cervical Cancer Epidemic With Current Lifestyles." *Family Practice News* 14:15 (August 1-14, 1984).
606. Krantz, Kermit E., M.D.; Litt, D.; Magrina, Javier F., M.D.; Capen, C. V., M.D. "Sexual Risk Factors for Developing Cervical Cancer." *Medical Aspects of Human Sexuality* 18:11 (November 1984).
607. Fenaglio, Cecilia M., M.D. "CIN or Not to Sin." *Journal of the American Medical Association* 252:21:3012 (December 7, 1984). (CIN = Cervical intraepithelial neoplasia.)
608. "Condyloma virus may be associated with cervical carcinogenesis." *Sexually Transmitted Diseases Bulletin* 4:4 (August 1984).
609. "Risk of Cervical Cancer May Depend on a Partner's Sexual Behavior." *Family Practice News,* April 1-14, 1983.
610. Piver, M. Steven, M.D. "Early Diagnosis and Treatment of Vulvar Cancer," *Hospital Medicine,* February 1984.
611. "Assessing Baby Boom Generation Effect on STD." *Family Practice News* 14:19 (October 1-14, 1984).
612. Haggard, Howard W. *Devils, Drugs and Doctors.* New York: Harper Brothers Publishers, 1929.
613. Fiumara, Nicholas J., M.D., M.P.H. "Infectious Syphilis." *Dermatologic Clinics* 1:1 (January, 1983).
614. "Violence Among the Ancients." *Medical Tribune,* November 27, 1985, p. 27, col. 1, 305. Haggard, Howard W. *Devils, Drugs and Doctors.* New York: Harper Brothers Publishers, 1929.
615. "Sexually Related Disorders." *Merck Manual.* Thirteenth edition, chapter 21. Rahway, NJ: Merck Sharp & Dohme Research Laboratories, 1977.
616. Weber, Deborah E., M.D.; Parish, Lawrence Charles, M.D.; Witkowski, Joseph A., M.D. "Syphilis Part 1. Clinical Manifestations." *Drug Therapy,* August 1986.
617. Kampmeier, R. H., M.D. "Late and Congenital Syphilis." *Dermatologic Clinics* 1:1 (January, 1983).
618. Method of Thomas A. Chapel, M.D. "Cardiovascular Syphilis." *Medical Aspects of Human Sexuality* 16:12 (December 1982).
619. "Neurosyphilis Signs Similar to Those of Psychiatric Disorders." *Psychiatric News,* May 17, 1985.
620. Thomas, E. W. *Syphilis: Its Course and Management.* New York: Macmillan, Inc., 1949. Noted by R. H. Kampmeier, M.D. "Late and Congenital Syphilis." *Dermatologic Clinics* 1:1 (January 1983).
621. STD Statistical Letter, 1983. Atlanta Centers of Disease Control, in press. Noted by H. Hunter Handsfield, M.D., and Sheila A. Lukehart, Ph.D. "Prevention of Congenital Syphilis." *Journal of the American Medical Association* 252:13 (October 5, 1984).
622. Mascola, Laurene, M.D., MPH; Pelosi, Rocco; Blount, Joseph H., MPH; Binkin, Nancy J., M.D., MPH; Alexander, Charles E., M.D., DPH; and Cates, Willard, Jr., M.D., MPH. "Congenital Syphilis: Why Is It Still Occurring?" *Journal of the American Medical Association* 252:13 (October 5, 1984).
623. Spence, Michael R., M.D., MPH. "Pelvic Inflammatory Disease." *Dermatologic Clinics* 1:1 (January 1983).
624. Nguyen, Duong, M.D., MPH. "Gonorrhea in Pregnancy and in the Newborn." *American Family Physicians* 29:1 (January 1984).
625. "Spreading the Word on Disseminated Gonorrhea." *Emergency Medicine,* May 15, 1983.
626. Duncan, W. Christopher, M.D. "Gonorrhea 1983." *Dermatologic Clinics* 1:1 (January 1983).
627. Rosoff, Maxine H., M.D. "Gonococcal Endocarditis: New Detectors of an Old Disease." *Primary Cardiology,* August 1984.
628. Henahan, John. "Gonorrhea Resurgent." *Medical Tribune,* October 22, 1986.
629. "Penicillin-Resistant Strain of Gonorrhea Seen in U.S." *Family Practice News* 13:15 (August 1-14, 1983).
630. Sexually Transmitted Diseases Statistical Letter, 1981. Atlanta, Centers for Disease Control, 1982. Noted by Thomas P. Bronken, M.D., John W. Dyke, Ph.D., and Mary H. Andruszewski, B.S. "A Solid-Phase Enzyme Immunoassay in Detection of Cervical Gonorrhea in a Low-Prevalence Population." *Journal of Family Practice* 20:1 (1985).
631. Fiumara, Nicholas J., M.D., MPH. "Trichomoniasis." *Medical Aspects of Human Sexuality* 20:2 (February 1986).
632. Greydanus, Donald E., M.D.; McAnarney, Elizabeth R., M.D. "Vulvovaginitis in the Adolescent. Part 1. Leukorrhea and Vaginitis." *Dermatology,* August 1983.
633. Hume, John C., M.D. "Trichomoniasis, Candidiasis and Gardnerella Vaginalis Vaginitis as Sexually Transmitted Diseases." *Dermatologic Clinics* 1:1 (January 1983).
634. Dabice, Rita Lazarony. "Trichomoniasis Tied to Infertility." *Medical Tribune,* May 22, 1985.
635. Sherman, K. J., et al. "Sexually Transmitted Diseases and Tubal Infertility." *Sexually Transmitted Disease,* January to March 1987, 14(1):12-16. Reported in "Sexually Transmitted Disease." *Today in Medicine* 2:2 (April 1987).
636. Modern Medicine interview with Masood A. Khatamee, M.D. "Chlamydia, Mycoplasma: What are the hidden risks of these STDs?" *Modern Medicine,* February 1984.
637. Bowie, William R., M.D. "Nongonococcal Urethritis." *Dermatologic Clinics* 1:1 (January 1983).
638. Quinn, Patricia A., Ph.D. "Mycoplasmas: What Kind of Association with Non-gonococcal Urethritis?" *Sexually Transmitted Diseases Bulletin* 21, 4:5 (October 1984).
639. Toth, Attila, M.D. "The Role of Infection in Infertility." *Female Patient* 9 (July 1984).
640. Calin, Andrei, M.A., MRCP. "Reiter's Syndrome." *Hospital Medicine,* November 1983.

641. Orkin, Milton, M.D., and Maibach, Howard I., M.D. "Scabies and Pediculosis Pubis." *Dermatologic Clinics* 1:1 (January 1983).

642. Richey, Hobart K., M.D.; Fenske, Neil A., M.D.; and Cohen, Laura E., M.D. "Scabies: Diagnosis and Management." *Hospital Practice,* February 15, 1986.

643. Adapted from a CME lecture by Kenneth A. Arndt, M.D. "Battling Sexually Transmitted Diseases." *Patient Care,* April 15, 1983.

644. 1 Corinthians 6:18, New International Version.

645. Calderwood, Deryck. *About Your Sexuality.* Boston: Beacon Press, 1983.

646. Thompson, Doug Cooper. *Mutual Caring/Mutual Sharing.* Dover, NH: Strafford County Prenatal and Family Planning Program, 1988.

647. Roach, Nancy, and Benn, LeAnna. *Teen-Aid.* Spokane, WA: Teen-Aid Inc., 1987.

648. Mast, Coleen Kelly. *Sex Respect.* Bradley, IL: Respect, Inc., P. O. Box 349, 1986. Revised, expanded and updated, 1990. (Also: Project Respect, P. O. Box 97, Golf, IL.)

649. Coulson, William R. "On Being Lobbied." Unpublished memorandum to the Technical Advisory Panel on Drug Education Curricula, April 1988.

650. U.S. Department of Education. "AIDS and the Education of Our Children." A pamphlet published in Washington, D.C., 1987.

651. Anchell, Melvin, M.D. *Sex and Insanity.* Portland, OR: Halcyon House, 1983.

652. Coulson, W. R., and J. D. "Confessions of an Ex-Sexologist." *Social Justice Review,* March/April 1988, pp. 43-47.

653. Masters, W. H.; Johnson, V. E.; and Kolodny, R. C. *Crisis: Heterosexual Behavior in the Age of AIDS.* New York: Grove Press, 1988. Referred to in Robert C. Kolodny, M.D., and Virginia E. Johnson, DSc. "New Directions in the AIDS Crisis: The Heterosexual Community." *Medical Aspects of Human Sexuality,* April 1988.

654. Kloser, Patricia, M.D. "AIDS News: Highlights: Fifth International AIDS Conference: Montreal, June 4-9." *Medical Aspects of Human Sexuality,* August, 1989.

655. Kloser, Patricia, M.D. "AIDS News: Special Report From the Fourth International AIDS Conference. Stockholm, June 12-16." *Medical Aspects of Human Sexuality,* August 1988.

656. Samuels, Sandra, M.D. "Chlamydia: Epidemic Among America's Young." *Medical Aspects of Human Sexuality,* December 1989.

657. Wright, V. Cecil, M.D., FACOG, FRCS(C), and FSOGC. "Link between cervical cancer and early coitus." *Medical Aspects of Human Sexuality,* March 1989.

658. Goldsmith, Marsha F. " 'Silent Epidemic' of 'Social Disease' Makes STD Experts Raise Their Voices." *Journal of the American Medical Association* 261:24 (June 23/30, 1989).

659. Gordan, Alan N., M.D. "New STD Menace: HPV Infection." *Medical Aspects of Human Sexuality,* February, 1990.

660. "Continuing Increase in Infectious Syphilis – United States." *Journal of the American Medical Association* 259:7 (February 19, 1988).

661. Martens, Mark G., M.D., and Faro, Sebastian, M.D., Ph.D. "Update on Trichomoniasis: Detection and Management." *Medical Aspects of Human Sexuality,* January 1989.

662. Hanson, Sandra L., et al. "The Role of Responsibility and Knowledge in Reducing Teenage Out-of-Wedlock Childbearing." *Journal of Marriage and the Family* 49 (May 1987). (Includes #179.)

663. "Correspondence." *New England Journal of Medicine* 322:11 (March 15, 1990). (Includes: Hearst, N., and Hulley, S. B. "Preventing the heterosexual spread of AIDS: are we giving our patients the best advice?" *Journal of the American Medical Association* 259, 1988. Fox, M. "Asking the right questions." *Health,* February 1988. Potterat, J. J.; Phillips, L.; and Muth, J. B. "Lying to military physicians about risk factors for HIV infections." *Journal of the American Medical Association* 257, 1987.)

664. Hogan, Dennis P., and Kitagawa, Evelyn M. "The Impact of Social Status, Family Structure, and Neighborhood on the Fertility of Black Adolescents." *American Journal of Sociology,* 1985.

665. Talbert, Chuck. "Sexually Transmitted Diseases – What Teachers, Counselors, and Parents Should Know." *Adolescent Counselor,* February/March 1990, pp. 33-37.

666. Grant, George. *Grand Illusions: The Legacy of Planned Parenthood.* Brentwood, TN: Wolgemuth & Hyatt Publishers, Inc., 1988, p. 30.

667. Hanson, Myers, Ginsburg Study. Published in *Journal of Marriage and Family,* May 1987, pp. 241-56.

668. Planned Parenthood *Insider* newsletter, Spring 1988.

669. Kirby, Douglas; Alter, Judith; and Scales, Peter. "An Analysis of U.S. Sex Education Programs and Evaluation Methods: Executive Summary." U.S. Department of Health, Education and Welfare. Study performed by Mathtech, Inc., July 1979.

670. Smith, Richard. "To Abstain, or Not to Abstain – That Is the Answer!" Public Education Committee, P. O. Box 33082, Seattle, WA 98133-0082.

671. Goedert, J. J. "What Is Safe Sex? Suggested Standards Linked to Testing for Human Immunodeficiency Virus." *New England Journal of Medicine,* May 21, 1987, p. 1339.

672. Anderson, Virginia, and Wright, Randall Allen. *The Impact of Media on the Sexual Attitudes of Adolescents.* Research paper presented at the National Council on Family Relations Annual Conference, New Orleans, Louisiana, November 5-8, 1989.

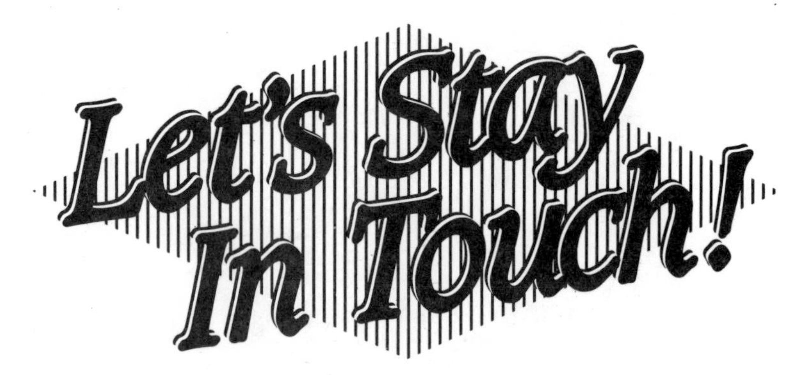

If you have grown personally as a result of this material, we should stay in touch. You will want to continue in your Christian growth, and to help your faith become even stronger, our team is constantly developing new materials.

We publish a monthly newsletter called **5 Minutes with Josh** which will:

1) tell you about those new materials as they become available,
2) answer your tough questions,
3) give creative tips on being an effective parent,
4) let you know our ministry needs, and
5) keep you up-to-date on my speaking schedule (so you can pray).

If you would like to receive this publication, simply fill out the coupon below and send it in. By special arrangement **5 Minutes with Josh** will come to you regularly – <u>no charge</u>.

Let's keep in touch!

Josh

Yes! I want to receive the free subscription to **5 Minutes with JOSH**

Name________________________________

Address____

City______________________ State______ Zip __________

Mail to: Josh McDowell Ministry, **5 Minutes with Josh**,
Box 1000, Dallas, TX 75221